INTERNATIONAL REVIEW OF CHILD NEUROLOGY SERIES

MOVEMENT DISORDERS IN CHILDREN

EMILIO FERNANDEZ-ALVAREZ
Head, Department of Paediatrics
Hospital Sant Joan de Déu
Barcelona, Spain

JEAN AICARDI
Consultant, Child Neurology Unit
Hôpital Robert Debré
Paris, France
and
Honorary Professor of Child Neurology
Institute of Child Health, University College
London, England

with contributions from

N Bathien	Isidro Ferrer
Diane C Chugani	Gurutz Linazasoro
Harry T Chugani	José A Obeso
Natalio Fejerman	Pilar Póo
Pierre Rondot	

2001
MAC KEITH PRESS
for the
INTERNATIONAL CHILD NEUROLOGY ASSOCIATION

THE INTERNATIONAL REVIEW OF CHILD NEUROLOGY SERIES

CONTENTS

FOREWORD

Movement disorders in childhood constitute a complicated and multifaceted subject, dificult to define and to clarify. Presentations and patterns of disease differ not only from those traditionally met in adult neurology but also within the individual child, where considerable changes occur with age and developmental stage. The authors of this comprehensive volume, two very learned and experienced child neurologists, have undertaken the huge work to collect and systematically sort, describe and present the widespread material and knowledge from literature and from their own experiences through many decades of clinical work. Most impressive are the many diagnostic problems – the 'difficult cases' – they have trawled from case reports in medical journals across decades. For the busy clinician with the odd and puzzling 'case for diagnosis' this book is a goldmine to dig in. For the paediatric neurology library, the volume is a 'must'!

BENGT HAGBERG
Göteborg, Sweden

PREFACE

Movement disorders in childhood have received little attention, especially when compared with such conditions as epilepsy or neuromuscular disorders. The information on movement disorders in childhood is mostly scattered in multiple neurological and paediatric journals. This book attempts to put together information from these various sources in a form accessible to clinically oriented paediatric and adult neurologists, and paediatricians.

We shall first outline the limits of the contents of this volume.

Only disorders of children and adolescents under 18 years of age are dealt with. The differences in movement disorders between children and adults are striking. The clinical manifestations of extrapyramidal disease are profoundly influenced by the age of onset. A good example is the difference between Huntington disease in adults and children. Moreover, a number of disease processes occur almost exclusively in the paediatric age, e.g. transient disorders. So the prevalence of the various movement disorders in children, their clinical presentation, course, prognosis and management differ considerably from those in adults. As an example, the space dedicated to hypokinetic–rigid syndromes is much more limited than in similar books of adult neurology.

The definition of the term 'disorders of movement' can be more or less comprehensive. The conditions included in this book are expressed clinically by the occurrence of abnormalities of movement and posture, often in association with alterations of muscular tone. These are involuntary but conscious, and are, generally, due to anomalies of CNS neurotransmitter function, often in the basal ganglia. Disorders of movement caused by pyramidal tract lesions (e.g. hemiplegia or paraplegia), or by lesions of the peripheral nervous system, and those resulting from cerebellar dysfunction are excluded as well as those resulting from epileptic discharges and some defects of eye movements.

Other terms have also been used to designate these conditions. 'Extrapyramidal diseases' is the oldest but has fallen into disuse because of its lack of precision. The term includes other systems of control of movement that are not usually termed extrapyramidal, for example the cerebellum (Fénelon and Percheron 1997).

'Disorders of the basal ganglia' is also inadequate as not all abnormal movements are the result of involvement of these structures, and, conversely, lesions of the basal ganglia can manifest with cognitive deficit rather than with movement disorders. For these reasons, the term 'movement disorders' seemed least inadequate, as it is merely descriptive and does not imply any hypothesis regarding the anatomical location of defects.

This book is essentially clinically oriented. It is written mostly by clinicians and is meant to help clinicians. The clinical features are its basic concern and are complemented by a description of the investigations that allow confirmation of diagnosis and guidance of treatment. We have elected to organize its chapters according to the predominant clinical feature, such as hypokinetic–rigid syndrome, tremor, chorea, dystonia or paroxysmal dyskinesia, thus enabling the reader to rapidly access the information pertinent to a particular patient. A special chapter deals with those disorders that usually manifest with several different types of abnormal movements. The introductory chapter deals with general concepts and the final chapter is dedicated to ancillary investigations as they apply to children.

Since Sydenham in 1686 identified the first disease characterized by a movement disorder, a long time has elapsed and, especially in the past 25 years, knowledge of the pathophysiology of abnormal movements has increased extraordinarily as a result of better understanding of neurotransmitter functions, of modern neuroimaging techniques (especially MRI but also functional neuroimaging with MR spectroscopy, PET and functional MR), and of the advent of molecular genetics. This last not only provides new bases for nosological classification, previously based exclusively on clinical/pathological data, but also raises the hope of prevention and possible cure of genetically determined movement disorders.

Although new disorders are being identified with such methods, progress in patient care has remained rather patchy, and much has to be done to improve the management of many movement disorders. Therapeutic difficulties are even greater where children are concerned. The consequences on learning, and on the neurological and psychological development of children with chronic movement disorders are largely unknown. Even drug doses are often poorly established and extrapolated from adult practice, even though there are well-known differences in the handling of pharmacological agents between children and adults.

REFERENCE

Fénelon G, Percheron G (1997) Revision of the International Classification of Diseases *Mov Disord* 12: 256–7.

1
GENERAL CONCEPTS*

Human beings think and move. The most characteristic movement of *Homo sapiens* is bipedal ambulation. It has allowed the development of hand use and, indirectly, of the most recently acquired cerebral structures, and thus of intellectual capabilities.

The disorders studied in this book are expressed clinically by alterations of muscular tone and the presence of abnormal movements.

The elements necessary to perform the simplest motor act include the muscle, its effector neuron and its connections (nerve end plate, receptors, etc.). Such an act would lack finality, usefulness, efficacy and control in the absence of other functional structures such as the pyramidal tracts, the extrapyramidal and cerebellar systems, proprioception and other sensory afferences which control, adjust and coordinate the act. In addition, motor activity is integrated in the behaviour of individuals, and is in large part genetically determined, but has a capacity (in large part acquired) for autoregulation and automatization.

Abnormal movements are difficult to define, and it is simpler to describe the various types of abnormal movement and analyse their characteristics (Jankovic 1997). Abnormal movements are often involuntary and nonintentional. They do not include automatic movements such as respiration or those of a person who is walking in a well-known place while reading a newspaper. Abnormal movements are, usually, involuntary, but involuntary movements are not always abnormal. An example of normal involuntary movement is yawning. One essential difference between involuntary and automatic movement is that the former cannot be initiated or interrupted voluntarily. This difference is not absolute and a certain amount of voluntary control, however partial and transient, can be exerted on several involuntary movement disorders, such as tics or chorea.

Another valuable distinction is between voluntary and nonvoluntary movements. The latter are often automatic but not necessary so. We can walk automatically concentrating our mind on other actions, but we can, at will, interrupt, re-initiate or accelerate ambulation.

Differentiation between voluntary and intentional movements is also useful, even though these terms are often considered synonymous. An intentional movement is one that has been desired or planned. Some involuntary actions and movements can be intentional. However, the distinction may not be absolute, as tics, for instance, may result

---

*Written in collaboration with José A Obeso and Gurutz Linazasoro, Centro de Neurología y Neurocirugía Funcional, Clínica Quirón, San Sebastian, Spain.

from lack of voluntary inhibition of planned movements. Conversely, a voluntary movement may not be intentional as in the case with some automatic movements.

Abnormal involuntary movements are symptoms and not diseases, although in certain cases (e.g. Sydenham chorea, torsion dystonia) a particular type of movement is so predominant as to come to designate a disease. This is unfortunate, as various types of movement, either simultaneously or in succession, often occur in the same disease process.

Rondot (1983) subdivides involuntary movements into arrhythmical (chorea, ballismus, athetosis, arrythmical myoclonus and tics) and rhythmical (tremor and rhythmical myoclonus). The presence of a rhythm implies the participation of a synchronizing mechanism of motor units and may thus be of pathophysiological significance.

FUNCTIONAL ORGANIZATION OF THE BASAL GANGLIA IN HEALTH AND MOVEMENT DISORDERS

Movement disorders may be divided into three major categories, all of which have in common a defect in the speed and accuracy of voluntary actions in the absence of muscular weakness or the presence of unwanted muscle activity. These categories are: (1) hypokinetic–rigid syndromes (parkinsonism); (2) dyskinesias (dystonia, chorea–ballism, tics, myoclonus and tremor); (3) ataxia.

In this introductory chapter, we shall concentrate on the pathophysiology of the basal ganglia and its typical clinical manifestations.

NORMAL FUNCTIONAL ORGANIZATION

Current views about the function of the basal ganglia have been greatly influenced over many years by clinicopathological correlation. Thus, the widely accepted role of the basal ganglia in the control of movement has largely derived from the study of patients with, for example, substantia nigra degeneration as in Parkinson disease, putaminal lesions producing dystonia, and subthalamic nucleus lesions inducing hemiballism.

The basal ganglia are currently conceived of as part of a distributive system involved in many functions. Studies in monkeys have allowed us to identify and isolate multiple, functionally segregated circuits running through the basal ganglia (Alexander et al. 1986). The best defined circuits are the motor, oculomotor, associative and limbic circuits which form parallel cortex–basal ganglia–thalamus–cortex loops that provide the anatomo-functional basis for motor, cognitive and associative functions. Disruption of such circuits can give rise to a diversity of problems ranging from the more common parkinsonian syndrome and dyskinesias (chorea, dystonia, etc.) to complex neuropsychological disorders such as Tourette syndrome (tics and obsessive–compulsive syndrome), disinhibition, depression and abulia (Bathia and Marsden 1994).

Of all circuits passing through the basal ganglia, the 'motor circuit' is the most relevant in the pathophysiology of movement disorders. This 'motor loop' includes the precentral motor areas (areas 4 and 6, supplementary motor area) and postcentral sensory

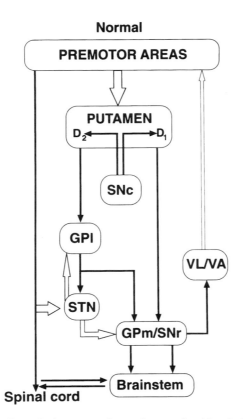

Fig. 1.1. Putaminal output pathways (see text for abbreviations).

fields (3a,b, 2, 1), which project to the putamen in a somatotopically organized fashion. Detailed anatomo-chemical studies have shown that putaminal output reaches the medial globus pallidus (GPm) and the substantia nigra reticulata (SNr) through two different projections, which arise from separate putaminal neuronal populations (Fig. 1.1). There is a direct monosynaptic pathway from putamen to GPm that uses GABA and co-localized substance P (SP) and dynorphin (Dyn) as neurotransmitters, and an indirect pathway that arises from GABA/encephalinergic putaminal neurons and projects to the lateral globus pallidus (GPl). Dopamine exerts an excitatory effect through D-1 receptors on the GABA-SP-Dyn neurons and produces inhibition, through D-2 receptors, of the GABA-encephalin neurons (Gerfen et al. 1990). The GPl sends a GABAergic inhibitory projection to the sensorimotor region of the subthalamic nucleus (STN) and also to the GPm. The STN exerts a powerful excitatory drive onto the GPm and SNr, which finally project to the ventrolateral thalamus 'en route' to the premotor cortices. The output from the GPm (through the ansa lenticularis) and SNr to the thalamus is GABAergic and, therefore, inhibitory. Basal ganglia output is also directed to the brainstem. The GPm also projects to the non-cholinergic portion of the pedunculopontine nucleus, and the SNr sends its efferents to the superior colliculus and mesopontine tegmentum.

Electrophysiological studies in monkeys have consistently shown that neurons in GPm and SNr exhibit high tonic neuronal firing. Phasic inhibition of discharging is associated with movement facilitation, while increases in neuronal discharge are associated with movement inhibition (De Long 1990). The general concept of the physiology of the 'motor circuit' can be summarized as follows:

(1) Cortico-striatal activation of the direct pathway will produce a GABA-mediated inhibition of GPm/SNr neurons which in turn will disinhibit their thalamic target, thus facilitating the thalamic projection to the precentral motor fields. The net effect of this sequence would be positive feedback for cortically initiated movements.

(2) Cortico-striatal stimulation of the GABA-encephalin neurons in the indirect pathway will produce inhibition of GPl and, secondarily, facilitation of the STN. The latter will result in increased excitatory drive onto the GPm/SNr, which will increase their output, thus over-inhibiting their thalamic and brainstem targets. The net effect of this sequence would be a negative feedback for movement, which could be functionally translated into inhibition of undesired muscle contraction or as a signal to halt movement.

This oversimplified scheme will have to be modified to accommodate new observations. One important point that requires refinement is to ascribe specific functions to particular circuits. For instance, it is conceivable that posture and locomotion depend more on basal ganglia–brainstem connections, while control of hand movements or speech will be under basal ganglia–thalamo-cortical control. Similarly, some movement disorders could depend more on the dysfunction of certain components of the basal ganglia.

PATHOPHYSIOLOGY OF MOVEMENT DISORDERS

Parkinsonism

Parkinsonian manifestations are rare in childhood. Current understanding of the model is mainly based on studies conducted in animals with lesions of the nigrostriatal pathway. The major features of the parkinsonian syndrome are a poverty of spontaneous movements (akinesia), impaired initiation resulting in slowness of movement (bradykinesia) and reduced amplitude of intended movements (hypokinesia), muscular rigidity and tremor at rest.

The basic mechanisms underlying the cardinal features of the parkinsonian syndrome are now relatively well understood as a result of studies using the model of 1,2,3-methyl-phenyl-tetrahydropyridine (MPTP) induced parkinsonism in monkeys. Loss of dopaminergic neurons in the substantia nigra compacta (SNc) reduces the normal inhibition of the nigrostriatal pathway on GABA-encephalin neurons, which increases their activity, thus overinhibiting the GPl. The inhibitory tone of GPl on the STN is reduced and the STN increases its activity well over normal to excite the GPm/SNr. Hyperactivity of the STN and overexcitation of its efferent targets can now be considered as the pathophysiological hallmark of the parkinsonian state. This has been shown by microelectrode recording and metabolic studies such as 2-deoxyglucose uptake and mRNA glutamine acid dehydrogenase (mRNA GAD) 'in situ' hybridization in MPTP monkeys. The pivotal role of increased STN activity in the origin of parkinsonism was further demonstrated by lesioning the STN in MPTP monkeys. A unilateral STN lesion induced a marked improvement in the contralateral limbs, but also in facial expression, flexor posture, spontaneous activity and even, albeit to a minor extent, in the limb ipsilateral to the STN lesion. In addition to the behavioural observations, it was also shown that the STN lesion restored the GABA activity in both the GPm and SNr towards normal levels as judged by the expression of mRNA GAD (Guridi et al. 1996). Increased activity of GPm/SNr leads to excessive inhibition of the thalamus and reduced thalamo-cortical activation. This probably accounts for the hypokinetic features of the disease.

Chorea and ballism

These dyskinesias differ only by the intensity and amplitude of the movements and appear to be a consequence of functional inactivation or lesion of the STN leading to reduced activity of the GPm. As a result, pallidal inhibitory output onto the thalamo-cortical projection is reduced (as opposed to increased in the parkinsonian state) and involuntary movements arise. Crossman et al. (1987) reported augmented 2-deoxyglucose uptake in the STN and physiological inhibition of this nucleus after blocking the striato-pallidal (GPl) projection. This explains why chorea may arise after lesioning or dysfunction of several basal ganglia nuclei.

Dystonia

The origin of dystonia has resisted most attempts to find a simple working hypothesis similar to those suggested above for chorea/ballism and parkinsonism. The complexity of the clinical features of dystonia may explain these difficulties. We believe, however, that dystonia is the movement disorder that best represents the pathological deviation of the normal motor function of the basal ganglia. In spite of the substantial achievements that have taken place in the study of dystonia, its pathophysiology is not entirely known.

Excessive co-contraction of agonist and antagonist muscles is one of the physiological hallmarks of dystonia. When executing repetitive alternating movements at a single joint, contractions of antagonist muscles typically alternate. The physiological basis of this organization is reciprocal inhibition. Co-contraction, the essential feature of the dystonic phenomenon, may be understood as a defect in reciprocal inhibition. Reciprocal inhibition can be studied in humans by studying the effect of stimulating the radial nerve at various times prior to producing the H-reflex with median nerve stimulation. The radial nerve afferents come from muscles that are antagonist to muscles innervated by the median nerve. Normal subjects show three periods of inhibition: the initial phase is believed to represent the disynaptic inhibition and the later inhibitory periods probably depend on presynaptic mechanisms (Day et al. 1984). Disynaptic inhibition is normal in dystonia, but presynaptic inhibition is clearly reduced. Other spinal and brainstem reflexes, such as the blink reflex, perioral reflexes, etc., have been extensively studied and a common result is that inhibitory processes are reduced. Accordingly, several observations suggest that reduction of spinal cord and brainstem inhibition is an important mechanism in dystonia.

The results of PET scan studies were at first equivocal, but recent studies suggest that there is an increased activation of the supplementary motor area (SMA) and lateral prefrontal cortex during the performance of voluntary movements with the dystonic arm (Ceballos-Baumann et al. 1995), and glucose utilization was enhanced in the lentiform nucleus and premotor cortices bilaterally in patients with dystonia. This pattern of cortical hyperactivity is the opposite to what is seen in parkinsonism, and may explain some of the clinical differences observed between the two conditions.

At present, and in spite of its imperfections, the dopamine agonist induced dystonia in MPTP treated monkeys is probably the best animal model for understanding the neural basis of dystonia. Animals, rendered parkinsonian after MPTP administration, develop choreic and dystonic dyskinesias after chronic levodopa treatment. Neuronal metabolic studies (using radioactively labelled 2-deoxyglucose (2-DG) are a measure of cell metabolism. 2-DG uptake reflects afferent activity more than nuclear neuronal activity. One study performed in animals with dystonia after chronic administration of levodopa or a dopamine agonist demonstrated only a partial reversal of the pattern of 2-DG uptake seen in parkinsonism (in parkinsonism 2-DG activity is increased in the GPl and GPm, and decreased in STN). Thus, the brain of these dystonic animals showed reduced 2-DG in GPl and increased 2-DG in STN, but in GPm the isotope uptake is increased and not decreased, as might be expected. This difference in the degree of GPm activity could explain the well known observation that thalamotomy is effective in alleviating levodopa induced choreic dyskinesias in patients with parkinsonism, but that larger thalamic lesions should be performed in order to ameliorate dystonic dyskinesias. Alternatively, the projection from the GPm to the pedunculopontine nucleus may be important for the mediation of dystonia.

According to the model presented here, the idea emerges that in dystonia the primary disorder would be overactivity of the direct pathway (striatum–GPm/SNr) and a secondary disorder shared with parkinsonism would be overactivity of the indirect (striatum–GPl–STN–GPm/SNr) pathway. This mechanism would explain some of the similarities and differences between dystonia and parkinsonism.

Tics and Tourette syndrome
Tics are the second major category of movement disorders that can appear during childhood. Tics are one of the most fascinating and complex movement disorders because of the combination of voluntary and involuntary, psychic and purely motor manifestations, and because of the association with some psychopathological problems. Tics are highly prevalent in the general population. While once considered psychogenic in origin,

it is now recognized that almost all tic disorders occur on an hereditary basis, although the detailed genetic transmission remains to be determined. This fact, and the increasingly recognized clinical heterogeneity of the disorder, has led to all types of tics being considered under the same umbrella. The term 'tic disease' has recently been coined to include transient tic disorder, chronic motor or vocal tic disorder, single tics and Tourette syndrome. Specific behavioural dysfunction, including obsessive–compulsive disorder and attention deficit–hyperactivity disorder, occurs commonly in association with tics and may represent alternative expressions of the same condition. These behavioural problems are the main cause of school difficulties in children with tics. The pathophysiology of tics remains largely unknown. Based on the therapeutic efficacy of neuroleptics, disturbance of dopaminergic neurotransmission has been suspected in the pathogenesis of tics. On the other hand, study of the pre- and postsynaptic nigrostriatal dopaminergic pathway has failed to show any consistent abnormality. In the few pathological studies available, a decrease in dynorphin inmunoreactivity in GPl has been the only abnormality observed.

No animal model is available for increasing our understanding of Tourette syndrome. The major clinical feature of Tourette syndrome is the difficulty or inability to suppress a motor activity that is inadequate in time and space or lacks specific purposes. This inability encompasses the whole range of the motor spectrum, from simple fragments of movement (tics) to complex motor acts to obsessive behaviour. The model shown above suggests that one plausible explanation for Tourette syndrome would be an abnormality in the control exerted by the basal ganglia onto cortical areas particularly involved in the decision processes, such as the prefrontal cortex. In a recent study, Wolf et al. (1996) measured the binding of iodobenzamide, a dopamine (D-2 receptors) antagonist, in the striatum of twins with Tourette syndrome. Binding in the caudate nucleus was significantly increased in the more affected twin but was normal in the putamen. Thus, differences in D-2 receptor binding in the head of the caudate nucleus correlated with the degree of severity as judged clinically. This work suggests that an as yet undeciphered dopamine abnormality of the caudate nucleus could be where the pathophysiology of Tourette syndrome lies. However, it still remains to be explained how the different motor, associative and limbic projections of the basal ganglia, all of which should be involved in Tourette syndrome, might be affected by dysfunction of the head of the caudate nucleus.

Summary

Despite substantial advances in the understanding of movement disorders in recent years much remains to be clarified. Particularly relevant to the field of neuropediatrics is how congenital and early acquired lesions, even asymptomatic ones, may influence motor function and behaviour in adulthood. Another crucial challenge in childhood is improvement of pharmacological management of severe motor problems and understanding of the development of functional compensation for acquired motor deficits. Clinical assessment and carefully documented observations from well studied cases will remain the primary source of information and progress.

MAIN TYPES OF MOVEMENT ABNORMALITIES

From a clinical viewpoint, the disorders of movement can be divided into two broad groups of (1) hypokinetic–rigid syndromes, and (2) dyskinesias.

HYPOKINETIC–RIGID SYNDROME

In the hypokinetic–rigid syndrome the fundamental disturbances consist of hypokinesia or/and bradykinesia, i.e. difficulty and/or slowness in initiating and completing movements.

Hypokinesia etymologically means rarity of movement, i.e. a decrease in the number of voluntary and automatic movements such as blinking, arm swinging during ambulation, etc. Bradykinesia refers to slowness in initiation and completion of movement in the absence of paralysis.

Hypokinesia is generally, but not always, associated with a peculiar form of hypertonia, termed rigidity. This is a type of hypertonia in which there is increased resistance to passive movements or articulations that is uniform regardless of the speed and direction of movement (flexion or extension), traditionally compared to the resistance of a lead pipe. This is in contrast with spasticity, in which hypertonicity predominates in flexor and pronator muscles in the upper limbs, and resistance is at onset of movement and then increases with the speed of passive motion (the so-called 'jack-knife' phenomenon). In rigidity, resistance can be rhythmically interrupted resulting in the 'cogwheel phenomenon'. Rigidity is best perceptible with slow movements.

Rigidity, bradykinesia and hypokinesia are usually associated, but one may predominate. Another symptom of the rigid akinetic syndrome is rest tremor (see below).

DYSKINESIAS

There is now a trend towards simplification of the classification of the dyskinetic syndromes, largely due to the work of Marsden who considers only five types: tremor, chorea, dystonia, tics and myoclonus. Precise definition of terms is necessary. The following example quoted by Quinn et al. (1988) illustrates the difficulties encountered. In the first description of a family with a movement disorder, Refsum and Sjaastad (1972) wrote that "[the] propositus presented generalised choreiform or myoclonic movements, mainly localised to the head, trunk and proximal parts of the extremities." In a subsequent paper (Sjaastad et al. 1983) on the same family, the authors comment: "Whereas the hyperkinetic events in the original description were interpreted as choreatic, we have been more inclined to interpret the movements as myoclonic. . . We . . . showed a movie of the proband to Professor Biemond, who felt very strongly that our patient demonstrated the same type of involuntary movements as [his patients with] paramyoclonus multiplex . . . Professor M.D. Yahr was also shown this film. . . he had also seen some cases [of] benign, non progressive chorea, and felt that the involuntary movements in our proband mimicked those. . ."

Video recording, which is better than any description, now makes analysis of abnormal movements much easier and is generating a consensus regarding the terms used.

For instance, the journal *Movement Disorders* includes videotapes in addition to conventional articles. In our opinion, the five categories mentioned above are not sufficient to describe the full spectrum of abnormal movements. Thus athetosis, a term virtually unused by Marsden and other modern authors, and dystonia are, probably, semiologically distinct expressions of the same physiopathological disturbance.

The major dyskinesias are defined below.

Tremor

Rhythmicity is the most useful characteristic for identification of tremor, although myoclonus may also be rhythmical. Tremor is a rhythmical oscillation of a part of the body around a fixed point or place, which results from alternating synchronous contractions of antagonist muscles reciprocally innervated (Jankovic and Fahn 1980).

Pathological tremors are defined in part by their conditions of occurrence. They include:

(1) *Rest tremor* (rare in childhood) that occurs in the absence of volitional muscle activity and ceases or decreases with intentional movement. Its frequency is 4–5 Hz. It usually occurs with the rigid–hypokinetic syndrome.

(2) *Postural tremor* (static or attitude tremor) appears when a part of the body (the arms for example) are maintained in a posture against gravity.

(3) *Action tremor* (kinetic or intention tremor) occurs with voluntary movement that it disturbs. It increases when the moving limb approaches its target ('terminal tremor'—Davis and Kunkle 1951). It is often due to cerebellar dysfunction. A special type of action tremor is 'task specific tremor' that only occurs during the performance of highly skilled activities.

(4) *Rubral tremor* or mesencephalic tremor applies to large amplitude tremor (2–5 Hz) that is present at rest, increases with posture and further aggravates with movement. Formerly, it was thought that lesions of the red nucleus were responsible, but it is now known that it is due to lesions of the superior cerebellar peduncle in the vicinity of the red nucleus. Focal lesions as produced by multiple sclerosis or infarctions are common causes.

In practice the circumstances of occurrence (rest, posture, action) and the frequency (high, more than 6 cycles per second; or low, less than 6 cycles/s) suffice to define a tremor.

Chorea and ballismus

Choreic movements are involuntary, non-propositional (although patients often try to dissimulate them by prolonging them with a propositional activity), arrhythmical, asymmetrical, sudden and brief movements which occur at rest or parasite voluntary movements. They predominate in the proximal limbs, neck, trunk and facial muscles. They may extend to other areas such as the oropharyngeal muscles, then generating swallowing difficulties.

The Research Group on Extrapyramidal Disorders of the World Federation of Neurology (Lakke et al. 1981) defined chorea as "a state of excessive, spontaneous movements, irregularly timed, non-repetitive, randomly distributed and abrupt in character" occurring haphazardly with variable frequency and intensity. This may result in simple restlessness with mild intermittent exaggeration of gestures or expressions and walking motions like those of a dancer, or produce a continuous flow of violent and incapacitating movements. Deep reflexes are pendular. The abnormal movements are exacerbated by action, tension or mental concentration. In the mildest cases, chorea may be difficult to differentiate from other abnormal movements such as myoclonus or tics. Repetitive contractions can be felt by introducing fingers into the hand of the patient, the so-called 'milking movements'. They disappear or decrease considerably during sleep.

Ballismus is probably a severe form of chorea (Marsden 1986), consisting of extremely violent uncontrollable movements of excessive amplitude of the proximal muscles of the limbs. Indeed, one of the present authors (EF-A) has observed it in severe cases of rheumatic chorea, and ballistic movements when the patient improves may become typically choreic.

Chorea is most commonly generalized but may be unilateral in classic choreic or ballistic forms. The electromyographic activity in chorea is similar to that of voluntary movements, albeit often more fragmented and less regular (Rondot 1983). Choreic movements are often regarded as resulting from overactivity of the dopaminergic system (see p. 3).

Despite many neuropathological studies (see Padberg and Bruyn 1986), structural lesion common to the various forms of chorea has not been identified. The most common lesions involve the striatum, subthalamic nucleus and ventral thalamic nucleus.

Hemiballismus is often produced by a lesion of the contralateral subthalamic nucleus.

In children a form of postural instability has been termed 'choreiform syndrome' (Prechtl and Stemmer 1962, Wolff and Hurtwitz 1966). It is usually associated with so-called 'minimal cerebral dysfunction'. The term is better avoided as this syndrome has no pathological or physiopathological relationship to chorea.

Dystonia and athetosis
These movements result from an abnormal muscle activity characterized by (1) the simultaneous and sustained tonic contraction of both agonist and antagonist muscles; and (2) the diffusion of contraction to muscles that would not normally participate in the assumption or maintenance of a given posture (overflow contraction). Some investigators regard dystonia and athetosis as different expressions of the same phenomenon (e.g. "athetosis refers to distal dystonic movements in the limbs"—Marsden and Harrison 1974).

Others, while accepting a relationship, maintain the distinction that dystonia applies to posture, while athetosis designates the abnormal movements often associated ("When abnormal involuntary movements occur in the course of a dystonia, they are usually of

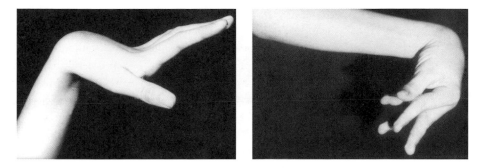

Fig. 1.2. Athetoid movements of the left hand in a girl with ataxia–telangiectasia.

an athetosic type"—Rondot 1983). Denny-Brown (1968) defined dystonia as a fixed or relatively fixed attitude. Rondot et al. (1988) maintain that dystonia means a disturbance of muscular tone, especially marked in maintenance of attitudes and not movement.

It may be that dystonia in the maintenance of postures and dystonia in movement are not independent phenomena since movement is a prerequisite to the realization of a posture. A posture would thus be an 'arrested movement' or movement would be the succession in time of changing postures. The Scientific Advisory Board of the Dystonic Medical Research Foundation proposed that dystonia "is a syndrome of sustained muscle contractions, frequently causing twisting and repetitive movements, or abnormal postures" (Fahn 1988).

From a purely semiological viewpoint, athetosis is different from dystonia. Athetotic movements are complex, wormlike, irregular, non-propositional, and predominate over postural anomalies and on the distal parts of limbs and face. Athetosis can be a mixed disturbance with both dystonia and choreic features, the so-called choreo-athetosis (Fig. 1.2).

In children up to 5 years of age, certain dystonic attitudes can occur normally while maintaining a posture requiring tension such as holding the hands in a position facing the thorax.

Dystonia may manifest itself with variable severity. *Action dystonia* (Zeman and Dyken 1967) is not manifest at rest and appears only on performing voluntary movements (external facilitation, according to Rondot et al. 1988) that it modifies. Movements at a distance can precipitate the disturbance in the affected body part (overflow). Generally, the precipitating movement is specific, such as writing, whereas the same extremity can be used normally for other activities such as sewing (paradoxical kinesia). Examples of action dystonia include flexion of the wrist on attempted writing, plantar flexion and inversion of the foot in ambulation, and opening of the jaw and protraction of the tongue on attempted talking.

Postural dystonia is characterized by the appearance of abnormal sustained postures that may last from half a minute to many hours or days (Weiner and Lang 1989). These postures disappear during sleep. While awake, the patients can discover tricks whereby

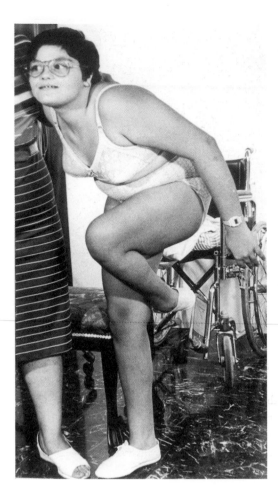

Fig. 1.3. Dystonic posture in a 16-year-old girl. Note hyperextension of the neck and abnormal posture of the left lower limb with flexion on the thigh and internal rotation of the foot.

the dystonia can be suppressed for a brief period of time, such as pressing a finger on the chin in cases of torticollis. With progression of the disorder, however, the abnormal postures tend to become fixed. The most common dystonic postures include flexion or extension of fingers, flexion of the wrist, plantar flexion of feet, retrocollis and tortipelvis. When extreme, they realize grotesque attitudes such as camel posture (hyperextension of the head and extreme tortipelvis) or flamingo posture (flexion of the thigh with cephalic hyperextension) (Fig. 1.3). Muscular hypertrophy with absent subcutaneous fat is often a consequence of continuous muscle contraction.

Dystonic patients can show myoclonus as an associated sign (myoclonic dystonia). This can be difficult to differentiate from *dystonic spasms*: rapid spasmodic movements that may be localized, intermittent and brief (Fig. 1.4). They may be repeated alternately (e.g. extension and flexion of the fingers) and are sometimes rhythmical, resembling tremor. When generalized they can make the patients fall from their chair. In some cases

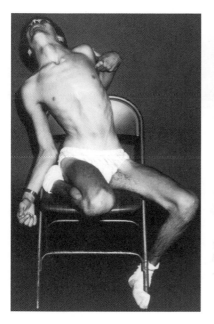
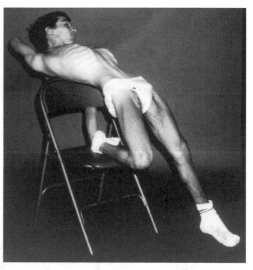

Fig. 1.4. Dystonic spasms in a 17-year-old boy with idiopathic torsion dystonia.

they represent 'dystonic storms' (also termed status dystonicus) with continuous spasmodic activity.

Although dystonia may severely disrupt voluntary function when severe, the motor impairment is often less than would be expected. Dystonia, whether of movement or posture, disappears with sleep. The amplitude of diurnal fluctuation is generally modest but can be extremely marked in particular forms. Gentle stimulation of the skin in the affected region may reduce intensity of the dystonia. Intermittent forms (paroxysmal dystonias) exist.

Various scales have been devised for comparison of results of multicentric studies. Coleman (1970) recognized seven grades depending on tone, movement, speech, locomotion and feeding ability. The scale of Burke et al. (1985) is based on both movement characteristics and the degree of resulting disability.

We consider in our clinical practice several levels of dystonia:
• level 1 = dystonia only with specific movements;
• level 2 = fixed but reducible dystonic posture;
• level 3 = irreducible dystonic posture;
• level 4 = massive dystonic spasms.

Such levels occur generally in succession in cases of idiopathic dystonia but symptomatic dystonias can begin at levels 2 or 3.

According to extension of dystonia, cases can be divided into:
• focal dystonias, when limited to a single muscle group such as in blepharospasm or dystonic dysphonia);

- segmental dystonias when involving two contiguous segments or a whole extremity;
- hemidystonia when involving a half of the body;
- multifocal dystonia when two or more non-contiguous parts are affected;
- generalized dystonia.

From the electrophysiological point of view, dystonia and athetosis are identical: both involve tonic activity simultaneously involving agonists and antagonists.

The pathophysiological basis of dystonia is probably multiple. For instance, in idiopathic torsion dystonia (see Chapter 5, p. 82) the dystonia may selectively appear only for certain movements, whereas other movements that involve the same muscle groups are not disturbed. By contrast, in transient idiopathic dystonia of infancy (Chapter 5, p 91) dystonia is only postural, disappearing when the infant engages in a propositional activity. This strongly suggests that the programme of movement is altered. Remarkably, automatic or often rehearsed movements are often more disturbed than unusual ones (for example, forward more than backward walking).

Some other abnormal movements may resemble dystonia. Slow tics, known as dystonic tics, differ from dystonia by their variability with time and by the temporary control the patient may exert on them. Choreic movements do not result from muscular tensions but may coexist with athetosis. Paretic–spastic syndromes can produce attitudes similar to those in dystonia (Manfredi et al. 1975), and this may also occur in muscular or neuropathic disorders. Psychiatric disturbances may be quite difficult to distinguish from dystonia, and dystonia is often mistaken for hysteria.

Tics

Tics are repetitive movements of skeletal or pharyngo-laryngeal muscles; the latter are responsible for emission of sounds or noises. They are considered as stereotyped, involuntary, sudden, inopportune, non-propositional, absurd, irresistible movements, of variable intensity (Shapiro and Shapiro 1986). The involuntary character is not absolutely clear. The patients are able to exert some control on the movement. Moreover, sometimes they explain that they are 'urged' to do it as a compulsive action. The voluntary suppression of tics generates an unpleasant feeling, that is relieved with the execution of the tic (Leckman et al. 1992). Frequent tics can produce pain (Riley and Lang 1989).

Tics (Table 1.1) can be divided into:

(a) *simple motor tics* that involve a single muscle or group of muscles, e.g. eye blink, shoulder shrug or twitch of the nose;

(b) *complex motor tics* that result in elaborate movements involving several muscle groups. Although essentially involuntary they may have a degree of intentionality and a great variety of expression, such as scratching one's nose or jumping;

(c) *phonatory tics* can express as vocalization or simpler noises such as throat clearing, grunts or sounds imitating animal cries, e.g. barking. They may utilize articulate language. They include echolalia (repetition of the words of an interlocutor), palilalia (repetition of one's last words) and coprolalia (emission of obscene language). This last modality,

TABLE 1.1
Various types of tics

Simple motor tics (eye closure, head turns)
Complex motor tics (scratching, jumping)
Elaborate motor tics (cycle walking)
Dystonic tics (sustained movement)
Simple phonatory tics (coughing, sniffing, throat cleaning)
Complex phonatory tics
Verbal outbursts (coprolalia, echolalia)
Sensory tics

TABLE 1.2
Characteristics of tics that permit differentiation from other abnormal movements

The patient can reproduce tics voluntarily
The patient can partially control them
Tics do not interfere with voluntarily activity (e.g. do not alter handwriting or prevent drinking out of a glass)
Tics predominate in facial muscles, trunk and proximal parts of limbs (the further from the face, the rarer the involvement)
Tics may persist during sleep

although uncommon (8% of adult cases according to Goldenberg et al. 1994) is of historical interest as it was one of the remarkable features mentioned in the original description by Itard (1825) of the case of the Marquise de Dampierre who said "extraordinary words which make deplorable contrast to her distinguished manner. Those words are mostly rude oaths, obscene adjectives . ."

Echopraxia (imitation of gesture) and copropraxia (obscene gestures) are rare.

Sensory tics (Shapiro et al. 1988, Kurlan et al. 1989) are recurrent somatic sensations, in the form of feelings of pressure, heat, cold or pain in localized body areas, that are temporarily suppressed by movement. The patient feels a need to execute the movement that suppresses the abnormal sensation and so this is, in a sense, a compulsive phenomenon.

Other difficulties in the analysis of tics, in addition to their variable expression, are the fact that they 'come and go', that is their expression and location change without apparent reason, and that the patient can inhibit them for some time especially in front of witnesses and the physician. In one study (Goetz et al. 1987) with video recording, there was a 27% reduction when the subject was facing the examiner. The patients recognize the imminence of their tics and may mask them by giving them a propositional appearance. Although tics are generally easy to identify, even for lay persons, they may sometimes be difficult to distinguish from other abnormal movements (Table 1.2).

Complex tics should be differentiated from choreic movements, dystonia and stereotypies, and simple tics from myoclonus.

For each patient there exist specific situations in which the frequency of tics increases or decreases (e.g. watching television, concentrating attention, pleasurable situations, etc.). Especially, events causing anxiety, emotional trauma, and social gatherings increase tics (Silva et al. 1995). Tics are not precipitated by stimuli as occurs in some forms of myoclonus. Although it is generally held that tics disappear during sleep, it is now clear that many patients continue to have tics in some stages of sleep (Glaze et al. 1983).

From an electromyographic viewpoint, tics are indistinguishable from normal voluntary contractions. The pathophysiology of tics is dealt with in Chapter 9.

Myoclonus
Myoclonus is defined as the occurrence of sudden, brief involuntary contractions of a muscle or group of muscles. They look like contractions produced by electrical shock in a peripheral nerve (Marsden et al. 1982).

Myoclonic contractions may be isolated or repetitive. They may be focal, involving a single muscle or muscle group, multifocal or generalized. According to their pattern of repetition one can distinguish rhythmical and arrhythmical myoclonus. Rare cases of oscillatory myoclonus are on record (Fahn and Sing 1981). Myoclonus can be spontaneous, without any precipitating factor, or precipitated by stimuli (reflex myoclonus) such as sudden unexpected noises, light, voluntary movement, intention to move or even the command not to move.

The intensity of the phenomenon is variable, from massive contraction (generalized myoclonus) producing large movements or falls, to localized (focal myoclonus), minimal discharges that do not result in segmental displacement. Myoclonus can be present only at rest or only when the patient engages in a delicate task. For these reasons, myoclonus is easily confused with other abnormal movements. If arrhythmical, it can be mistaken for simple motor tics, but it is not even partially controllable.

Fasciculations and minipolymyoclonus (Spiro 1970) also should be distinguished from arrhythmical myoclonus. Rhythmical myoclonus has to be separated from tremor. The latter is a sinusoidal movement, whereas in myoclonus there are silent intervals between individual contractions. Rapid, jerk-like movements can occur in some cases of dystonia and be difficult to differentiate from rhythmical myoclonus (see above).

Asterixis (flapping tremor) is the term introduced by Adams and Foley (1949) to designate brief and sudden interruptions of muscular contraction that result in the fall of a member or part of a member maintained in an antigravity posture. It represents an inverse phenomenon to myoclonus, hence the term negative myoclonus (Shahani and Young 1976). Since other myoclonic phenomena may feature a silent period in both agonist and antagonist muscles on electromyographic recordings there is no essential difference. The main distinction may be in duration of the silent period. Asterixis is observed in Angelman syndrome (Guerrini et al. 1996), diffuse encephalopathies from renal, hepatic or pulmonary failure, in some malabsortion syndromes and in some cases of hydantoin toxicity (Murphy and Goldstein 1974).

Myoclonus is the most protean of all abnormal movements (Obeso et al. 1988). It can be a normal phenomenon (termed 'physiological') or a sign of dysfunction at multiple CNS levels.

Myoclonus classification is discussed in Chapter 8.

Other types of abnormal movements
Akathisia (from the Greek kathisis: sitting down) is an 'internal anxiety' that forces the subject to constantly change postures. It can be controlled temporarily by will. It is different from hyperkinesia in which the child maintains a constant level of general hyperactivity rather than just constant changes in posture. Akathisia is considered an extrapyramidal disturbance, whereas hyperkinesia is an abnormality of higher level functions possibly due to a reduced level of attention (Fejerman 1997).

Opsoclonus, described by Orzechowski (1927) is a disorder of eye movement characterized by discharges of rapid involuntary and chaotic movements in all directions of the eyes. Although the eye movements appear to be conjugate, analysis has shown that they are not (Vignaendra and Lim 1977). Opsoclonus is often associated with rapid fluttering movements of the eyelids.

The term *stereotypy* refers to repetitive, often rhythmical, voluntary (can be initiated or interrupted by the subject) but non-propositional movements. Common examples include head rolling, head banging, and knitting movements of the hands.

CLINICAL CONTEXT OF ABNORMAL MOVEMENTS
HISTORY-TAKING
History-taking is an essential step in the orientation of investigations and diagnosis. The following aspects are especially important in movement disorders. A positive family history suggestive of dominant genetic disorder, or the presence of consanguinity that may suggest a recessive condition, are to be carefully looked for, taking into account the marked variation of expressivity of many dominant conditions. The presence of perinatal antecedents of neonatal encephalopathy or neonatal icterus is also of interest as it may explain such disorders as athetosis or dystonia.

However, only well-documented antecedents should be relied upon. A history of 'difficult birth' does not signify that a movement disorder is the result of hypoxia and/or ischaemia. Such diagnosis should be accepted only when, in addition to documented symptoms and signs of perinatal distress, neurological signs of encephalopathy, especially convulsions, in the neonatal period are well established.

Information about the age of onset of the disorder, its initial manifestations and course (acute onset, slow progressivity, spontaneous improvement) is essential, even though the precise date of onset of certain symptoms such as tremor may be difficult to document so that the parents often wrongly indicate that it has always been present.

Attention should also be given to the possibility of precipitating factors (drugs, infections, muscular exercise) or of aggravating (effect of fatigue, diurnal fluctuation) or ameliorating factors (sleep, alcohol).

The description given by the child is often more precise than that of the parents and an effort to obtain it is worthwhile. Description of the abnormal movements by lay persons and even by physicians is often unreliable. Photographs and, especially, videotapes of patients are of extreme value and every effort should be made to look at these.

CLINICAL EXAMINATION

The child should be observed carefully in spontaneous and required activities rather than interfered with for a 'formal' neurological examination. The characteristics, topography and modifying factors of the abnormal movements should be carefully noted. The presence of abnormal movements should be investigated in imposed attitudes such as extension of both arms and in the classical tests such as finger-to-nose test. Ambulation is particularly important to observe not only in regular forward walking but also in toe- and heel-walking, tandem walking and backward ambulation, which may paradoxically improve gait in cases of dystonia. In older children, drawing and writing are especially sensitive tests. Search for associated movements is important. Looking for the distant effects of movements to detect overflow movement is important in dystonia and athetosis.

Asking the patient to press gently her/his extended hands on those of the examiner while her/his attention is distracted is a useful manoeuvre to detect mild choreic or myoclonic movements, and requesting the patient to engage in fine activities such as threading pearls makes many abnormal movements appear or increase.

Standard neurological examination is necessary to rule in or out involvement of other systems. Some movement disorders, especially dopa-sensitive dystonia (see Chapter 5), are especially associated with marked hyperreflexia and often with extension of the great toes, the so-called 'striatal toe', wrongly suggesting involvement of the pyramidal tract.

DISTRIBUTION, STATISTICAL DATA

Personal experience (of EF-A) with dyskinesias beginning before 18 years of age, not including dyskinetic forms of cerebral palsy, cerebellar tremor, epileptic myoclonus and iatrogenic dyskinesias, is summarized in Figures 1.5–1.7. Cases of delayed onset dystonia are included.

This series is not necessarily representative of population frequency as it was collected in a referral centre.

The factors responsible for age of onset and sex distribution are unknown. Cerebral influence of steroids has been suggested on the basis of animal studies (Loscher et al. 1995).

CLASSIFICATION OF THE MOVEMENT DISORDERS

Any classification of movement disorders is made difficult by the lack of a pathological

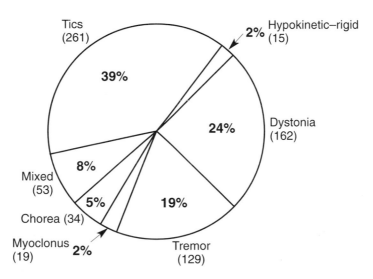

Fig. 1.5. Absolute values (in brackets) and percentages in personal (EF-A) series of 684 patients under 18 years of age with movement disorders. 'Mixed' refers to cases with two or more types of movement. Cases of cerebral palsy and iatrogenic movement disorders are not included.

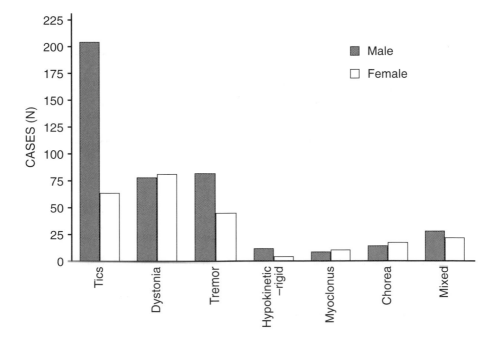

Fig. 1.6. Distribution of sexes and types of abnormal movements in personal series of movement disorders.

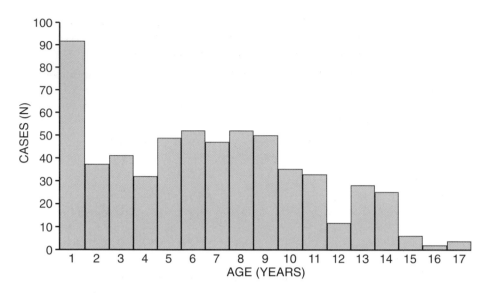

Fig. 1.7. Age of onset in 550 patients with movement disorders in whom this was known. Cases of cerebral palsy and iatrogenic movement disorders are not included.

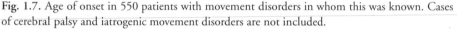

TABLE 1.3
Transient movement disorders in children

Essential palatal tremor
Jitteriness
Shuddering
Transient idiopathic dystonia of infancy
Transient paroxysmal dystonia of infancy
Spasmus nutans
Benign paroxysmal torticollis of infancy
Benign paroxysmal tonic upgaze
Benign myoclonus of the newborn
Benign myoclonus of infancy
Transient tic

and biochemical basis in the majority of diseases. The most used is the ICD (Jankovic 1995).

Based on aetiology one can distinguish idiopathic (or essential) diseases when the movement disorder is the only feature of the disease, and secondary forms in the remaining cases. Secondary forms may be of known or unknown (cryptogenic) cause. Marsden and Quinn (1990) term 'primary or idiopathic' all cases in which no cause is found.

According to evolution, movement disorders can be separated into transient, chronic and paroxysmal. The term *chronic* applies to cases in which abnormal symptoms persist uninterrupted for more than a year. *Paroxysmal* disorders means diseases in which the disturbance is episodic (even if the episodes last several days) and between the episodes the patient is free of symptoms. The term *transient* is used in two circumstances: for those that can be chronic but last less than a year (e.g. tic); and those lasting longer but disappearing without leaving residua (Table 1.3).

All transient movement disorders are idiopathic and unassociated with other neurological disease (Fernández-Alvarez 1998). Many of them have only been identified in recent years. The investigations always prove to be normal; there are no specific markers, which means that the only diagnostic tool is clinical experience. Knowledge of these conditions is important because it avoids not only unnecessary tests and treatment but also familial anxiety.

REFERENCES

Adams RD, Foley J (1949) Neurological changes in more common types of severe liver disease. *Trans Am Neurol Ass* 74: 217–9.

Alexander GE, De Long MR, Strick PL (1986) Parallel organization of functionally segregated circuits linking basal ganglia and cortex. *Ann Rev Neurosci* 9: 357–81.

Bathia KP, Marsden CD (1994) The behavioural and motor consequences of focal lesions of the basal ganglia in man. *Brain* 117: 859–76.

Burke RE, Fahn S, Marsden CD, et al. (1985) Validity and reliability rating scale for the primary torsion dystonias. *Neurology* 35: 73–7.

Ceballos-Bauman AO, Passingham RE, Warner T, et al. (1995) Overactive prefrontal and under-active motor cortical areas in idiopathic dystonia. *Ann Neurol* 37: 363–72.

Coleman M (1970) Preliminary remarks on the L-dopatherapy of dystonia. *Neurology* 20: 114–21.

Crossman AR (1987) Primate models of dyskinesia: the experimental approach to the study of basal ganglia-related involuntary movement disorders. *Neurosci* 21: 1-40.

Davis CH, Kunkle EC (1951) Benign essential (heredo-familial) tremor. *Arch Int Med* 87: 808–16.

Day BL, Marsden CD, Obeso JA, Rothwell JC (1984) Reciprocal inhibition between the muscles of the human forearm. *J Physiol* 349: 519–34.

De Long MR (1990) Primate models of movement disorders of basal ganglia origin. *Tins* 13: 281–5.

Denny-Brown D (1968) Clinical symptomatology of diseases of the basal ganglia. In: Vinken PD, Bruyn GW (eds) *Handbook of Clinical Neurology, Vol. 6.* Amsterdam: North Holland.

Fahn S (1988) Concept and classification of dystonia. In: Fahn S, Marsden CD, Calne DB (eds) *Advances in Neurology, Vol. 50, Dystonia 2.* New York: Raven Press, pp. 1–9.

— Sing N (1981) Oscillatory myoclonus. *Neurology* 31: 80.

Fejerman N (1997) Trastornos del desarrollo y disfunción cerebral mínima. In: Fejerman N, Fernández-Alvarez E (eds) *Neurología Pediátrica, 2nd edn.* Buenos Aires: Panamericana, pp. 653–82.

Fernández-Alvarez E (1998) Transient movements disorders in children. *J Neurol* 245: 1–5.

Gerfen CR, Engber TR, Mahan LC, et al. (1990) D1 and D2 dopamine receptor-regulated gene expression of striatonigral and striatopallidal neurons. *Science* 250: 1429–32.

Glaze DG, Frost JD, Jankovic J (1983) Sleep in Gilles de la Tourette syndrome: disorder of arousal. *Neurology* 3: 586–92.

Goetz CG, Tanner CM, Wilson RS, Shanon KM (1987) A rating scale for Gilles de la Tourette's syndrome: description, reliability and validity data. *Neurology* 37: 1542–4.

Goldenberg JN, Brown SB, Weiner WJ (1994) Coprolalia in younger patients with Gilles de la Tourette syndrome. *Mov Disord* 9: 622–5.

Guerrini R, De Lorey TM, Bonanni P, Moncla A (1996) Cortical myoclonus in Angelman syndrome. *Ann Neurol* 39: 699–708.

Guridi J, Herrero MT, Luquin MR, et al. (1996) Subthalamotomy in parkinsonian monkeys. Behavioural and biochemical analysis. *Brain* 119: 1717–27.

Jankovic J (1995) International Classification of Diseases, 10th Revision: Neurological adaptation (ICD-10 NA): extrapyramidal and movement disorders. *Mov Disord* 10: 533–40.

— (1997) Phenomenology and classification of tics. *Neurol Clin NA* 15: 267–75.

— Fahn S (1980) Physiologic and pathologic tremors: diagnosis, mechanism, and management. *Ann Intern Med* 93: 460–5.

Kurlan R, Lichter D, Hewitt D (1989) Sensory tics in Tourette's syndrome. *Neurology* 39: 731–4.

Lakke PWF, Barbeau A, Duvoisin RC, et al. (1981) Classification of extrapyramidal disorders. Proposal for an international classification and glossary of terms. *J Neurol Sci* 51, 311–27.

Leckman JF, Pauls DL, Peterson BS, et al. (1992) Pathogenesis of Tourette syndrome: Clues from the clinical phenotype and natural history. In: Case TN, Friedhoff AJ, Cohen DJ (eds) *Advances in Neurology, Vol. 58.* New York: Raven Press, pp. 15–25.

Loscher W, Blanke T, Richter A, Hoppen HO (1995) Gonadal sex hormones and dystonia: Experimental studies in genetically dystonic hamsters. *Mov Disord* 10: 92–102.

Manfredi M, Sacco G, Sideri G (1975) The tonic ambulatory foot response: A clinical and electro-myographic study. *Brain* 98: 167–80.

Marsden CD (1986) Movement disorders and the basal ganglia. *Trends Neurosci* 9: 512–5.

— Harrison JG (1974) Idiopathic torsion dystonia (dystonia musculorum deformans). A review of forty-two patients. *Brain* 97: 793–810.

— Quinn NP (1990) The dystonias. Neurological disorders affecting 20,000 people in Britain. *BMJ* 300: 139–44.

— Hallett M, Fahn S (1982) The nosology and pathophysiology of myoclonus. In: Marsden CD, Fahn S (eds) *Movement Disorders.* London: Butterworth Scientific, pp. 196–248.

Murphy MJ, Goldstein MN (1974) Diphenylhydantoin induced asterixis: a clinical study. *JAMA* 1111 330 40.

Obeso JA, Artieda J, Marsden CD (1988) Different clinical presentations of myoclonus. In: Jankovic J, Tolosa E (eds) *Parkinson's Disease and Movement Disorders.* Baltimore/Munich: Urban & Schwarzenberg, pp. 263–74.

Orzechwoski C (1927) De l'ataxie dysmétrique des yeux. *J Psychol Neurol* 35: 1–18.

Padberg G, Bruyn GW (1986) Chorea: differential diagnosis. In: Vinken PJ, Bruyn GN, Klawans HL (eds) *Handbook of Clinical Neurology, Vol. 49.* Amsterdam: Elsevier, pp. 549–64.

Prechtl HFR, Stemmer CHJ (1962) The choreiform syndrome in children. *Dev Med Child Neurol* 4: 119–27.

Quinn NP, Rothwell JC, Thompson PD, Marsden CD (1988) Hereditary myoclonic dystonia, hereditary torsion dystonia and hereditary essential myoclonus: an area of confusion. In: Fahn S, Marsden CD, Calne DB (eds) *Advances in Neurology, Vol. 50, Dystonia 2.* New York: Raven Press, pp. 391–402.

Refsum S, Sjaastad O (1972) Hereditary non-progressive involuntary movements with early onset and intentional tremor, without dementia. *Acta Neurol Scand* 51 (suppl.): 489–91.

Riley DE, Lang AE (1989) Pain in Gilles de la Tourette syndrome and related tic disorders. *Can J Neurol Sci* 16: 439–41.

Rondot P (1983) Involuntary movements and neurotrasmitters. *Neuropediatrics* 14: 59–65.

— Bathien N, Ziegler M (1988) *Les Mouvements Anormaux*. Paris: Masson.

Shahani BT, Young RR (1976) Physiological and pharmacological aids in the differential diagnosis of tremor. *J Neuro Neurosurg Psychiat* 39: 772–83.

Shapiro AK, Shapiro ES, Young JG, Fenberg TE (1988) *Gilles de la Tourette Syndrome, 2nd edn.* New York: Raven Press.

Shapiro E, Shapiro AK (1986) Semiology, nosology and criteria for tic disorders. *Rev Neurol* 142, 824–32.

Silva RR, Munoz DM, Barickman J, Friedhoff AJ (1995) Environmental factors and related fluctuation of symptoms in children and adolescents with Tourette's disorder. *J Child Psychol Psychiat* 36: 305–12.

Sjaastad O, Sulg I, Refsum S (1983) Benign familial myoclonus-like movements, partly of early onset. *J Neurol Transm* 19 (suppl.): 291–301.

Spiro AJ (1970) Minipolymyoclonus. A neglected sign in childhood spinal muscular atrophy. *Neurology* 20: 1124–6.

Vignaedra V, Lim CL (1977) Electro-oculographic analysis of opsoclonus: Its relationship to saccadic and nonsaccadic eye movement. *Neurology* 27: 1129–33.

Weiner WJ, Lang AE (1989) *Movement Disorders. A Comprehensive Survey.* Mont Kisco, NY: Futura.

Wolf S, Jones DW, Knable MB, et al. (1996) Tourette syndrome: Prediction of phenotypic variation in monozygotic twins by caudate nucleus D2 receptor binding. *Science* 273: 1225–7.

Wolff PH, Hurwitz I (1966) The choreiform syndrome. *Dev Med Child Neurol* 8: 160–5.

Zeman W, Dyken P (1967) Dystonia musculorum dephormans. Clinical, genetic and pathoanatomical studies. *J Psychiat Neurol Neurochir* 70: 77–121.

2

DISORDERS IN WHICH A HYPOKINETIC–RIGID SYNDROME IS THE PREDOMINANT FEATURE

Disorders expressed as a hypokinetic–rigid syndrome (H-RS) are rare in childhood, and exceptional in infants. Among 673 cases of disorders of movement seen at Hospital Sant Joan de Deu (Barcelona), only 14 (2%) had an H-RS. The average age of onset of such cases (Fig. 2.1) was 11.3 years (range 4–15 years).

Interestingly, when H-RS does occur in children it is frequently associated with dystonic features. It has been speculated that the deficiency in dopamine transmission responsible for H-RS in adults may be expressed in children by dystonia (Katchen and Duvoisin 1986). Thus, Hallervorden–Spatz disease begins in childhood with dystonia and in the adult with a parkinsonian syndrome, and in early-onset of parkinsonism there is a high incidence of dystonic phenomena, sometimes predating the onset of the parkinsonian syndrome.

A list of disorders that can present with such a syndrome appears in Table 2.1.

The term *parkinsonism* is used in the literature with variable significance. We use it here to designate the H-RS when it is not due to Parkinson disease. The term *Parkinson disease* applies to a specific condition observed mainly in adults. Parkinsonism can be 'pure' or associated with other movement disorders, and idiopathic or secondary to known (infective, toxic, tumoral, etc.) causes.

Two practical points should be mentioned. First, Wilson disease can present with rigidity. Because this disorder can be effectively treated, especially when recognized early, it is important to diagnose it. Second, even if the H-RS syndrome is related to dopamine deficit, the response to treatment with L-dopa is variable. It is usually non-responsive in many metabolic or degenerative diseases, possibly because they are due a postsynaptic lesion. When the cause is a lesion of the nigrostriatal neurons (presynaptic lesion) as occurs in Parkinson disease, there is a significant response to the therapy but it can be followed by the appearance of motor side-effects: fluctuating disability, end-of-dose deterioration, and 'on-off' phenomenon. In dopa-responsive dystonia the benefit of treatment with L-dopa is not associated with motor side-effects because the defect is purely one of dopamine synthesis.

JUVENILE IDIOPATHIC PARKINSONISM (JIP)
JIP refers to an idiopathic (no Parkinson disease) H-RS with onset before the age of 20

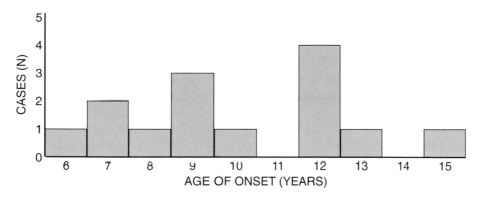

Fig. 2.1. Age of onset of 14 cases with hypokinetic–rigid syndrome as main clinical movement disorder. Hallervorden–Spatz disease (4 cases), Wilson disease (3), Huntington disease (2), neuronal intranuclear disease (2 cases), GM2 gangliosidosis (1), Gaucher disease (1) and subacute sclerosing panencephalitis (1).

TABLE 2.1
Disorders with H-RS in childhood

Early onset Parkinson disease
Parkinsonism
    Juvenile idiopathic parkinsonism
    X-linked dystonia parkinsonism
    Rapid onset dystonia parkinsonism
    Secondary
        Hydrocephalus
        Hypoparathyroidism and pseudohypoparathyroidism
        Intoxications
        Drugs
        Infections
        Basal ganglia tumours
Other diseases with H-RS
    Huntington disease
    Wilson disease (see Chapter 6)
    Juvenile GM2 gangliosidosis (see Chapter 5)
    Niemann–Pick type C (see Chapter 5)
    Multiple-system atrophies (see Chapter 6)
    Neuronal intranuclear inclusion disease
    Hallervorden–Spatz disease (see Chapter 6)
    Machado–Joseph disease (see Chapter 6)
    Mitochondrial cytopathies (see Chapter 6)
    Phenylketonuria
    Neuroacanthocytosis (see Chapter 6)
    Subacute sclerosing panencephalitis (Sawaishi et al. 1999)

years. JIP cases can be sporadic or familial with various types of inheritance. Pathology and response to L-dopa are also variable. In children, 'idiopathic' parkinsonism is often associated with dystonic signs. Therefore the term 'dystonia–parkinsonism' is nonspecific and, when used to designate a disease, easily causes confusion. In fact the best known disease with dystonia and parkinsonism is dopa-responsive dystonia (see Chapter 5).

This heterogeneous group can be subdivided into two main subgroups: progressive pallidal atrophy, and JIP from miscellaneous other causes.

PROGRESSIVE PALLIDAL ATROPHY

One group of JIP is related to *progressive pallidal lesions*. In 1917, Ramsay Hunt described four sporadic cases of 'paralysis agitans of the juvenile type'. In two of these the age of onset was 13 and 15 years of age. The disease was progressive with parkinsonian signs and dystonic features and with an intact intellect. Autopsy at age 30 years of one of these cases, with onset at 15 years, showed a selective atrophy of the motor neurons of the globus pallidus, a lesion different from that seen in Parkinson disease. Hunt considered that all these patients had the same disease, termed 'primary atrophy of the pallidal system'. One of the remaining three cases he reported later developed pyramidal tract signs and was reported by Davison (1954) with other cases under the term 'pallidopyramidal disease'. Cases of 'pure' and 'combined' (associated with corpus Luysi and/or substantia nigra lesions) pallidal atrophy, both sporadic and familial, have been reported (Ota et al. 1958, Jellinger 1986). Whether the cases reported as 'juvenile paralysis agitans' or 'Ramsay Hunt syndrome' could be considered as a specific disease entity is doubted by some authors (Lyon et al. 1996).

MISCELLANEOUS CASES OF JIP

Other cases of JIP begin with tremor and/or dystonia by 6–16 years of age, with subsequent development of parkinsonism with a normal intellect. Ancillary investigations are normal. Some patients show atypical signs, e.g. the case of Naidu et al. (1978) with right-sided dystonia. Some cases are sporadic (Gershanik and Leist 1986) but a majority are familial. Familial cases may have an autosomal dominant inheritance with incomplete penetrance (Spellman 1962, Allen and Knop 1976). Cases with autosomal recessive inheritance are less rare (Martin et al. 1971, Sachdev et al. 1977, Carlier and Dubru 1979).

Most patients treated with L-dopa are reported to have improved significantly, but similar to what occurs in Parkinson disease but not in dopa-responsive dystonia, soon developed fluctuations and abnormal involuntary movements (Martin et al. 1971, Kilroy et al. 1972, Carlier and Dubru 1979). Similarities in both clinical manifestations and therapeutic response makes it difficult to differentiate JIP from early-onset Parkinson disease.

EARLY-ONSET PARKINSON DISEASE (EOP)

Parkinson disease is usually a disorder of the second half of life. Its aetiology is unknown.

Its basic physiopathologic defect is a loss of dopaminergic nigral neurons and the presence of Lewy bodies (concentric hyaline cytoplasmic inclusions) that cause a decreased dopaminergic activity. Because of the progressively reduced capacity to produce dopamine, a progressively larger dose of L-dopa treatment is necessary and frequent motor fluctuation appears.

Parkinson disease starting between 20 and 40 years is sometimes termed 'young onset Parkinson disease'. Cases with clinical similarities to Parkinson disease but with the onset before 20 years of age are often termed 'juvenile parkinsonism' (Quinn et al. 1987, Golbe 1991) but different terms have been used (see Gershanik 1988). To avoid confusion, we prefer to term all such cases 'early-onset Parkinson disease'. EOP may be a different entity from adult-onset Parkinson disease because of clinical and genetic differences (Muthane et al. 1994).

Cases of EOP constitute a highly heterogeneous group. Narabayashi et al. (1986) collected eight cases (two in siblings of different sex) that they denominate 'juvenile Parkinson disease' with onset between 6 and 16 years. Rest tremor, depressive states and seborrhoeic facies were less marked than in the adult-onset Parkinson disease. They responded to small doses of L-dopa, regardless of the interval between onset of the disease and treatment. Abnormal movements, mainly dystonia (more frequent in the feet), tremor, often as the first manifestation, and spontaneous diurnal fluctuations with marked improvement after sleep were frequent features. In a 6-year-old girl (a patient's younger brother was also affected), described in detail, the onset was with asymmetrical rigidity and mild dystonia of the feet. The disease progressed to invalidity by age 24. The patient responded spectacularly to L-dopa initiated at 30 years of age and was able to walk almost normally. One year later, however, she developed ballismus despite a minimal dose of L-dopa. Following thalamotomy, she could resume L-dopa treatment associated with a low dose of bromocriptine which permitted normal activity. She died of paralytic ileus at 39 years.

Familial cases of EOP are more frequent than sporadic ones (Yokochi et al. 1984, Narabayashi et al. 1986). Of special interest are the 14 members of a single family, all of whom had gradual onset of symptoms between 5 and 39 years. Dystonia (inconstant) affected only the legs and feet (Dwork et al. 1993). A distinct form of familial Parkinson disease, called also 'autosomal recessive juvenile parkinsonism', characterized by early onset, temporary improvement following sleep, and good dopa responsiveness but with motor fluctuations after L-dopa treatment has been reported (Yamamura et al. 1973, Ishikawa et al. 1996). Pathological studies showed loss of neurons in the substantia nigra but without Lewy bodies (Takahashi et al. 1994). A gene responsible for this form of Parkinson disease (called *Parkin* gene) has been identified (Kitada et al. 1998, Wang et al. 1999).

Pathological studies in other forms of juvenile parkinsonism showed lesions similar to those of idiopathic Parkinson disease with reduced pigmentation of the substantia nigra and even a few Lewy bodies (familial case reported by Yokochi et al. 1984, later by Narabayashi et al. 1986, and restudied by Gibb et al. 1991).

Cases of EOP and JIP have many similarities to dopa-responsive dystonia especially as some cases of dopa-responsive dystonia do not feature diurnal fluctuation. However, fluorodopa PET scanning show reduced fixation of fluorodopa in basal ganglia in patients with juvenile parkinsonism or EOP in contrast to dopa-responsive dystonia in which the fluorodopa uptake is normal (Snow et al. 1993, Turjanski et al. 1993). Moreover, initial levodopa response is similar in these diseases but (with very few exceptions – Rajput et al. 1997) EOP and JIP are progressive disorders and prolonged dopa therapy leads to a failure of response. These data suggest different pathogenic mechanisms for EOP and dopa-responsive dystonia. In the latter there would be a presynaptic dysfunction of dopamine nerve terminals without anatomical lesion, whereas in juvenile parkinsonism and Parkinson disease a progressive loss of dopaminergic neurons in the substantia nigra (Rondot and Ziegler 1983) would be present.

The differential diagnosis of JIP includes Wilson disease, the rigid form of Huntington disease and dopa-responsive dystonia as well as cases of secondary parkinsonism. In the latter cases the H-RS is usually associated with other 'non-extrapyramidal' neurological signs ('parkinsonism-plus' – Pranzatelli et al. 1994).

X-LINKED DYSTONIA–PARKINSONISM
(X-linked parkinsonism, 'Lubag' disease)
This disorder is encountered in the island of Panay (Philippines) (Lee et al. 1976). The mean age of onset is 31 years, but despite this the disease tends to become generalized. X-linked inheritance of ITD has been mapped to the pericentromeric region of the X chromosome (Wilhelmsen et al. 1991).

RAPID-ONSET DYSTONIA PARKINSONISM
Although only three families with this disorder are known (Dobyns et al. 1993, Brashear et al. 1996, Webb et al. 1999), the clinical peculiarities make it of special interest. The most remarkable characteristic was the very rapid development of dystonia and parkinsonism. In half the cases, the clinical picture was completed within a single day or was even found by the patient on awakening. Both dystonic and parkinsonian features are generalized even though they can be localized at onset. In all cases the face and upper limb are less involved than the rest of the body.

The disorder appears to be transmitted as an autosomal dominant trait and begins between 15 and 45 years of age. All investigations remain negative except a low CSF level of HVA. The disorder is not linked to either *DYT1* gene or the locus of dopa-responsive dystonia.

Treatment with L-dopa or other antiparkinsonian drugs is of limited efficacy.

JUVENILE HUNTINGTON DISEASE
The interesting history of Huntington disease (HD) (a better term than Huntington chorea as chorea is not a constant feature, especially in children) is detailed by Bruyn and

Went (1986). In 1872, Huntington described the major features of the disorder including "its hereditary nature" without skipped generations and the mental disorder that some-times led to suicide, but he considered erroneously that the disease was limited to adults. The prevalence of the disease varies with country and race. In Caucasians, it varies between 16 and 92 per million (Bruyn and Went 1986). A lower rate is seen in Japanese, Jewish and Black populations. The disorder is genetically determined with an autosomal dominant inheritance. The genetic abnormality in HD has been identified as an intra-genic expansion of a CAG trinucleotide repeat (Gusella et al. 1983, Wesler et al. 1985) in the distal part of the short arm of chromosome 4. All HD patients tested have had at least 37 CAG repeats. The mutation rate is unknown but it is very low. The product of the gene is a 348-Kd protein named 'huntingtin'. It is widely expressed, and expression is high in the brain (Strong et al. 1993). Its physiological role is as yet unknown.

HD could be considered in different chapters of this book (chorea, multysystemic diseases) but is included here because the hypokinetic–rigid form occurs predominantly in childhood.

CLINICAL FEATURES
HD has a highly variable expression between and within families and even between monozygotic twins (Oepen 1973).

The disease has an insidious onset which makes it difficult to determine the age of first manifestations. The mean age of onset of symptoms is between 35 and 51 years (Myers et al. 1988). Arbitrarily, forms that begin before 10 years or before 20 years are considered as juvenile (Bruyn and Went 1986, Byers et al. 1973). Early-onset forms in children (Markhan and Knox 1965, Hansotia et al. 1968, Fernández-Alvarez 1972, Jongen et al. 1980, Osborne et al. 1982) have attracted attention during the last few decades. To our knowledge the earliest onset reported was at age 2 years (Went et al. 1984). The reported frequency in children under age 10 varies between 1% (Stevens 1976), 4.7% (Hayden and Beighton 1982) and 6.8% (Dewhurst and Oliver 1970) of total HD cases. Other studies found 3% of cases beginning under 15 years (Caviness 1985) and 10% before 20 years (Bruyn and Went 1986).

The type of onset is variable. Some patients first show neurological signs and later psychiatric symptoms, while in others the opposite occurs. For many patients, the first clinical disturbances are non-propositional movements that, even if initially difficult to differentiate from normal motor activity, increase in frequency to realize a full-fledged chorea in a few years. Walking becomes abnormal because of choreic movements, or lordotic or flexion postures. Dysarthria and dysphagia are frequent in advanced disease. Abnormalities of eye movements, especially of vertical saccades (Leigh et al. 1983), are common. Ataxia, amyotrophy and pyramidal tract signs may be seen (Young et al. 1986). Psychiatric disturbances with eventual dementia are an essential part of the picture but are quite variable in type. Rarely only one category of anomalies (motor or psychiatric) is present. Progression is variable with individual cases. Suicide is frequent being the cause of death in 6–7% of adult patients (Conneally 1984). The median survival time after onset ranges between 14 and 17 years (Myers et al. 1982, Farrer et al. 1984) but the course tends to be more rapid in childhood onset than in adult cases, with a mean age at death of 9.3 years (11.0±5.1 in rigid juvenile forms) (Vegter-van der Vlis et al. 1976, Osborne et al. 1982). In rare cases the course is slower: Brooks et al. (1987) reported on a patient who had disturbances of conduct and mental regression starting at 11 years, developed ataxia and "abrupt jerking movements" at 25 years and died at 27 years.

Juvenile cases share with adult forms slow progressivity, and the presence of disorders of conduct and of movement (Campbell et al. 1961, Bittenbender and Quadfasel 1962) but differ by several features. The disease may also begin with rest or action tremor, epilepsy, intellectual regression (Lenti and Bianchini 1993) or conduct disorder (Brooks et al. 1987). In the latter case, the diagnosis can only be suggested by a positive family history. A rigid form (originally described by Westphal in 1813, before Huntington's description) is more frequent in juvenile than in adult cases. It was found in 29 of 43 reviewed by Osborne et al. (1982). Chorea was seen in only 12 of 43 juvenile cases (Osborne et al. 1982). Epilepsy is a feature in 40% of infantile cases. Oculomotor abnormalities similar to those in adults have been reported (Bird and Paulson 1971).

DIAGNOSIS

The diagnosis of HD should be thought of in children with a family history of the disease who present with any neurological or psychiatric disturbance not clearly attributable to another cause. Penetrance of the gene is complete, and spontaneous mutations are virtually unheard of. However, clinical normality of parents does not exclude the diagnosis as the disease can manifest in offspring before it does in a parent (Erdohazi and Marshall 1979). Diagnostic certainty can now be obtained by techniques of molecular genetics in 96% of cases (Schömig-Spingler et al. 1989, Craufurd et al. 1989, Skraastad et al. 1991). In suspect cases for which molecular studies do not confirm the diagnosis of HD, that of dentato-rubro-pallidal atrophy (Chapter 6) should be considered.

The possible psychological consequences of presymptomatic screening are a matter for discussion. Some investigators (Wiggins et al. 1992) and even associations of affected persons (Hayes 1992) argue that it may maintain or even improve the psychological well-being of people at risk, as the very basic risk of 50% is in itself hard to accept and the diagnosis can be firmly excluded.

The phenomenon of anticipation, common to genetic disorders due to expansion of trinucleotide repeats, is typically seen in HD. In childhood cases the size of the repeat is usually larger than in the affected parent, and the size of the repeat tends to increase in the spermatic rather than the oocyte lineage (Duyao et al. 1993). In childhood and juvenile cases, the disease is paternally inherited 4–7 times more frequently than maternally (Bruyn 1969, Osborne et al. 1982, Conneally 1984) but this seems to apply only to the subgroups with rigidity as a dominant feature (van Dijk et al. 1986). Currently, demonstration of the trinucleotide expansion on chromosome 4p16.3 is the ultimate diagnostic test. Normal individuals have repeats in the range of 11 to 31. The average number of CAG repeats in patients is 44 (range 36–121) (Duyao et al. 1993). Cases with severe early onset and/or fast rate of progression tend to have the greatest number of repeats (Snell et al. 1993, Stine et al. 1993, Illarioshkin et al. 1994). However, correlation between the size of the trinucleotide expansion and the severity of the disease is controversial (Snell et al. 1993, Andrew et al. 1993, Furtado et al. 1996).

The possibility of 'very benign' forms that may even present as benign chorea has been reported in patients with repeat expansions within the range of HD (McMillan et al. 1993, Britton et al. 1995).

Except for the DNA studies, laboratory investigations are unhelpful. The EEG usually shows an increased proportion of slow waves. When epilepsy is present paroxysmal discharges are seen (Sishta et al. 1974).

The differential diagnosis includes cases of rigid akinetic syndrome and other forms of chorea, especially dentato-rubro-pallido-luysian atrophy (which is due to a different trinucleotide repeat) and benign familial chorea (see Chapter 4).

Neuroimaging is normal early in the illness but in advanced cases it shows ventricular dilatation and decreased volume of the head of the caudate nucleus with resulting increase in the bicaudate diameter (Jernigan et al. 1991). Areas of increased attenuation may be present in the basal nuclei (Kuhl et al. 1982). MRI better demonstrates atrophy of the caudate and putamen (Harris et al. 1992, Ho et al. 1995). In addition, it may show increased signal from the basal ganglia on T_2-weighted sequences (Ho et al. 1995).

PET scanning has shown a decreased utilization of glucose in the caudate nucleus (Reid et al. 1988), and this was suggested as a diagnostic tool in the presymptomatic stage (Hayden et al. 1987). This finding has not been confirmed (Young et al. 1987) but is now of no practical interest since the advent of DNA studies.

PATHOLOGY

Macroscopically, there is obvious atrophy of the head of the caudate nucleus with ventricular dilatation (Byers et al. 1973). Histologically, there is a marked loss of neurons in the caudate and cortical layers III, V and VI, especially in the frontal and parietal lobes, less severe in the putamen and pallidum (Markhan and Knox 1965, Roos 1986). There is, in addition, marked gliosis of the striatum, which may not be secondary, but could play a role in neuronal death (Martin and Gusella 1986). Golgi studies showed selective involvement of medium size spinous neurons (Graveland et al. 1985). Whether there are neuropathological differences between adult and juvenile cases Is controversial (Goebel et al. 1978, Myers et al. 1988) but no consistent relation between clinical severity and pathology is evident: asymptomatic cases may show obvious lesions (Carrasco and Mukherji 1986), while clinical cases may not show pathological damage.

PATHOGENESIS

Despite isolation of the protein encoded by the HD gene (*huntingtin*), the relationship between the abnormal gene product of the mutant gene and the disease is as yet unexplained (Landwehrmeyer et al. 1995). The lesions in the basal ganglia that could be reproduced in mice might correspond to excitotoxic damage similar to that induced by kainic acid. There may be an increased concentration of GABA especially in the striate cortex (Brodman area 17) (Storey et al. 1992). Recently it has been suggested that mutant huntingtin might induce defective mitochondrial function (Koroshetz et al. 1997). This defect of energy metabolism may mediate cell death through cytotoxicity. A decrease in the activities of complexes II and III of the mitochondrial respiratory chain has been reported in the caudate nuclei (Gu et al. 1996).

TREATMENT

Unfortunately there is currently no neuroprotective treatment effective against the neuronal degeneration in HD. Attempts at compensation of the biochemical disturbances of the CNS by increasing GABA transmission have no proven efficacy (Tell et al. 1981). Agents claimed to improve mitochondrial metabolism such as ubiquinone (coenzyme Q10) or L-acetyl carnitine have been tried (Koroshetz et al. 1997, Goetz et al. 1990). The therapy of HD is disappointing and limited to symptomatic treatment (Nutt et al. 1978, Perry et al. 1979, Shoulson 1981). When rigidity predominates, anticholinergic drugs (see below) can be used although the benefit is very limited. When chorea is the predominant manifestation, antidopaminergic agents such as haloperidol and pimozide are partially helpful and may also have an effect on associated conduct disorders.

Serious behavioural disturbances or depression may benefit from antipsychotic neuroleptic therapy or antidepressants such as clomipramine, fluoxetine (Prozac) or paroxetine (Paxil). Psychological and family support is necessary

NEURONAL INTRANUCLEAR INCLUSION DISEASE (NIID)
CLINICAL FEATURES

NIID is a slowly progressive disorder that variably features: H-RS, behaviour disturbances, abnormal ocular movements, ataxia, pyramidal tract signs and dysfunction of the anterior horn cells of the spinal cord (Sung et al 1980, Patel et al. 1985, Garen et al. 1986). The disease affects children more than adults.

NIID was first reported in 1968 by Lindenberg et al. who demonstrated the characteristic eosinophilic inclusions in the nuclei of neurons. According to Goutières et al. (1990) 11 childhood cases had been published at that date. Some cases are familial (sibs or identical twins) (Schuffler et al. 1978, Janota 1979, Haltia et al. 1984) and autosomal recessive transmission is probable. The age of onset in children is between 3 and 12 years, mainly between 9 and 12 years. Usually initial symptoms include a slow cognitive and behavioural regression and change of mood. Parkinsonism (Fig. 2.2), tremor, choreoathetosis or ataxia appear later but the clinical spectrum is varied as shown by the case reported by Sloane et al. (1994) with onset at 2 years of age and death at 4, with a picture of rapidly progressive cerebellar ataxia, internuclear ophthalmoplegia and intrac-

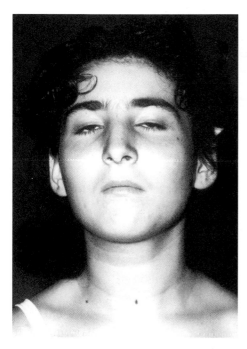

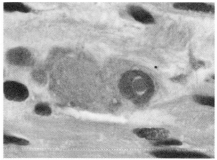

Fig. 2.2. Neuronal intranuclear inclusion disease. Onset at age 9 years with cognitive regression, behavioural changes, difficulties in deglutition, cephalic and tongue fine tremor, oculogyric crises and hypokinetic–rigid syndrome. MRI normal. EMG neurogenic. At age 16 years an appendix study (above) showed typical intranuclear eosinophilic inclusions in the neurons. At 21 years she was wheelchair-dependent. She died age 22 years.

table epilepsy. Intestinal pseudoobstruction has been reported as a presenting symptom (Schuffler et al. 1978). Oculogyric crises are frequent. Involvement of spinal anterior horn cells and bulbar neurons may result in fasciculations and articulatory difficulties. Epilepsy is infrequent. Cardiomyopathy has been reported. Death occurs before age 30 years.

Diagnosis during life has been made by study of rectal biopsy sample (Goutières et al. 1990) or of the appendix (personal case, EF-A). The disorder has to be differentiated from other degenerative disorders. It can mimic juvenile parkinsonism (see below), spino-cerebellar degeneration (Soffer 1985), GM2 gangliosidosis or infantile neuroaxonal dystrophy (see Chapter 5).

Neuroimaging studies are usually unremarkable. The EMG may demonstrate anterior horn cell disease. Severe mixed peripheral neuropathy has been reported (Patel et al. 1985).

PATHOLOGY

Ubiquitous intranuclear neuronal, eosinophilic hyaline inclusions, neuronal loss and gliosis are the main pathologic findings. The neuronal inclusions (Fig. 2.2) are auto-fluorescent with ultraviolet light. Ultrastructurally they show haphazardly arranged, uniform, fine straight filaments. Severe cerebellar cortical atrophy involving chiefly the vermis has been reported (Sloane et al. 1994). In non-neuronal tissue, similar inclusions can be found (Schuffler et al. 1978). The origin and nature of the inclusions are unknown.

OTHER DISEASES WITH HYPOKINETIC–RIGID SYNDROME.

AROMATIC L-AMINO ACID DECARBOXYLASE DEFICIENCY

Deficit of aromatic L-amino acid decarboxylase (AADC), an enzyme that catalyses the decarboxylation of both L-dopa to dopamine and of 5-hydroxytryptophan to serotonin, causes oculogyric crises, tremor of the arms, rigidity, ophthalmoplegia, mental retardation and vegetative symptoms (sweating, temperature dysregulation) (Hyland et al. 1992, Korenke et al. 1997). Symptoms begin during the first month of life. Elevated concentration of homovanillic acid in urine, reduced AADC activity and elevated levels of L-dopa in plasma are the biochemical abnormalities. Patients treated within the first year of life with pyridoxine, bromocriptine and trancylpromine (MAO inhibitor) showed a striking clinical improvement (Hyland et al. 1992).

POST-ENCEPHALITIC PARKINSONISM

Parkinsonism as a sequela of encephalitis is well known and was frequent following the pandemics of lethargic encephalitis in the 1920s. Cases of transient or chronic parkinsonism possibly due to other infections (Kilroy et al. 1972; case 3 of Sachdev et al. 1977; Alves et al. 1992; Pranzatelli et al. 1994; Picard et al. 1996) such as *mycoplasma infection* (Al-Mateen et al. 1988, Kim et al. 1995), *influenza virus* (Isgreen et al. 1976), and HIV-related *progressive multifocal leukoencephalopathy* (Singer et al. 1993) are on record. Parkinsonism can be also a symptom in infantile bilateral striatal or thalamic necrosis (see Chapter 5)

COMMUNICATING HYDROCEPHALUS OR AQUEDUCTAL STENOSIS

Communicating hydrocephalus or aqueductal stenosis may cause parkinsonism (Lang et al. 1982, Brazin and Epstein 1985) that can be improved by shunting and L-dopa. In such cases, some patients have remained dopa-dependent (Curran and Lang 1994). *Central pontine myelinolysis*, although it is more usually associated with dystonia or chorea, may rarely cause parkinsonism (Sadeh and Goldhammer 1993).

MISCELLANEOUS

Miscellaneous patients, mostly adults, with idiopathic *pseudohypoparathyroidism* and less frequently *hypoparathyroidism* may demonstrate parkinsonism and bilateral calcification of the basal ganglia, easily detected by CT scanning (Illum and Dupont 1985).

Eaton et al. (1939) have described a 13-year-old boy with hypoparathyroidism, hypomimia, shuddering and rigidity, and the patient of Evans and Donley (1988) presented at 12 years of age with rigidity and tremor, although without the basal ganglia calcification usually present in this condition. Slit lamp examination in search of cataracts, blood and urine levels of calcium and phosphorus, determination of parathyroid hormone level and of urinary cyclic AMP permit the diagnosis.

Hypokinesia and rigidity have been reported, although rarely, as the predominant clinical manifestation of other metabolic diseases such as mitochondrial cytopathies

(Leigh syndrome – van Erven et al. 1989; MELAS – De Coo et al. 1997). Some patients with *phenylketonuria* can develop a parkinsonian syndrome (McLeod et al. 1983). A patient with *Niemann–Pick C disease* developed a parkinsonian syndrome by age 5 years (Coleman et al. 1988). *GM2 gangliosidosis* can produce a parkinsonian syndrome with bradykinesia and tremor (see p. 104).

Intoxications by *mercury*, *manganese* (Barron et al. 1994) and *methanol* can produce a parkinsonian syndrome. *Carbon monoxide poisoning* can be responsible for an akinetic–rigid syndrome either in the initial phase (Ringel and Klawans 1972) or as a sequela (Choi 1983). This is associated with images of low density in the pallidum.

Neoplastic lesions of the basal ganglia are not generally associated with parkinsonian anomalies of movement, but this has been reported in some cases of tumour (Pranzatelli et al. 1994).

The H-RS, like virtually any type of extrapyramidal syndrome, can be caused by *drugs* that interfere with the synthesis, storage or release of dopamine or prevent its fixation on post-synaptic receptors. Such syndromes usually appear some time after onset of administration. The symptoms and signs are symmetrical and usually disappear upon discontinuation of the medicines (see Chapter 10).

A leukoencephalopathy with parkinsonism has been reported in leukaemic children, having received a bone marrow transplant, treated with high-dose *amphotericin B*. Neuroimaging studies showed basal ganglia atrophy and other signs of cerebral and cerebellar involvement (Mott et al. 1995). It has been suggested that similar lesions can be due to *cytosine-arabinoside* (Chutorian 1997). Parkinsonism has also been observed following *open-heart surgery** (Straussberg et al. 1993).

SYMPTOMATIC TREATMENT OF H-RS

Although the best known mechanism of H-RS is defective dopaminergic activity, not all cases will respond to the administration of dopamine agonists. Some cases of idiopathic juvenile parkinsonism are clearly improved or even completely corrected by L-dopa. This also applies to some secondary cases (Picard et al. 1996) such as post-hydrocephalic parkinsonism. Dopamine agonists are a more effective treatment for the bradykinesia and rigidity than for tremor. This drug should always be tried, usually in association with a peripheral decarboxylase inhibitor (carbidopa or benserazide). The dose will depend on individual response. A reasonable strategy in children is to try the administration of 12.5 mg of L-dopa (use of the 25/100 Sinemet preparation is recommended for children – Pranzatelli 1996) three times daily for one week, then double the dose if there is clinical improvement and according to tolerance. Usually, the drug is well tolerated. Side-effects may include nausea, vomiting and choreatic movements. However, many conditions, e.g. neuronal inclusion disease, do not respond to L-dopa. Disorders that may respond to L-dopa are listed in Table 2.2.

*Can also cause chorea (see p. 70).

TABLE 2.2
Disorders of movement that may respond to L-dopa

Dopa-responsive dystonia
Juvenile idiopathic parkinsonism
Dystonia–parkinsonism
Machado–Joseph disease (striatonigric degeneration) (Chapter 6) (some cases)
Benign paroxysmal tonic upgaze in infancy (Chapter 7) (some cases)
Parkinsonism secondary to hydrocephalus (some cases)
Pallidopyramidal syndrome (some cases)

Bromocriptine and lysuride are agonists of dopaminergic receptors used mainly in the treatment of idiopathic Parkinson disease. There is little paediatric experience with these drugs.

In case of inefficacy of L-dopa, anticholinergic agents may be used. The most commonly used is trihexyphenidyl (Artane) in slowly increased doses, starting at 1–2 mg/d and increasing by 1–2 mg weekly to a maximum of 15–20 mg/d. Fahn (1983) utilizes much higher doses (up to 70 mg/d) that the present authors have not used personally. Biperidine (Akineton) can be used at slightly lower doses to a maximum of 10–15 mg/d. Secondary effects of anticholinergic agents include drowsiness and dryness of mouth. At high doses they can induce psychosis. For treatment of tremor, ethopropazine (Pranzatelli 1996) or propranolol can be tried (see p. 56). Surgical treatment by thalamotomy is rarely, if ever, indicated in paediatric patients.

Physiotherapy and psychological support are necessary in all cases.

REFERENCES

Allen N, Knopp W (1976) Hereditary parkinsonism-dystonia with sustained control by L-dopa and anticholinergic medication. *Adv Neurol* 14: 201–13.

AleMurreu M, Giblw M, Dierrich R, or al. (1988) Encephalitic lethargica like illness in a girl with mycoplasma infection. *Neurology* 38: 1155–8.

Alves R, Barbosa ER, Scatt M (1992) Postvaccinal parkinsonism. *Mov Disord* 7: 178–80.

Andrew SE, Goldberg YP, Kremer B, et al. (1993) The relationship between trinucleotide (CAG) repeat length and clinical features of Huntington's disease. *Nature Genet* 4: 398–403.

Barron TF, Devenyi AG, Mamourian AC (1994) Symptomatic manganese neurotoxicity in a patient with chronic liver disease: Correlation of clinical with MRI findings. *Pediatr Neurol* 10: 63–5.

Bird MT, Paulson GW (1971) The rigid form of Huntington's chorea. *Neurology* 21: 271–6.

Bittenbender JB, Quadfasel FA (1962) Rigid and akinetic forms of Huntington's chorea. *Arch Neurol* 7: 275–88.

Brashear A, Farlow MR, Butler IJ, et al. (1996) Variable phenotype of rapid-onset dystonia parkinsonism. *Mov Disord* 11: 151–6.

Brazin ME, Epstein LG (1985) Reversible parkinsonism from shunt failure. *Pediatr Neurol* 1: 306–7.

Britton JW, Uitti RJ, Ahlskog JE, et al. (1995) Hereditary late-onset chorea without significant dementia: Genetic evidence for substantial phenotypic variation in Huntington's disease. *Neurology* 45: 443–7.

Brooks DE, Murphy D, Janota I, Lishman WA (1987) Early onset Huntington's chorea. *Br J Psychiatry* 151: 850–2.

Bruyn GW (1969) The Westphal variant and juvenile type of Huntington's chorea. In: Barbeau A, Brunette JR (eds) *Progress in Neurogenetics, Vol. 1.* Amsterdam: Excerpta Medica, pp. 666–76.

Bruyn GW, Went CN (1986) Huntington's chorea. In: Vinken PJ, Bruyn GW, Klawans HL (eds) *Handbook of Clinical Neurology. Vol. 5, no 49.* Amsterdam: North Holland, pp. 267–314.

Byers RK, Gilles FH, Fung C (1973) Huntington's disease in children. Neuropathologic study of four cases. *Neurology* 25: 561–9.

Campbell AMG, Corner B, Norman RM, et al. (1961) The rigid form of Huntington's disease. *J Neurol Neurosurg Psychiatry* 24: 71–7.

Carlier G, Dubru JM (1979) Familial juvenile parkinsonism. *Acta Pediat Belg* 32: 123–7.

Carrasco LH, Mukherji CS (1986) Atrophy of corpus striatum in normal male at risk of Huntington's chorea. *Lancet* 1: 1388–9 (letter).

Caviness VS (1985) Huntington's disease. *Dev Med Child Neurol* 27: 826–9.

Choi IS (1983) Delayed neurologic sequelae in carbon monoxide intoxication. *Arch Neurol* 40: 433–5.

Chutorian A (1997) Síndromes parkinsonianos en la infancia. *Rev Neurol* 25: 954–65.

Coleman RJ, Robb SA, Lake BD, et al. (1988) The diverse neurological features of Niemann–Pick disease type C: A report of two cases. *Mov Disord* 3: 295–9.

Conneally PM (1984) Huntington's disease: Genetics and epidemiology. *Am J Hum Genet* 36: 506–26.

Craufurd D, Dodge A, Kerzin-Storrar L, Harris R (1989) Uptake of presymptomatic predictive testing for Huntington's disease. *Lancet* 2: 603–5.

Curran T, Lang A (1994) Parkinsonian syndromes associated with hydrocephalus: Case report, a review of the literature and pathophysiological hypothesis. *Mov Disord* 9: 508–20.

Davison CH (1954) Pallido-pyramidal disease. *J Neuropath Exp Neurol* 13: 50–9.

Dewhurst K, Oliver J (1970) Huntington's disease of young people. *Europ Neurol* 3: 278–89.

De Coo IFM, Renier WO, Ruitenbeek W, et al. (1997) A 4bp deletion in the mitochondrial cytochrome b gene associated with Parkinsonism–MELAS overlap syndrome. *Europ J Paediatr Neurol* 2/3: A-27 (abstract).

Dobyns WB, Farlow MR, Butler IJ (1991) Rapid-onset dystonia-parkinsonism with partial response to L-dopa. *Ann Neurol* 30: 504.

— Ozelius LJ, Kramer PL et al. (1993) Rapid-onset dystonia parkinsonism. *Neurology* 43: 2596–602.

Duyao M, Ambrose C, Myers RH, et al. (1993) Trinucleotide repeat length instability and age of onset in Huntington's disease. *Nature Genet* 4: 387–92.

Dwork AJ, Balmaceda C, Fazzini FA, et al. (1993) Dominantly inherited, early-onset parkinsonism: Neuropathology of a new form. *Neurology* 43: 69–74.

Eaton L, Camp JD, Love JG (1939) Symmetric cerebral calcifications particularly of the basal ganglia demonstrable radiographically. *Arch Neurol Psych* 41: 921–42.

Erdohazi M, Marshall P (1979) Striatal degeneration in childhood. *Arch Dis Child* 54: 85–91.

Evans BK, Donley DK (1988) Pseudohypoparathyroidism, Parkinsonism syndrome, with no basal ganglia calcification. *J Neurol Neurosurg Psychiatry* 51: 709–13.

Fahn S (1983) High dose anticholinergic therapy in dystonia. *Neurology* 33: 1255–61.

Farrer LA, Conneally PM, Yu PL (1984) The natural history of Huntington's disease. *Am J Med Genet* 18: 115–23.

Fernández–Alvarez, E (1972) Forma infantil de enfermedad de Huntington. *Rev Esp Ped* 28: 809–12.

Furtado S, Suchowersky O, Rewcastle B, et al. (1996) A relationship between trinucleotide repeats and neuropathological changes in Huntigton's disease. *Ann Neurol* 39: 132–6.

Garen PD, Powers JM, Young GF, Lee V (1986) Neuronal intranuclear hyaline inclusion disease in a nine year old. *Acta Neuropathol* 70: 327–32.

Gershanik OS (1988) Parkinsonism of early onset. In: Jankovic J, Tolosa E (eds) *Parkinson Disease and Movement Disorders.* Baltimore, Munich: Urban & Schwarzenberg, pp. 191–204.

— Leist A (1986) Juvenile onset Parkinson's disease. In: Yahr MD, Bergmann KJ (eds) *Advances in Neurology, Vol. 45.* New York: Raven Press, pp. 213–6.

Gibb WRG, Narabayashi H, Yokochi M, et al. (1991) New pathologic observations in juvenile onset parkinsonism with dystonia. *Neurology* 41: 820–2.

Goebel MH, Heipertz R, Scholz W, Telleznagel I (1978) Juvenile Huntington chorea, clinical, ultrastructural and biochemical studies. *Neurology* 28: 23–31.

Goetz CG, Tanner CM, Cohen JA, et al. (1990) L-Acetyl-carnitine in Huntington's disease: double blind placebo controlled crossover study of drug effects on movement disorders and dementia. *Mov Disord* 5: 263–5.

Golbe LI (1991) Young-onset Parkinson's disease: A clinical review. *Neurology* 41: 168–73.

Goutières F, Mikol J, Aicardi J (1990) Neuronal intranuclear inclusion disease in a child: Diagnosis by rectal biopsy. *Ann Neurol* 27: 103–6.

Graveland GA, Williams RS, DiFiglia M (1985) Evidence for degenerative and regenerative changes in neostriatal spiny neurons in Huntington's disease. *Science* 22: 770–3.

Gu M, Cooper JM, Gash M, et al. (1996) Mitochondrial defect in Huntington's disease caudate nucleus. *Ann Neurol* 39: 385–9.

Gusella JF, Wexler NS, Conneally PM, et al. (1983) A polymorphic DNA marker genetically linked to Huntington's disease. *Nature* 306: 234–8.

Haltia M, Somer H, Palo J, Johnson WG (1984) Neuronal intranuclear inclusion disease in identical twins. *Ann Neurol* 15: 316–21.

Hansotia P, Cleeland CS, Chun RN (1968) Juvenile Huntington's chorea. *Neurology* 18: 217–24.

Harris GJ, Pearlson GD, Peyser CE, et al. (1992) Putamen volume reduction on magnetic resonance imaging exceeds caudate changes in mild Huntington's disease. *Ann Neurol* 31: 69–75.

Hayden MR, Beighton PH (1982) Genetic aspects of Huntington's chorea. *Am J Med Genet* 11: 135–41.

Hayden MR, Hewitt BS, Stoessl AJ, et al. (1987) The combined use of positron emission tomography and DNA polymorphisms for preclinical detection of Huntington's disease. *Neurology* 37: 1441–7.

Hayes CV (1992) Genetic testing for Huntington's disease – A familial issue. *New Engl J Med* 327: 1449–51.

Ho VB, Chuang S, Rovira MJ, Koo B (1995) Juvenile Huntington disease: CT and MR features. *Am J Neuroradiol* 16: 1405–12.

Hyland K, Surtees RAH, Rodeck C, Clayton PT (1992) Aromatic amino acid decarboxylase deficiency: Clinical features,diagnosis, and treatment of a new inborn error of neurotransmitter amine synthesis. *Neurology* 42: 1980–8.

Illarioshkin SN, Igarashi S, Onodera O, et al. (1994) Trinucleotide repeat length and rate of progression of Huntington's disease. *Ann Neurol* 36: 630–5.

Illum F, Dupont E (1985) Prevalence of CT detected calcification in the basal ganglia in idiopathic hypoparathyroidism and pseudohypoparathyroidism. *Neuroradiology* 27: 32–7.

Isgreen WP, Chutorian AM, Fahn S (1976) Sequential parkinsonism and chorea following 'mild' influenza. *Trans Amer Neurol Assoc* 101: 56–60.

Ishikawa A, Tsuji S (1996) Clinical analysis of 17 patients in 12 Japanese families with autosomal recessive type juvenile parkinsonism. *Neurology* 47: 160–6.

Janota I (1979) Widespread intranuclear intraneuronal corpuscles (Marinesco bodies) associated with a familial spinal degeneration with cranial and peripheral nerve involvement. *Neuropathol Appl Neurobiol* 5: 311–7.

Jellinger K (1986) Pallidal, pallidonigral and pallidoluysionigral degenerations including association with thalamic and dentate degenerations. In: Vinken PJ, Bruyn GW, Klawans HL (eds) *Handbook of Clinical Neurology, Vol. 5, no 49. Extrapyramidal Disorders.* Amsterdam: Elsevier, pp. 445–63.

Jernigan TL, Salmon DP, Butters N, et al. (1991) Cerebral structure on MRI. Part II: Specific changes in Alzheimer's and Huntington's diseases. *Biol Psychiatry* 29: 68–81.

Jongen PJH, Renier WO, Gabreëls FJM (1980) Seven cases of Huntington's disease in childhood and levodopa induced improvement in the hypokinetic rigid form. *Clin Neurol Neurosurg* 82: 251–61.

Katchen M, Duvoisin RC (1986) Parkinsonism following dystonia in three patients. *Mov Disord* 1: 151–7.

Kilroy AW, Paulsen WA, Fenichel GM (1972) Juvenile parkinsonism treated with levodopa. *Arch Neurol* 27: 350–3.

Kim JS, Choi ILS, Lee MC (1995) Reversible parkinsonism and dystonia following probable *Mycoplasma pneumoniae* infection. *Mov Disord* 10: 510–2.

Kitada T, Asakawa S, Hattori N et al. (1998) Mutations in the *Parkin* gene cause autosomal recessive juvenile parkinsonism. *Nature* 392: 605–8.

Korenke GC, Christen H-J, Hyland K, et al. (1997) Aromatic L-amino acid decarboxylase deficiency: An extrapyramidal movement disorder with oculogyric crises. *Europ J Paediatr Neurol* 2/3: 67–71.

Koroshetz WJ, Jenkins BG, Rosen BR, Beal MF (1997) Energy metabolism defects in Huntington's disease and effects of coenzyme Q10. *Ann Neurol* 41: 160–5.

Kuhl DE, Phelps ME, Markhand CH, et al. (1982) Cerebral metabolism and atrophy in Huntington's disease determined by 18FDG and computed tomographic scan. *Ann Neurol* 12: 425–34.

Landwehrmeyer GB, McNeil SM, Dure LS, et al. (1995) Huntington's disease gene: regional and cellular expression in brain of normal and affected individuals. *Ann Neurol* 37: 218–30.

Lang AE, Meadows JC, Parkes JD, Marsden CD (1982) Early onset of the 'on-off' phenomenon in children with symptomatic parkinsonism. *J Neurol Neurosurg Psychiatry* 45: 823–5.

Lee LV, Pascasio FM, Fuentes FD, Viterbo GH (1976) Torsion dystonia in Panay Philippines. In: Elridge R, Fahn S (eds) *Advances in Neurology, Vol. 14. Dystonia.* New York: Raven Press, pp. 137–51.

Leigh R, Newman S, Folstein A, et al. (1983) Abnormal oculomotor control in Huntington's disease. *Neurology* 33: 1268–75.

Lenti C, Bianchini E (1993) Neuropsychological and neuroradiological study of a case of early-onset Huntington's chorea. *Dev Med Child Neurol* 35: 1007–14.

Lindenberg R, Rubinstein LJ, Herman MM, Haydon GB (1968) A light and electron microscopy study of an unusual widespread nuclear inclusion body disease. A possible residuum of an old herpesvirus infection. *Acta Neuropathol* 10: 54–73.

Lyon G, Adams RD, Kolodny EH (1996) *Neurology of Hereditary Metabolic Diseases of Children.* New York: McGraw-Hill.

MacMillan JC, Morrison PJ, Nevin NC, et al. (1993) Identification of an expanded CAG repeat in the Huntington's disease gene (*IT15*) in a family reported to have benign hereditary chorea. *J Med Genet* 30: 1012–3.

Markhan CH, Knox JW (1965) Observations on Huntington's chorea in childhood. *J Pediatr* 67: 46–57.

Martin JB, Gusella JF (1986) Huntington's disease. Pathogenesis and management. *New Engl J Med* 315: 1267–75.

Martin WE, Resch JA, Baker AB (1971) Juvenile parkinsonism. *Arch Neurol* 25: 494–500.

McLeod MD, Munro JF, Ledingham JG, et al. (1983) Management of the extrapyramidal manifestations of phenylketonuria with L-dopa. *Arch Dis Child* 58: 457–8.

Mott SH, Packer RJ, Vezina LG, et al. (1995) Encephalopathy with parkinsonian features in children following bone marrow transplantations and high-dose Amphotericin B. *Ann Neurol* 37: 810–4.

Muthane UB, Swamy HS, Satishchandra P, et al. (1994) Early onset Parkinson's disease: Are juvenile- and young-onset different? *Mov Disord* 9: 539–44.

Myers RH, Madden JJ, Teague JL, Falek A (1982) Factors related to onset age of Huntington's disease. *Am J Hum Genet* 34: 481–8.

Myers RH, Vonsattel JP, Stevens TJ, et al. (1988) Clinical and neuropathological assessment of severity in Huntington's disease. *Neurology* 38: 341–7.

Naidu S, Wolfson LI, Sharpless NS (1978) Juvenile parkinsonism: A patient with possible primary striatal dysfunction. *Ann Neurol* 3: 453–8.

Narabayashi H, Yokochi M, Iizuka R, Nagatsu T (1986) Juvenile parkinsonism. In: Vinken PJ, Bruyn GW, Klawans HL (eds) *Handbook of Clinical Neurology, Vol. 49. Extrapyramidal Disorders.* Amsterdam: Elsevier, pp. 153–65.

Nutt JG, Rosin A, Chase TN (1978) Treatment of Huntington's disease with a cholinergic agonist. *Neurology* 28: 1061–4.

Oepen H (1973) Discordant features of monozygotic twin sisters with Huntington's chorea. *Adv Neurol* 1: 199–201.

Osborne JH, Munson P, Burman D (1982) Huntington's chorea. Report of 3 cases and review of the literature. *Arch Dis Child* 57: 99–103.

Ota Y, Miyoshi S, Ueda O, et al. (1958) Familial paralysis agitans juvenilis: A clinical, anatomical and genetic study. *Folia Psychiatr Neurol Jap* 12: 112–21.

Patel H, Norman MG, Perry TL, Berry KE (1985) Multiple system atrophy with neuronal intra-nuclear hyaline inclusions. Report of a case and review of the literature. *J Neurol Sci* 67: 57–65.

Perry TL, Wright JM, Hansen S, et al. (1979) Isoniacid therapy of Huntington's disease. *Neurology* 29: 370–75.

Picard F, Hirsch E, Salmon E, et al. (1996) Syndrome Parkinsonien et mouvements involontaires stéréotypés post-encéphalitiques, sensible à la L-dopa. *Rev Neurol* 152: 267–71.

Pranzatelli MR, Mott SH, Pavlakis SG, et al. (1994) Clinical spectrum of secondary parkinsonism in childhood: A reversible disorder. *Pediatr Neurol* 10: 131–40.

Pranzatelli MR (1996) Antidyskinetic drug therapy for pediatric movement disorders. *J Child Neurol* 11: 355–69.

Quinn N, Critchley P, Marsden CD (1987) Young onset Parkinson's disease. *Mov Disord* 2: 73–91.

Rajput A, Kishore A, Snow B, et al. (1997) Dopa-responsive, nonprogressive, juvenile parkinsonism: Report of a case. *Mov Disord* 12: 453–6.

Reid JC, Besson JAO, Best PV, et al. (1988) Imaging of cerebral blood flow markers in Huntington's disease using single photon emission computed tomography. *J Neurol Neurosurg Psychiatry* 51: 1264–8.

Ringel SP, Klawans HL (1972) Carbon monoxide-induced parkinsonism. *J Neurol Sci* 16: 245–51.

Rondot P, Ziegler M (1983) Dystonia-L-dopa responsive or juvenile parkinsonism? *J Neural Transm Suppl* 19: 273–81.

Roos RAC (1986) Neuropathology of Huntington's chorea. In: Vinken PJ, Bruyn GW, Klawans HL (eds) *Handbook of Clinical Neurology, Vol. 49.* Amsterdam: Elsevier, pp. 315–26.

Sachdev KK, Singh N, Krishnamoorty MS (1977) Juvenile parkinsonism treated with levodopa. *Arch Neurol* 34: 244–5.

Sadeh M, Goldhammer Y (1993) Extrapyramidal syndrome responsive to dopaminergic treatment following recovery from central pontine myelinolysis. *Eur Neurol* 33: 448–50.

Sawaishi Y, Yano T, Watanabe Y, Takada G (1999) Migratory basal ganglia in subacute sclerosing panencephalitis (SSPE): Clinical implications of axonal spread. *J Neurol Sci* 168: 137–40.

Schömig-Spingler M, Hammer J, Kruse K (1989) DNA analysis in juvenile Huntington disease. *Eur J Pediatr* 48: 447–9.

Schuffler MD, Bird TD, Sumi SM, Cook A (1978) Familial neuronal disease presenting as intestinal pseudobstruction. *Gastroenterology* 75: 889–98.

Shoulson I (1981) Care of patients and families with Huntington's disease. In: Marsden CD, Fahn S (eds) *Movement Disorders.* London: Butterwoth, pp. 277–90.

Singer C, Berger JR, Bowen BC, et al. (1993) Akinetic–rigid syndrome in a 13-year-old girl with HIV-related progressive multifocal leukoencephalopathy. *Mov Disord* 8: 113–6.

Sishta SK, Troupe A, Marszalek KS, Kremer LM (1974) Huntington's chorea: An electroencephalographic and psychometric study. *EEG Clin Neurophysiol* 36: 387–93.

Skraastad MI, Verwest A, Bakker E, et al. (1991) Presymptomatic, prenatal, and exclusion testing for Huntington disease using seven closely linked DNA markers. *Am J Med Genet* 39: 217–22.

Sloane AE, Becker LE, Ang LC, et al. (1994) Neuronal intranuclear hyaline inclusion disease with progressive cerebellar ataxia. *Pediatr Neurol* 10: 61–6.

Snell RG, Macmillan JC, Cheadle JP, et al. (1993) Relationship between trinucleotide repeat expansion and phenotypic variation in Huntington's disease. *Nature Genet* 4: 393–97.

Snow BJ, Nygaard TG, Takahashi H, Calne DB (1993) Positron emission tomographic studies of dopa-responsive dystonia and early onset idiopathic parkinsonism. *Ann Neurol* 34: 733–8.

Soffer D (1985) Neuronal intranuclear hyaline inclusions presenting as Friedreich's ataxia. *Acta Neuropathol* 65: 322–9.

Spellman GG (1962) Report of familial cases of parkinsonism. *JAMA* 179: 372–4.

Stevens DL (1976) Huntington's chorea: a demographic, genetic and clinical study. MD thesis, University of London.

Stine OC, Pleasant N, Franz ML, et al. (1993) Correlation between onset age of Huntington's disease and length of the trinucleotide repeat in IT-15. *Hum Mol Genet* 2: 1547–9.

Storey E, Kowall NW, Finn SF, et al. (1992) The cortical lesion of Huntington's disease: Further neurochemical characterization, and reproduction of some of the histological and neurochemical features by N-methyl-D-aspartate lesions of rat cortex. *Ann Neurol* 32: 526–34.

Straussberg R, Shahar E, Gat R, Brand N (1993) Delayed parkinsonism associated with hypotension in a child undergoing open-heart surgery. *Dev Med Child Neurol* 35: 1011–4.

Strong TV, Tagle DA, Valdes JM, et al. (1993) Widespread expression of the human and rat Huntington's disease gene in brain and nonneural tissues. *Nat Genet* 5: 259–65.

Sung JH, Ramirez-Lassepas M, Mastri AR, Larkin SM (1980) An unusual degenerative disorder of neurons associated with a novel intranuclear hyaline inclusion (neuronal intranuclear hyaline inclusion disease): A clinicopathological study of a case. *J Neuropathol Exp Neurol* 39: 107–30.

Takahashi H, Ohama E, Suzuki S, et al. (1994) Familial juvenile parkinsonism: clinical and patho-logical studies in a family. *Neurology* 44: 437–41.

Tell G, Bohlen P, Schechter PJ, et al. (1981) Treatment of Huntington's disease with gamma-acetylenic GABA, an irreversible inhibitor of GABA-transaminase: Increased CSF GABA and homocarnosine without clinical amelioration. *Neurology* 31: 207–11.

Turjanski N, Bhatia K, Burn DJ, et al. (1993) Comparison of striatal [18F] DOPA uptake in adult-onset dystonia–parkinsonism, Parkinson's disease, and DOPA-responsive dystonia. *Neurology* 43: 1563–8.

van Dijk JG, van der Velde EA, Roos RA, et al. (1986) Juvenile Huntington's disease. *Hum Genet* 73: 235–9.

van Erven PMM, Renier WO, Gabreëls FJM, et al. (1989) Hypokinesia and rigidity as clinical manifestations of mitochondrial encephalomyopathy: report of three cases. *Dev Med Child Neurol* 31: 81–97.

Vegter-van der Vlis M, Volkers MS, Went IN (1976) Ages of death of children with Huntington's chorea and of their affected parents. *Ann Hum Genet* 39: 329–34.

Wang M, Hattori N, Matsumine H, et al. (1999) Polymorphism in the *Parkin* gene in sporadic Parkinson's disease. *Ann Neurol* 45: 655–8.

Webb DW, Broderick A, Brashear A, Dobyns WB (1999) Rapid onset dystonia–parkinsonism in a 14-year-old girl. *Eur J Paediatr Neurol* 3: 171–3.

Went LN, Vegter-van der Vlis M, Bruyn GW (1984) Parenteral transmission in Huntington's disease. *Lancet* 1: 1100–2.

Wesler NS, Conneally PM, Housman D, Gusella JF (1985) A DNA polymorphism for Hunting-ton's disease marks the future. *Arch Neurol* 42: 20–4.

Wiggins S, Whyte P, Huggins M, et al. (1992) The psychological consequences of predictive testing for Huntington's disease. *New Engl J Med* 327: 1401–5.

Wilhelmsen K, Weeks DE, Nygaard TG, et al. (1991) Genetic mapping of 'Lubag' (X-linked dys-tonia parkinsonism) in a Filipino kindred to the pericentromeric region of the X chromosome. *Ann Neurol* 29: 124.

Yamamura Y, Sobue I, Ando K, et al. (1973) Paralysis agitans of early onset with marked diurnal fluctuation of symptoms. *Neurology* 23: 239–44.

Yokochi M, Narabayashi H, Izuka R, Nagatsu T (1984) Juvenile parkinsonism. Some clinical, pharmacological and neuropathological aspects. In: Hassler RG, Christ JF (eds) *Advances in Neurology, Vol. 40.* New York: Raven Press, pp. 407–13.

Young AB, Shouldson I, Penney JB, et al. (1986) Huntington's disease in Venezuela. Neurologic features and functional decline. *Neurology* 36: 247–9.

— Penny JAB, Starosta-Rubinstein S, et al. (1987) Normal caudate glucose metabolism in persons at risk for Huntington's disease. *Arch Neurol* 44: 254–7.

3

MOVEMENT DISORDERS WITH TREMOR AS THE MAIN CLINICAL MANIFESTATION

INTRODUCTION AND CLASSIFICATION

Although it is possible that the cerebellum or cerebellar pathways are involved in any type of tremor, only tremor unassociated with cerebellar syndrome is considered here.

In childhood, non-cerebellar tremor is not rare although few publications are available (Paulson 1976, Franz 1993, Fernández-Alvarez and Lopez-Casas 1996). There are various classification schemes for tremor (Findley and Cleeves 1989).

According to circumstances of occurrence it can be divided into: (1) rest tremor; (2) postural tremor; (3) action tremor.

According to aetiology two groups exist: (1) idiopathic, and (2) secondary tremor (Table 3.1). The term idiopathic applies to those cases in which tremor is the only manifestation of the disorder, that have no recognizable cause (e.g. drugs, infections, etc.) and that occur in patients with normal biochemical and neuroimaging investigations. Secondary tremor refers to cases that do not fulfil these conditions.

According to evolution, tremor can be transient, when it disappears spontaneously without sequelae, or chronic.

Tremor can cause severe functional impairment or constitute only a minor, hardly recognizable, symptom (see p. 9). However, a mild tremor to which an adult would easily adapt may cause problems (writing, drawing, eating) more difficult for a child to compensate.

In 129 (19%) of 673 personal (EF-A) cases of movement disorder with onset before age 18 years, tremor was the sole or predominant feature (see Fig. 1.5, p. 19). Overall, tremor was more frequent in males (2:1). The mean age of onset was 5.98 years, slightly earlier in boys (5.74y) than in girls (6.46y).

Physiological tremor is present in normal children, as in adults, but with such a low amplitude and fast frequency that it is not visible under normal circumstances (see Chapter 1). Its frequency is slower (about 6 cycles/s) in children up to the age of 9 than in adults (Marshall 1959). Thereafter the frequency changes fairly abruptly, and by the age of 16 years most children have a physiological tremor frequency similar to that of adults (8–12 c/s).

TABLE 3.1
Classification of non-cerebellar tremors

Idiopathic
Chronic
    Enhanced physiological
    Essential
        Familial
        Sporadic
    Trembling of the chin
Transient
    Jitteriness
    Shuddering spells
    Palatal essential
    Spasmus nutans

Secondary
Parkinsonian (sometimes idiopathic)
Essential-like, associated with:
    Neuromuscular diseases
    Drugs
    Metabolic diseases
    Endocrinopathies
    Other disorders
Coarse cephalic
    Bobble-head doll syndrome

In healthy children, physiological tremor may occur with fear, anxiety and fatigue, while excitation can cause visible tremor. The same can occur with the action of drugs such as theophylline and metaproterenol, toxic agents (mercury, bismuth) or stimulant drinks (coffee, tea, cola).

As with adults, some children can experience tremor in situations that in the general population do not generate tremor. This is termed 'exaggerated physiological tremor'. There is not a clear cut between normal and exaggerated physiological tremors caused in these circumstances We have several patients with mental retardation, in whom the exaggerated physiological tremor is so intense in stressing situations that tremor is more disabling than the mental retardation.

PRIMARY TREMORS
CHRONIC TREMORS
Essential tremor (ET)
Criteria and age of onset. The necessary criteria for ET include:
1. Visible and persistent postural tremor (sometimes also of action) permanently present although of variable intensity.

2. Prolonged duration of tremor (more than one year).

3. Absence of pyramidal, cerebellar and sensory anomalies and of involvement of the peripheral nervous system.

4. Normal intelligence.

5. No concurrent or recent exposure to tremorogenic drugs.

6. Absence of systemic disease potentially responsible for enhanced physiological tremor such as hyperthyroidism.

7. Normal neuroimaging study (only in non-familial cases).

8. No history of perinatal anomalies or abnormal psychomotor development.

Supportive criteria include:

1. A family history of tremor.

2. Benefit of alcohol ingestion (not applicable to children).

The onset of ET can be at any age (Critchley 1949, Findley and Koller 1987), and as early as 2 years (Bain et al. 1994, Fernández-Alvarez and Lopez-Casas 1966). Nineteen per cent of ET cases begin below age 20 years (Koller et al. 1994). The age of onset may vary even in the same family. In one study (Bain et al. 1994), six of 14 first-degree relatives of ET patients less than 15 years of age (range 2–13 years) were possibly affected. However, there is only one publication dealing exclusively with ET in childhood (Paulson 1976). As a result, aspects of special interest at this age such as consequences on learning and attitude of relatives are often underestimated and therapy is poorly documented. The prevalence of ET in childhood is unknown. Epidemiological studies in the adult population have given widely discrepant estimates of prevalence varying between 4.1 and 39.2 per 1000 (Louis et al. 1998)

Inheritance. Many cases of essential tremor are transmitted as an autosomal dominant character (Critchley 1949), although penetrance and expressivity are contentious. Larsson and Sjogren (1960) and Bain et al. (1994) did not find families with skipped generations but Critchley (1972) and Findley (1984) recorded such pedigrees (Fig. 3.1). Approximately 60% of patients with essential tremor have affected relatives, so isolated cases are not uncommon (Rautokorpi et al. 1982, Rajput et al. 1984) . In a study of childhood ET, that included 28 patients under 16 years, tremor was familial in 20 cases, and sporadic in eight (Fernández-Alvarez and Lopez-Casas 1966). Because the age of onset is very variable within the same family (Larsson and Sjogren 1960) and can be as late as 75 years, the occurrence of missed generations could easily be only apparent. Truly isolated cases probably result from a new mutation. Genetic anticipation (onset at increasingly early age in successive generations) was recognized in some families (Critchley 1972, Jankovic et al. 1997). In a family with genetic anticipation of ET an ET susceptibility gene was localized on chromosome 2p22–p25 (Higgins et al. 1997).

In our own series, there is a clear male preponderance (female/male ratio of 0.25 for 28 cases) (Fernández-Alvarez and Lopez-Casas 1996), but in some adult series sex distribution is not significantly different (Bain et al. 1994, Koller et al. 1994), predominance

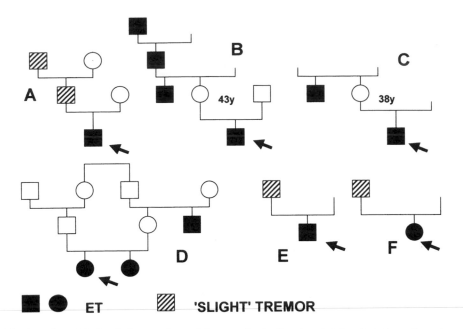

Fig. 3.1. Tree of six familial cases of essential tremor. In families B and C the clinical manifestations skip the mothers (aged 38 and 43 years respectively). In families A, E and F the father shows only a very slight tremor. Family D is more complex because there is consanguinity, but a maternal uncle shows obvious ET.

of males was found in Scandinavian studies (female/male ratios of 0.5 and 0.71 respectively) (Rautokorpi et al. 1982), and a predominance of females was found in the USA (Haerer et al. 1982).

Clinical features. The disturbance begins in a slow and subtle manner. Some parents indicate that their child "has always had tremor", but is worried about the symptom only when it interferes with writing; and sometimes teachers are the first to draw attention to the problem. Taking into account the difficulty in knowing the onset of tremor (Fig. 3.2), the mean age in paediatric patients for whom it could be ascertained was 3.81 years (Fernández-Alvarez and Lopez-Casas 1996).

In children, tremor is usually limited to the hands (flexion–extension, pronosupination). It is, usually, asymmetrical, predominating in the dominant hand (Biary and Koller 1985), and may even seem unilateral at onset (Critchley 1949, Findley and Koller 1987), although Larsson and Sjogren (1960) have claimed that symmetrical onset is more common. The tremor is of the postural type but sometimes is augmented by action. Its amplitude is low and the frequency varies between 8 and 10 Hz (Cleeves and Findley 1987). (Tremor amplitude is inversely proportional to tremor frequency.) It is normally

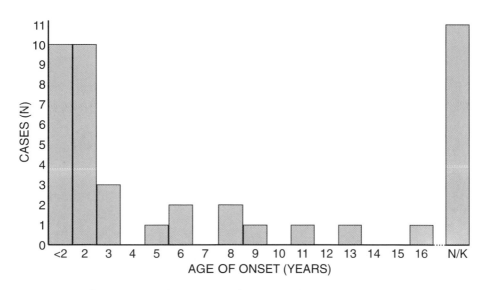

Fig. 3.2. Age of onset of 45 paediatric cases with ET. Note that in 11 cases (25%) the onset was so insidious that it was not known (N/K) at what age it occurred.

absent at rest, although Critchley (1972) mentioned that it was "occasionally present at rest". Tandem gait abnormalities are observed in 50% of adult ET patients (Singer et al. 1994) but this has not been studied in childhood cases.

Tremor in ET, like physiological exaggerated tremor, is often increased by fatigue, extremes of temperature and emotional tension, and disappears during sleep. The well-known effect of alcohol (Growdon et al. 1975, Findley 1987) has not been studied in children for obvious reasons. The disorder is usually slowly progressive. In rare cases childhood ET can remit (personal case, EF-A) or transiently disappear and reappear after a free interval (Paulson 1976).

The disability resulting from ET is variable. It is negligible in some children, limited to irregularities in handwriting and to some 'insecurity' in fine movements. In others there is marked interference with everyday life, for example in drinking out of a glass. Impairment is a function of the amplitude of the tremor but is often made worse by the anticipation of awkward situations. One of my (EF-A) adolescent patients had to stop going to restaurants because he would spill drinks there, which did not occur at home. ET does not affect life expectancy. Disability usually increases with the duration of tremor and age of the patient (Bain et al. 1994).

Tashimira et al. (1987) have found a high incidence of induced mirror writing: when asked to write with the non-dominant hand, 12 of 65 patients with ET had complete and four partial mirror writing. A high incidence of left-handedness has also been recorded (Biary and Koller 1985).

Sub-classification. Several sub-classifications of ET have been proposed (Marsden et al. 1983, Deuschl et al. 1987). Deuschl et al. (1987) suggested a classification based on the EMG pattern and the presence of abnormal long-latency reflex responses. However, other investigators (Elble 1986, Koller et al. 1992) deny the possibility of defining sub-types of ET.

Unusual clinical variants such as *manual tremor predominating on action, combined rest and postural tremor* (Critchley 1949, Koller and Rubino 1985), *isolated tremor of voice* (Koller et al. 1985), *jaw* (Rapoport et al. 1991) and *tongue* (Biary and Koller 1987), *orthostatic truncal tremor* (Pape and Gershanik 1988) have been described in adults but it is not known whether they also occur in children.

Primary writing tremor. Rothwell et al. (1979) reported the case of a 12-year-old girl who had sudden onset of bouts of tremor of pronosupination in the right forearm of such great amplitude as to suggest myoclonus, precipitated exclusively by active pronation. This resulted in considerable difficulties in writing or any activity involving pronation of this forearm (e.g. bringing a glass to her mouth). On EMG these movements displayed the characteristics of a tremor and the authors regarded the disturbance as a variant of ET. Later reports (Kachi et al. 1985, Ravits et al. 1985) defined the syndrome as (i) an action tremor induced only by specific tasks, (ii) without associated neurologic abnormalities. The nosological position of this syndrome is unclear. Some investigators regard it more as a variant of focal dystonia (Elble et al. 1994), and the patient of Ravits et al. (1985) also presented with writer's cramp.

Differential diagnosis. Differentiation of physiological, exaggerated physiological and essential tremor is, sometimes, clinically difficult. Tremor in ET is permanently present, although the amplitude can fluctuate. ET clinical variants create more diagnostic diffi-culties. Manual tremor predominating in action must be distinguished from cerebellar tremor, and from primary writing tremor myoclonus.

Not uncommonly, ET is regarded as the initial symptom of a cerebellar disease, as an incomplete form of cerebral palsy, or as a manifestation of anxiety. We have seen several children referred for psychological therapy in spite of a clear family history of ET. When there is no family history or when not all criteria are fulfilled, the possibility of a secondary tremor has to be considered (Table 3.2). Some conditions can present with a predomin-antly monosymptomatic tremor similar to ET: chronic hydrocephalus, hereditary motor and sensory neuropathy (HMSN), Wilson disease and Klinefelter syndrome. In case of doubt a slit-lamp examination, cupruria and ceruloplasmin blood levels will exclude the treatable Wilson's disease. CT or MRI will rule out hydrocephalus, and familial history and nerve conduction velocity measurements rule out a polyneuropathy.

Pathophysiology. The basic abnormality of ET is abnormal rhythmical alternation of motor unit activity during voluntary muscle contraction (Elble et al. 1994). The anatom-

TABLE 3.2
Secondary tremor

Neuromuscular diseases
Spinal muscular atrophy
Guillain–Barré syndrome
Hereditary motor and sensory neuropathies
  (Roussy–Lévy syndrome)*

Endocrinological disorders
Hyperthyroidism*
Pseudohyparathyroidism

Drug-induced (Chapter 10)
Antiasthmatic drugs: albuterol, procaterol,
  salbutamol (Mazer et al. 1990)
Sodium valproate (Karas et al. 1983)
L-Dopa
Overdose of iron (Aranda and Asenjo 1969)

Metabolic diseases
Lesch–Nyhan disease (Chapter 5)
Wilson disease (Chapter 6)*
Phenylketonuria (MacLeod et al. 1983)

Others
Dopa-responsive dystonia
Idiopathic torsion dystonia
Benign familial chorea
Essential myoclonus
Juvenile Huntington disease*
Hallervorden–Spatz disease

Juvenile idiopathic parkinsonism*
Delayed-onset dystonia
Psychogenic tremor
Chronic hydrocephalus (bobble-head doll
  syndrome)*
Subdural haematoma
Cranial trauma (Broggi et al. 1993)
Acute hemiplegia (Quaglieri et al. 1977)
Ataxia–telangiectasia (Chapter 5)
Hypomagnesaemia
Hypocalcaemia
Uraemia
Vitamin B_{12} deficiency
Kwashiorkor
Ceroid-lipofuscinosis (Greenwood and
  Nelson 1978)
Spasmus nutans*
Opsoclonus–myoclonus syndrome
Familial spastic paraplegia (Dick and
  Stevenson 1953)
Olivopontocerebellar atrophy
Cockayne disease
Pelizaeus–Merzbacher disease
Klinefelter syndrome*
Fetal alcohol syndrome
Intranuclear neuronal inclusion disease
  (Chapter 2)*

*Tremor can be the first symptom.

ical bases of ET are unknown. The few available pathological reports do not mention any consistent abnormality (Rajput et al. 1991).

The main issue is whether ET is due to central or peripheral dysfunction or involves both. A majority of authors favour a central origin on the basis of benefit from thalamotomy (Hirai et al. 1983), disappearance with the occurrence of ipsilateral hemiparesis (Young 1986), cerebellar stroke (Dupuis et al. 1989), and the effect of efficacious drugs (propranolol, alcohol) which seem to act at a central level.

There is increasing evidence that the cerebellum plays an important role in the physiopathology of ET. PET studies (Jenkins et al. 1993) have shown an increased cerebellar blood flow and glucose consumption rate presumed to be in the cerebellar olives, suggesting that ET might be due to overactivity within the olivocerebellar pathways. Abnormally increased cerebellar flow is also evident even in patients at rest (Willis et al. 1994).

Such an oscillating process could be transmitted to the thalamus – also active during tremor (Jenkins et al. 1993, Willis et al. 1994 – and then to motor cortex and from there to the spinal cord. This would explain the abolition of tremor as a result of cerebellar infarcts, hemiplegia or thalamotomy.

Treatment. Except in the unusual childhood cases in which ET causes marked disability, we do not favour pharmacological (beta-adrenergic receptor blocking agents, primidone) treatment (see later). Explanation, reassurance and psychological support to the child and family are usually sufficient.

Trembling of the chin (Laurance et al. 1968)
This is an intermittent involuntary tremor facilitated by emotional tensions involving cutaneous muscles of the chin in an up-and-down quivering as the patient starts crying. The episodes may last several minutes (Danek 1993). The condition is dominantly in-herited; a gene has been located in the 9q13–q21 region (Jarman et al. 1997). It appears usually shortly after birth or up to some years of age. It can occur spontaneously but is more often precipitated by emotional stimuli that are specific for each individual. The frequency of episodes decreases with age. It is a benign condition but it can interfere with speech and drinking and cause distress (Soland et al. 1996). The condition has been reported in association with disturbances of conduct and of sleep (Blaw et al. 1989). Al-though trembling of the chin has been regarded as a form of ET its peculiar characteristics set it apart as a different condition.

Differential diagnosis is easy, and only focal peribuccal epileptic myoclonus is to be considered. In most cases no treatment is necessary. Benzodiazepines (Johnson et al. 1971), phenytoin (Wadlington 1958) and haloperidol are ineffective. In exceptional cases when the trouble has been socially incapacitating, botulinum toxin has been useful (Soland et al. 1996)

TRANSIENT TREMORS
NEONATAL JITTERINESS
Almost one-half of normal term neonates exhibit, during the first days of life, when excited or crying (Levene et al. 1988, Parker et al. 1990), a particular tremor of high fre-quency and low amplitude known as jitteriness, involving the chin and extremities. It can persist in severe form in almost all arousal states. Jitteriness can also occur in infants with hypoxic–ischaemic encephalopathy, hypocalcaemia, hypoglycaemia and drug withdrawal (Volpe 1995). 'Essential' jitteriness usually disappears, without sequelae, in the neonatal period, but in a follow-up study (Kramer et al. 1994), 22% of cases persisted for up to two months. In addition, in some infants, jitteriness may reappear after an interval of up to six weeks but also disappear before the child is 1 year old (Shuper et al. 1991).

Jitteriness can be misdiagnosed as an epileptic phenomenon especially when it re-appears after a free interval. Differential features include precipitation by crying or by sudden movement, abolition by restraint or change of position of the affected limb, and absence of abnormal eye movements. In jitteriness, the EEG shows no paroxysmal activity. However, jitteriness and seizures can occur coincidentally and be difficult to differentiate.

Jitteriness can be regarded as a spontaneous clonus triggered by the infant's sudden movements.

Shuddering

Shuddering episodes consist of brief bursts (5–15 seconds) of rapid tremor of the head and arms reminiscent of a shiver (Vanasse et al. 1976). Such episodes can recur up to 100 times daily. They have their onset in the first months of life, although Holmes and Russman (1986) have described two patients with onset at 6 and 10 years. The EEG during these episodes showed no abnormalities (Holmes and Russman 1986). The course is benign. Such cases might be associated with those of 'benign myoclonus of infants' (Lombroso and Fejerman 1977). Vanasse et al. (1976) suggested that shuddering spells might be an early manifestation of essential tremor in the immature brain.

Essential Palatal Tremor

Also known as palatal myoclonus, palatal nystagmus, myorhythmias or oculopalatal myoclonus, this is a rare entity consisting of rhythmical twitching of the soft palate, pharynx and larynx, sometimes resulting in an audible click perceived by the patient. Occasionally it involves the extraocular and shoulder muscles. The term palatal myoclonus was used until recently, but tremor seems to be more accurate because of the rhythmical pattern (Herrmann and Brown 1967, Gresty and Findley 1984).

Two forms exist, symptomatic and essential (Deuschl et al. 1994). The symptomatic form occurs almost exclusively in adults, usually is associated with hemiplegia, cerebellar signs and diplopia, lasts for the rest of the patient's life, and does not disappear with sleep or even barbiturate anaesthesia or deep coma. It results from lesions of the brainstem or cerebellum with hypertrophy of the inferior olive (Lapresle 1979). A few symptomatic cases of palatal tremor have been reported in childhood, e.g. with Krabbe disease (Yamanouchi et al. 1991), cerebellar tumour (Nathanson 1956) and encephalitis (Baram et al. 1986).

The essential form mainly occurs in children. In 1923, WH Jewell reported on a child with tremor of the soft palate which disappeared following adenoidectomy. Age at onset of reported cases is most often between 6 and 10 years of age. Of 11 reported cases, seven started before the age of 18 years (Jacobs et al. 1981, Boulloche and Aicardi 1984, de Campos et al. 1986, Yokota et al. 1990). The youngest patient was in infancy (de Campos et al. 1986), the two oldest were 26 years of age (Yokota et al. 1990). At our (EF-A) institution, three patients with essential palatal tremor have been seen with onset at 6, 6 and 9 years respectively. All were referred because of an auditory click that could be perceived at auscultation. This is a rhythmical metallic sound that could even be heard at a distance. Familial cases has been reported (Klein et al. 1998).

Examination shows rhythmical contraction of the soft palate at a frequency of 4–5 Hz. The rhythmical movements may sometimes involve the submental muscles and lips (Jacobs et al. 1981). Other results of the neurological examination are negative as are those of ancillary investigations. The tremor usually disappears in all stages of sleep, but in some cases persisted during sleep (Boulloche and Aicardi 1984, de Campos et al. 1986, and one case seen by EF-A). A certain degree of voluntary control is possible for either inhibiting or provoking the abnormal movement. Sometimes, twitches cease completely when the patient is concentrating or, for instance, receiving an injection (Yokota et al. 1990). This has led to considering the phenomenon as of psychogenic origin and can explain why the condition is sometimes missed on a single otorhinolaryngological examination.

The movement usually persists for months or years (Jacobs et al. 1981). Cases with a good response to flunarizine (Cakmur et al. 1997), carbamazepine (Sakai et al. 1981), sumatriptan injections (Scott et al. 1996), sodium valproate (Borggreve and Hageman 1991), 5-hydroxytryptophan, tetrabenazine, clonazepam and botulinum toxin (Deuschl et al. 1991) have been reported. I (EF-A) have tried propranolol in three patients, with a disappearance of the tremor on some days. Because in some patients benefit may result from relaxation sessions (de Campos et al. 1986) or hypnosis, and, moreover, others can learn to voluntarily control the movement (Jacobs et al. 1981), it is difficult to assess the efficacy of drugs.

Deuschl et al. (1994) have shown that the symptomatic and essential forms affect different muscles. In the former, there is contraction of the levator veli palatini (innervated by the VIIth and IXth cranial nerves); in the later, the contraction involves the tensor veli palatini (innervated by the Vth nerve). According to these authors the essential form is bilateral and is the only one to be accompanied by auditory clicks.

The pathophysiology is unknown. At least some cases seem related to an oto-rhinolaryngological disturbance (de Campos et al. 1986). The ability to control the movements implies a degree of cortical influence

When suspected, the diagnosis is easy. Exceptionally, epilepsia partialis continua with 'palatal tremor' has been reported but is associated with perioral twitching, and twitching of the floor of the mouth and arm (Tatum et al. 1991, Noatchar et al. 1995). The diagnosis of essential palatal tremor avoids costly and invasive examinations and inappropriate treatments such as psychotherapy.

SPASMUS NUTANS

Spasmus nutans is a self-limited disorder of infants. It consists of a slow cephalic tremor (2–4 Hz), usually of negation, associated with pendular horizontal, rarely vertical (Norton et al. 1954, Gottlob et al. 1990), nystagmus that may be bilateral and asymmetrical but is often monocular (Antony et al. 1980), rapid and of small amplitude. Abnormal head positions are frequently present, as is strabismus.

TABLE 3.3
Differential diagnosis between congenital nystagmus and spasmus nutans

	Spasmus nutans	Congenital nystagmus
Onset	4 mo– 3 y (mainly before 12 mo)	Birth (but can be detected later)
Family history	Negative	Positive or negative
Nystagmus	Asymmetric (31% unilateral)	Bilateral symmetric
Cephalic movement	Usually previous to nystagmus	Simultaneous with nystagmus
Evolution	Disappearance in 36 months	Persistent

The onset is generally between 4 and 12 months of age and is exceptional after the third year of life. The disorder generally disappears in a few months but can last for years (Doummar et al. 1998). Its aetiology is unknown. Familial cases have been reported (Doummar et al. 1998).

Spasmus nutans should be distinguished from congenital nystagmus (Table 3.3). Visually impaired infants can present with oculocephalic movements similar to those of spasmus nutans (Jan et al. 1990). The common practice of neuroimaging has shown that optic nerve or chiasmatic gliomas can simulate spasmus nutans (Antony et al. 1980, Albright et al. 1984) so that Farmer and Hoyt (1984) recommend that a neuroimaging study always be obtained.

SECONDARY TREMORS

Tremor can accompany a vast number of diseases (see Table 3.2). Different from essential tremor, several of the causal disorders are associated with CNS lesions (Narabayashi 1986): substantia nigra and locus ceruleus, implicated in parkinsonism; red nucleus and surrounding area, implicated in Benedikt syndrome (unilateral tremor and contralateral oculomotor nerve palsy). In other disorders, the pathological basis of tremor is not known, e.g. bobble-head doll syndrome. Some cases cannot be differentiated from essential tremor on a semiological basis ('essential-like' tremor) and probably have a similar pathophysiological basis. Parkinsonian tremor has already been dealt with in Chapter 2.

Tremor and Hydrocephalus

In children, tremor (together with a large head) may be the only manifestation of chronic, apparently arrested, hydrocephalus. Two forms are possible. In one, the extremities, especially the hands, are involved in an 'essential-like' tremor. In the other the tremor is axial with resulting cephalic tremor, known as bobble-head doll syndrome (BHDS) (Benton et al. 1966).

In BHDS the movements are usually affirmative, very seldom negative (Nellhaus 1967, Kaplan et al. 1984) and slow (1–4 Hz). The name is due to their resemblance to

Chinese dolls with weighted heads and coil-spring necks. In some cases, the tremor extends to involve the trunk, shoulders or hands (Nellhaus 1967, Russman et al. 1975). It is interesting that the movement can be controlled for minutes by the patients voluntarily (Pollack et al. 1995) or when they concentrate their attention (Nellhaus 1967) or fixate their gaze on something. It disappears during sleep and in the lying position (Deonna and Dubey 1976). Other signs may include optic pallor, nystagmus, ocular flutter, intention or resting tremor of the hands, obesity and short stature.

According to the review of Mussell et al. (1997) the symptoms of BHDS have their onset before age 10 years (mean age of onset: 3 years 3 months), although one case had a late onset at 21 years.

The pathology of BHDS always includes a dilatation of the third ventricle although the actual cause is variable: hydrocephalus secondary to aqueductal stenosis, suprasellar arachnoid cyst (Wiese et al. 1985, Goikhman et al. 1998), colloid cyst of the third ventricle, third ventricular plexus papilloma or craniopharyngioma (Parizek et al. 1989, Pollack et al. 1995). The phenomenon has also been observed as a result of obstruction of ventricular shunt (Dell 1981).

The pathogenesis is obscure. The existence of a colloid cyst of the third ventricle had suggested the hypothesis of a learnt behaviour to alleviate the hydrocephalus, since movement of the head may relieve pressure in this condition (Wiese et al. 1985). More attractive is the opinion that the disorder results from compression on periventricular structures of the mesial part of the dorsomedial thalamic nucleus and/or dentate subthalamic pathways (Benton et al. 1966). A similar mechanism could be responsible for the rigid–akinetic syndrome of aqueductal stenosis (see Chapter 2). Surgical treatment of the hydrocephalus produces disappearance of the abnormal movement. but if delay from onset of head bobbing to neurosurgical treatment is more than six years head bobbing can persist (Rouberge et al. 1985, Wiese et al. 1985, Musell et al. 1997).

TREMOR OF NEUROPATHIES AND SPINAL MUSCULAR ATROPHIES

The Roussy–Lévy syndrome variably features signs of chronic polyneuropathy (Charcot–Marie–Tooth disease or HMSN type I) (Said et al. 1982, Barbieri et al. 1984, Cardoso and Jankovic 1993) and a tremor with the characteristics of ET. The syndrome is dominantly inherited and the tremor may be the predominant manifestation. Two main interpretations are possible: (1) the syndrome may result from a genetic defect that affects both the gene of HMSN type I and that of essential tremor; or (2) it may be due to peculiar characteristics of the peripheral nerve lesion (Salisachs 1976).

A fast tremor has been reported in HMSN type II (Harding and Thomas 1980), distal spinal muscular atrophies (Thomas 1975), Guillain–Barré syndrome, chronic inflammatory polyneuropathies (Dalakas et al. 1984), dysgammaglobulinic neuropathy (Dalakas et al. 1984) and diabetic, uraemic and amyloidosis neuropathies, and is attributed to a defect in the transmission of proprioceptive influxes.

The tremor of neuropathies may share its mechanism with the irregular, small amplitude movements observed in the spinal amyotrophies (Boyland and Cornblatt 1992) known as minipolymyoclonus (Spiro 1970) This is due to imperfect synchronization of the large motor units resulting from collateral adoption of fibres by remaining anterior horn cell neurons.

OTHER SECONDARY TREMORS

Vitamin B₁₂ (cobalamin) deficiency is probably a major factor in the 'infantile tremor syndrome' (Garg and Srivastava 1969), a self-limiting (within 4–6 weeks) syndrome of infants with malnutrition (but not marasmus) observed in India or in exclusively breast-fed infants of strict vegetarian mothers (Higginbottom et al. 1978). Symptoms commence between 4 and 8 months of age. Irritability and apathy are often the first manifestations, followed by regression. Pallor, lethargy, failure to thrive, hypotonia and brisk reflexes may occur. Tremor (sometimes with added myoclonus) varies in severity and timing. It may be the presenting manifestation or, more often, appears after institution of vitamin therapy. MRI shows apparent brain atrophy and sometimes delayed myelination (Grattan-Smith et al. 1997). Macrocytosis is always present and often also anaemia. Hyperglycinaemia with hyperglycinuria resulting from the metabolic defect are of diagnostic importance and may play a pathogenetic role. In spite of the risk of appearance of tremor, vitamin treatment produces dramatic improvement, both clinical and on neuroimaging (Graham et al. 1992)

In *kwashiorkor*, a fine tremor may be precipitated by stressful situations such as diarrhoea, pneumonia or pertussis. In some cases, tremor occurs within several days to weeks after starting renutrition (Kahn and Falcke 1956). This tremor is coarse, parkinsonian in type, and may be extremely intense. It affects most commonly the upper extremities but may involve also the legs, the tongue and the facial muscles and may be asymmetrical. It disappears after a few days to several weeks. It may be associated with diffuse, cogwheel hypertonia. The same type of tremor may occur at the time of recovery of any type of severe malnutrition and is seen in industrialized countries among children of migrants workers coming back after holidays at home during which severe diarrhoea with poor nutrition occurred.

Tetrahydrobiopterin (THB4) deficiency may result in hyperphenylalaninaemia. Neurological signs typically include developmental delay, hypotonia or spasticity, dystonia and epilepsy. Infants with coarse tremor have been reported (Butler et al. 1981). In one case, paroxysmal episodes of 'rubral-like' tremor in arms and legs, and orofacial dyskinesia, between the ages of 3 and 6 months and lasting several hours, were the main clinical signs. Treatment with L-dopa results in a dramatic improvement (Factor et al. 1991).

Postural tremor is common in patients with *Klinefelter syndrome* (Baughman 1969) and, in general, with syndromes of supernumerary X chromosome in males and also, probably, supernumerary Y chromosomes. Tremor (sometimes cerebellar) may occur following *head trauma* (Broggi et al. 1993), *CNS vascular accidents* (Ferbert and Gerwig 1993) and *multiple sclerosis* (Fig. 3.3) can also be accompanied by tremor.

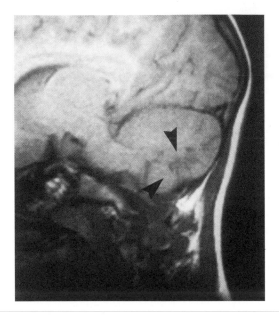

Fig. 3.3. Multiple sclerosis starting with focal tremor. In this patient, onset was sudden at 5 years with abnormal movements of the right hand for four months, referred by the parents as tremor. He became left-handed. At age 6 years he showed only light dystonia and tremor in the right hand. CT scan performed at that time was normal. MRI at 9 years showed right hemispheric cerebellar lesion. At 10 years he developed acute ophthalmoplegia. MRI then showed diffuse white matter lesions.

PSYCHOGENIC TREMOR

Hysterical or psychogenic tremor can be very difficult to diagnose. It often shows an inconsistent mixture of rest, postural and action components. Koller et al. (1989) consider that the main diagnostic features are: (1) abrupt onset; (2) static course; (3) occurrence of spontaneous remissions; (4) complex movements; (5) inconsistent features for ET, such as the occurrence of selective disabilities; (6) changing characteristics; (7) failure to respond to antitremorigenic drugs; (8) increase with attention; (9) decrease when attention is diverted; (10) response to placebo; (11) absence of neurological signs; (12) remission with successful psychotherapy. Many of these characteristics are non-specific.

SYMPTOMATIC TREATMENT OF TREMOR

When pharmacological treatment is indicated, currently popular drugs include: primidone (Findley et al. 1985), and beta-adrenergic blockers especially propranolol (Cleeves and Findley 1988).

Primidone seems to be better tolerated (Winkler and Young 1974). The usual dose is 20–30 mg/kg/d in two doses and should be reached progressively. Twenty per cent of patients suffer side-effects as nausea, vomiting, and sedation over the first days of treatment (Koller 1995).

Optimal doses of propranolol in adults range from 240 to 320 mg/d (Koller 1986, Rondot et al. 1988). There is no established dose for children but 60 mg/d seems a safe dose. The relationship between blood level and clinical effect remains questionable (Jefferson et al. 1979). Pulse rate is lowered in most patients (Koller 1995). Side-effects include fatigue, lethargy and hypotension, so the drug is relatively contra-indicated in patients with heart failure and insulin-dependent diabetes (in which propranolol may block the adrenergic manifestations of hypoglycaemia). It is absolutely contraindicated in asthma and other causes of bronchoconstriction. Its mechanism of action is unknown.

Both primidone and propranolol are usually only partially effective and their side-effects are often disproportionate so that they should be used only in severe cases.

Other drugs have been thought to be efficacious by some authors and useless by others. These include the benzodiazepines (Biary and Koller 1987, Huber and Paulson 1988), amantadine (Critchley 1972), trazodone (serotoninergic agent) (McLeod and White 1986), glutethimide (hypnotic and anticholinergic agent) (McDowell 1989), nadolol (Koller 1983), carbonic anhydrase inhibitors (Busenbark et al. 1993), nicardipine (Garcia-Ruiz et al. 1993) and flunarizine (Biary et al. 1991).

Botulinum toxin has been used in some extreme cases of cephalic or manual tremor (Jankovic and Schwartz 1991). Despite its favourable effect, alcohol cannot be used in children.

REFERENCES

Albright AL, Sclabassi RJ, Slamovits TL, et al. (1984) Spasmus nutans associated with optic gliomas in infants. *J Pediatr* 105: 778–80.

Antony JH, Ouvrier RA, Wise G (1980) Spasmus nutans, a mistaken identity. *Arch Neurol* 37: 373–5.

Aranda LC, Asenjo A (1969) Tremor induced by iron overloading. *J Neurosurg* 30: 35–7.

Bain PG, Findley LJ, Thompson PD, et al. (1994) A study of hereditary essential tremor. *Brain* 117: 805–24.

Baram TZ, Parke JT, Mahoney DH (1986) Palatal myoclonus in a child: Herald of acute encephalitis. *Neurology* 36: 302–3.

Barbieri F, Filla A, Ragno M, et al. (1984) Evidence that Charcot–Marie–Tooth disease with tremor coincides with the Roussy–Levy syndrome. *Can J Neurol Sci* 11: 534–40.

Baughman FA (1969) Klinefelter's syndrome and essential tremor. *Lancet* 2: 545.

Benton JW, Nellhaus G, Huttenlocher PR, et al. (1966) The bobblehead syndrome. Report of a unique truncal tremor associated with third ventricular cyst and hydrocephalus in children. *Neurology* 16: 725–9.

Biary N, Koller W (1985) Handedness and essential tremor. Arch Neurol 42: 1082–3.

— — (1987) Essential tongue tremor. *Mov Disord* 2: 25–9.

— Al Deeb SM, Langenberg P (1991) The effect of flunarizine on essential tremor. *Neurology* 41: 311–2.

Blaw MR, Leroy RF, Steinberg JB, Herman J (1989) Hereditary quivering chin and REM behavioral disorder. *Ann Neurol* 26: 471–3.

Borggreve F, Hageman G (1991) A case of idiopathic palatal myoclonus: treatment with sodium valproate. *Eur Neurol* 31: 403–4.

Boulloche J, Aicardi J (1984) Syndrome de myoclonies du voile du palais spontanément régressif chez l'enfant. *Arch Fr Pediatr* 41: 645–7.

Boylan KB, Cornblath DR (1992) Werdnig–Hoffmann disease and chronic spinal muscular atrophy with apparent autosomal dominant inherence. *Ann Neurol* 32: 404–7.

Broggi G, Brock A, Franzini A, Geminiani G (1993) A case of posttraumatic tremor treated by chronic stimulation of the thalamus. *Mov Disord* 8: 206–8.

Busenbark K, Pahwa R, Hubble J, Koller WC (1993) Double-blind controlled study of methazolamide in the treatment of essential tremor. *Neurology* 43: 1045–7.

Butler IJ, O'Flynn ME, Seifert WE, Howell R (1981) Neurotransmitter defects and treatment of disorders of hyperphenylalaninemia. *J Pediatr* 98: 729–33.

Cakmur R, Idiman E, Idiman F, et al. (1997) Essential palatal tremor successfully treated with flunarizine. *Eur Neurol* 38: 133–4.

Cardoso FE, Jankovic J (1993) Hereditary motor–sensory neuropathy and movement disorders. *Muscle Nerve* 16: 904–10.

Cleeves L, Findley LJ (1987) Variability in amplitude of untreated essential tremor. *J Neurol Neurosurg Psychiatry* 50: 704–8.

— — (1988) Propranolol and propranolol-LA in essential tremor: a double blind comparative study. *J Neurol Neurosurg Psychiatry* 51: 379–84.

Critchley E (1972) Clinical manifestations of essential tremor. *J Neurol Neurosurg Psychiatry* 35: 365–72.

Critchley McD (1949) Observations on essential (heredofamilial) tremor. *Brain* 72: 113–39.

Dalakas MC, Terevainene H, Engel WK (1984) Tremor as a feature of chronic relapsing and dysgammaglobulinemic polyneuropathies. Incidence and management. *Arch Neurol* 41: 711–4.

Danek A (1993) Geniospasm: Hereditary chin trembling. *Mov Disord* 8: 335–8.

de Campos CC, Campos CAH, Rosemberg S (1986) Tinitus objetivo e mioclonias velopalatinas na criança. Una análise de quatro casos. *Rev Bras Neurol* 22: 165–7.

Dell S (1981) Further observations on the "bobblehead doll syndrome". *J Neurol Neurosurg Psychiatry* 44, 1046–9.

Deonna T, Dubey B (1976) Bobblehead doll syndrome. Case report with a review on the different types of abnormal head movements in infancy and their clinical significance. *Helv Paediat Acta* 31, 221–7.

Deuschl G, Lucking CH, Schenk E (1987) Essential tremor: Electrophysiological and pharmacological evidence for a subdivision. *J Neurol Neurosurg Psychiatry* 50: 1435–41.

Deuschl G, Löhle E, Heinen F, Lücking CH (1991) Ear click in palatal tremor. Its origin and treatment with botulinum toxin. *Neurology* 41: 1677–9.

— Toro C, Hallett M (1994) Symptomatic and essential palatal tremor. Differences of palatal movements. *Mov Disord* 9: 676–8.

Dick AP, Stevenson CJ (1953) Hereditary spastic paraplegia. Report of a family with associated extrapyramidal signs. *Lancet* 1. 921–3.

Doummar D, Roussat B, Beauvais P, et al. (1998) Spasmus nutans: à propos de 16 cas. *Arch Pediatr* 5: 264–8.

Dupuis MJM, Delwaide PJ, Boucquey D, Gonsette RE (1989) Homolateral disappearance of essential tremor after cerebellar stroke. *Mov Disord* 4: 183–7.

Elble RJ (1986) Physiologic and essential tremor. *Neurology* 36: 225–31.

— Higgins C, Leffler K, Hugues H (1994) Factors influencing the amplitude and frequency of essential tremor. *Mov Disord* 6: 589–96.

Factor SA, Coni RJ, Cowger M, Rosenblum EL (1991) Paroxysmal tremor and orofacial dyskinesia secondary to a biopterin synthesis defect. *Neurology* 41: 930–2.

Farmer J, Hyot CS (1984) Monocular nystagmus in infancy and early childhood. *Am J Ophthalmol* 98: 504–9.

Ferbert A, Gerwig M (1993) Tremor due to stroke. *Mov Disord* 8: 179–82.

Fernández-Alvarez E, Lopez-Casas J (1996) Essential tremor (ET) in childhood. In: Arzimanoglou A, Goutières F (eds) *Trends in Child Neurology.* Paris: John Libbey Eurotext, pp. 147–55.

Findley LJ (1984) Essential tremor: introductory remarks. In: Findley LJ, Capildeo R (eds) *Movement Disorders: Tremor.* London: Macmillan, pp. 207–9.

— (1987) The pharmacology of essential tremor. In: Marsden CD, Fahn S (eds) *Movement Disorders.* London. Butterworths, pp. 438–58.

— Cleeves L (1989) Classification of tremor. In: Quinn NP Jenner PG (eds) *Disorders of Movement: Clinical, Pharmacological and Physiological Aspects.* London: Academic Press, pp. 505–19.

— Koller WC (1987) Essential tremor: A review. *Neurology* 37: 1194–7.

— Cleeves L, Calzetti S (1985) Primidone in essential tremor of hands and head: A double blind controlled clinical study. *J Neurol Neurosurg Psychiatry* 48: 911–5.

Franz DN (1993) Tremor in childhood. *Pediatr Annals* 22: 60–4.

Garcia-Ruiz PJ, Garcia De Yebenes Prous J, Jimenez-Jimenez J (1993) Effect of nicardipine on essential tremor: Brief report. *Clin Neuropharmacol* 16: 456–9.

Garg BK, Srivastava JR (1969) Infantile tremor syndrome. *Indian J Pediatr* 36: 213–8.

Goikhman Y, Zelnuk N, Peled N, Michowiz S (1998) Bobble-head doll syndrome: A surgical treatable condition manifested as a rare movement disorder. *Mov Disord* 13: 192–4.

Gottlob Y, Zubcov A, Catalano RA, et al. (1990) Signs distinguishing spasmus nutans (with or without central nervous system lesions) from infantile nystagmus. *Ophthalmology* 97: 166–75.

Graham SM, Arvela OM, Wise GA (1992) Long term neurological consequences of nutritional B12 deficiency in infants. *J Pediatr* 121: 710–4.

Grattan-Smith PJ, Wilcken B, Procopis PG, Wise GA (1997) The neurological syndrome of infantile cobalamin deficiency: Developmental regression and involuntary movements. *Mov Disord* 12: 39–46.

Greenwood RS, Nelson JS (1978) Atypical neuronal ceroid lipofuscinosis. *Neurology* 28, 710–7.

Gresty MA, Findley LJ (1984) Definition, analysis and genesis of tremor. In: Findley LJ, Capildeo R (eds) *Movement Disorders: Tremor.* London: Macmillan, pp. 15–26.

Growdon JH, Shahani BT, Young RR (1975) The effect of alcohol on essential tremor. *Neurology* 28, 259–62.

Haerer AF, Anderson DW, Schoenberg BS (1982) Prevalence of essential tremor. Results from the Copiah County Study. *Arch Neurol* 39, 750–1.

Harding AE, Thomas PK (1980) The clinical features of hereditary motor and sensory neuropathy types I and II. *Brain* 103: 259–80.

Herrmann C, Brown JW (1967) Palatal myoclonus: A reappraisal. *J Neurol Sci* 5: 473–92.

Higginbottom MC, Sweetman L, Nyhan WL (1978) A syndrome of methylmalonic aciduria, homocystinuria, megaloblastic anaemia and neurological abnormalities in a vitamin B_{12}-deficient breast-fed infant of a strict vegetarian. *N Engl J Med* 299: 317–23.

Higgins JJ, Pho LT, Nee LE (1997) A gene (*ETM*) for essential tremor maps to chromosome 2p22–p25. *Mov Disord* 12: 859–64.

Hirai T, Miyazaki M, Nakajima H, et al. (1983) The correlation between tremor characteristics and the predicted volume of effective lesions in stereoataxic nucleus ventralis intermedius thalamotomy. *Brain* 106: 1001–18.

Holmes GL, Russman BS (1986) Shuddering attacks. *Am J Dis Child* 140: 72–3.

Huber SJ, Paulson GW (1988) Efficacy of alprazolam for essential tremor. *Neurology* 38: 241–3.

Jacobs L, Newman RP, Bozian D (1981) Disappearing palatal myoclonus. *Neurology* 31: 748–51.

Jan JE, Groenveld M, Connolly MB (1990) Head shaking by visually impaired children: a voluntary visual adaptation which can be confused with spasmus nutans. *Dev Med Child Neurol* 32: 1061–6.

Jankovic J, Schwartz K (1991) Botulinum toxin treatment of tremors. *Neurology* 41: 1185–8.

— Beach J, Pandolfo M, Patel PI (1997) Familial essential tremor in 4 kindreds: Prospect for genetic mapping. *Arch Neurol* 54: 289–94.

Jarman PR, Wood NH, Davis MT, et al. (1997) Hereditary geniospasm: Linkage to chromosome 9q13–q21 and evidence for genetic heterogeneity. *Am J Hum Genet* 61: 928–33.

Jefferson D, Jenner P, Marsden CD (1979) Relationship between plasma propranolol concentration and relief of essential tremor. *J Neurol Neurosurg Psychiatry* 42: 831–7.

Jenkins IH, Bain PG, Colebatch JGM, et al. (1993) A positron emission tomography study of essential tremor: Evidence for overactivity of cerebellar connections. *Ann Neurol* 34: 82–90.

Johnson LF, Kinsbourne M, Renuart AW (1971) Hereditary chin trembling with nocturnal myoclonus and tongue-biting in dizygous twins. *Dev Med Child Neurol* 13: 726–9.

Kachi T, Rothwell JC, Cowan JMA, Marsden CD (1985) Writing tremor: Its relationship to benign essential tremor. *J Neurol Neurosurg Psychiatry* 41, 545–50.

Kahn E, Falcke HC (1956) A syndrome simulating encephalitis affecting children recovering from malnutrition (kwashiorkor). *J Pediatr* 49: 37–45.

Kaplan BJ, Mickle JP, Parkhurst R (1984) Cystoperitoneal shunting for congenital arachnoid cysts. *Child's Brain* 11: 304–11.

Karas BJ, Wilder BJ, Hammond EJ, Bauman AW (1983) Treatment of valproate tremors. *Neurology* 33, 1380–2.

Klein C, Gehsking E, Vieregge D (1998) Voluntary palatal tremor in two siblings. *Mov Disord* 13: 545–8.

Koller WC (1983) Nadolol in essential tremor. *Neurology* 33: 1076–7.

— (1986) Doseresponse relationship of propranolol in the treatment of essential tremor. *Arch Neurol* 43: 42–3.

— (1995) Treatment of tremor disorders. In: Kurlan R (ed) *Treatment of Movement Disorders.* Philadelphia: JB Lippincott, pp. 407–37.

— Rubino FA (1985) Combined resting–postural tremor. *Arch Neurol* 42: 683–4.

— Graner D, Mlcoch A (1985) Essential voice tremor: treatment with propranolol. *Neurology* 35: 106–8.

— Lang A, Veteroberfield B, et al. (1989) Psychogenic tremors. *Neurology* 39: 1094–9.

Burenbark K, Gray C, et al. (1992) Classification of essential tremor. *Clin Neuropharmacol* 15: 81–7.

— — Miner K (1994) The relationship of essential tremor to other movement disorders. A report of 678 patients. *Ann Neurol* 35: 717–23.

Kramer U, Nevo Y, Harel S (1994) Jittery babies: A short term follow-up. *Brain Dev* 16: 112–4.

Lapresle J (1979) Rhythmic palatal myoclonus and the dentato-olivary pathway. *J Neurol* 220: 223–30.

Larsson T, Sjogren T (1960) Essential tremor: a clinical and genetic population study. *Acta Psychiatr Neurol Scand* 36 (suppl 144): 1176.

Laurance BM, Matthews WB, Diggle JH (1968) Hereditary quivering of the chin. *Arch Dis Child* 43: 249–51.

Levene MI, Bennett MJ, Punt J (1988) *Fetal and Neonatal Neurology and Neurosurgery.* London: Churchill Livingstone.

Lombroso CT, Fejerman N (1977) Benign myoclonus of early infancy. *Ann Neurol* 1, 138–48.

Louis DE, Ottman R, Hauser A (1998) How common is the most common adult movement disorder? Estimates of the prevalence of essential tremor throughout the world. *Mov Disord* 13: 5–10.

Macleod MD, Munro JF, Ledingham JG, Farquhar JW (1983) Management of the extrapyramidal manifestations of phenylketonuria with L-dopa. *Arch Dis Child* 58: 457–66.

Marsden CD, Obeso JA, Rothwell JC (1983) Benign essential tremor is not a single entity. In: Yahr MD (ed) *Current Concepts in Parkinson's Disease.* Amsterdam: Excerpta Medica, pp. 31–46.

Marshall J (1959) Physiological tremor in children. *J Neurol Neurosurg Psychiatry* 22: 33–5.

Mazer B, Figueroa-Rosario W, Bender B (1990) The effect of albuterol on fine-motor performance in children with chronic asthma. *J Allergy Clin Immunol* 86: 243–8.

McDowell FH (1989) The use of glutethimide for treatment of essential tremor. *Mov Disord* 4, 75–80.

McLeod NA, White LE (1986) Trazodone in essential tremor. *JAMA* 256: 2675–6.

Mussell HG, Dure LS, Percy AK, Grabb PS (1997) Bobble-head doll syndrome: Report a case and review of the literature. *Mov Disord* 12: 810–4.

Narabayashi H (1986) Tremor: its generating mechanism and treatment. In: *Handbook of Clinical Neurology, Vol. 5, no 49. Extrapyramidal Disorders.* Vinken PJ, Bruyn GW, Klawans HL (eds) Amsterdam: Elsevier, pp. 597–608.

Nathanson M (1956) Palatal myoclonus. Further clinical and pathological observations. *Arch Neurol Psychiatry* 75: 285–96.

Nellhaus G (1967) The bobblehead doll syndrome: A "tic" with a neuropathologic basis. *Pediatrics* 40: 250–3.

Noatchar S, Ebner A, Witte OW, Seitz RJ (1995) Palatal tremor of cortical origin presenting as epilepsia partialis continua. *Epilepsia* 36: 207–9.

Norton EWD, Cogan DG (1954) Spasmus nutans: A clinical study of twenty cases followed two years or more since onset. *Arch Ophthalmol* 52: 442–6.

Pape SM, Gershanik OS (1988) Orthostatic tremor: An essential tremor variant. *Mov Disord* 3: 97–108.

Parizec J, Nemeckova J, Sercl M (1989) Bobble-head doll syndrome associated with III ventricular cyst. *Child's Nerv Syst* 5: 241–5.

Parker S, Zuckerman B, Bauchner H, et al. (1990) Jitteriness in full-term neonates: Prevalence and correlates. *Pediatrics* 85: 17–23.

Paulson GW (1976) Benign essential tremor in childhood. *Clin Ped* 15: 67–70.

Pollack IF, Schor NF, Martinez J, Towbin R (1995) Bobble-head doll syndrome and drop attacks in a child with a cystic choroid plexus papilloma of the third ventricle. *J Neurosurg* 83: 729–32.

Quaglieri RF, Chun RWM, Cleeland C (1977) Movement disorder as a complication of acute hemiplegia of childhood. *Am J Dis Child* 131: 1009–10.

Rajput AH, Offord KP, Beard CM, Kurland LT (1984) Essential tremor in Rochester, Minnesota: A 45-year study. *J Neurol Neurosurg Psychiatry* 47: 466–70.

Rajput AH, Rozdilsky B, Ang L, Rajput A (1991) Clinicopathological observations in essential tremor. Report of 6 cases. *Neurology* 41: 1422–4.

Rapoport A, Lampel Y, Sarova I (1991) Clinical and epidemiological features of essential tremor of the jaw. *Mov Disord* 6: 276–9.

Rautakorpi I, Takala J, Martila RJ, et al. (1982) Essential tremor in a Finnish population. *Acta Neurol Scand* 66: 58–67.

Ravits J, Hallett M, Baker M, Wilkins D (1985) Primary writing tremor and myoclonic writer's cramp. *Neurology* 35: 1387–91.

Rondot P, Bathien N, Ziegler M (1988) *Les Mouvements Anormaux.* Paris: Masson.

Rothwell JC, Traub MM, Marsden CD (1979) Primary writing tremor. *J Neurol Neurosurg Psychiatry* 42, 1106–14.

Rouberge A, Beauvais P, Richardet JM (1985) Syndrome de la poupée à tête ballotante. *Arch Fr Pediatr* 42: 377–8.

Russman BJ, Tucker SH, Shut G (1975) Slow tumor and macroencephaly: Expanded version of the bobblehead doll syndrome. *J Pediatr* 87: 63–6.

Said G, Bathien N, Cesaro P (1982) Peripheral neuropathies and tremor. *Neurology* 32: 480–5.

Sakai T, Shiraishi S, Murakami S (1981) Palatal myoclonus responding to carbamazepine. *Ann Neurol* 9: 199–200.

Salisachs P (1976) Charcot–Marie–Tooth disease associated with "essential tremor": Report of 7 cases and a review of the literature. *J Neurol Sci* 28: 17–40.

Scott BL, Evans RW, Jankovic J (1996) Treatment of palatal myoclonus with sumatriptan. *Mov Disord* 11: 748–51.

Shuper A, Zalzberg J, Weitz R, Mimouni M (1991) Jitteriness beyond the neonatal period: A benign pattern of movement in infancy. *J Child Neurol* 6: 243–5.

Singer C, Sanchez-Ramos J, Weiner WJ (1994) Gait abnormality in essential tremor. *Mov Disord* 9: 193–6.

Soland VL, Bhatia KP, Sheean GL, Marsden CD (1996) Hereditary geniospasm: Two new families. *Mov Disord* 11: 744–6.

Spiro AJ (1970) Minipolymyoclonus. A neglected sign in childhood spinal muscular atrophy. *Neurology* 20: 1124–6.

Tashimira K, Matsumoto A, Hamada T, Moriwaka F (1987) The aetiology of mirror writing: A new hypothesis. *J Neurol Neurosurg Psychiatry* 50: 1572–8.

Tatum WO, Sperling MR, Jacobstein JG (1991) Epileptic palatal myoclonus. *Neurology* 41: 1305–6.

Thomas PK (1975) Clinical features and differential diagnosis. In: Dick PJ, Thomas PK, Lamber EH (eds) *Peripheral Neuropathy.* Philadelphia: WB Saunders, pp. 495–512.

Vanasse M, Bedard P, Andermann F (1976) Shuddering attacks in children: An early clinical manifestation of essential tremor. *Neurology* 26: 1027–30.

Volpe JJ (1995) Neonatal seizures. In: *Neurology of the Newborn. 3rd edn.* Philadelphia: WB Saunders, pp. 172–207.

Wadlington WB (1958) Familial trembling of the chin. *J Pediatr* 53: 316–21.

Willi JM, Glenny LD, Manson AH (1985) Bobble-head doll syndrome: Review of the pathophysiology and CSF dynamics. *Pediatr Neurol* 1: 361–6.

Willis AJ, Jenkins IH, Thompson PD, et al. (1994) Red nuclear and cerebellar but not olivary activation associated with essential tremor: Evidence for overactivity of cerebellar connections. *Ann Neurol* 36: 636–42.

Winkler GF, Young RR (1974) Efficacy of chronic propranolol therapy in action tremors of the familial, senile or essential varieties. *N Engl J Med* 290: 984–8.

Yamanouchi H, Kasai H, Sakuragawa N, Kurokawa T (1991) Palatal myoclonus in Krabbe disease. *Brain Dev* 13: 355–8.

Yokota T, Hirashima F, Sto Y, et al. (1990) Idiopathic palatal myoclonus. *Acta Neurol Scand* 81: 239–42.

Young RR (1986) Essential–familial tremor. In: Vinken PJ, Bruyn GW, Klawans HL (eds) *Handbook of Clinical Neurology, Vol. 5, no 49. Extrapyramidal Disorders.* Amsterdam: Elsevier, pp. 565–82.

4

DISORDERS WITH CHOREA OR BALLISMUS AS PREDOMINANT CLINICAL FEATURES

INTRODUCTION AND CLASSIFICATION

Chorea is a relatively infrequent movement disorder in children. Its semiology has been discussed in Chapter 1. Various aetiological classifications of chorea exist (see Goetz et al. 1981); Table 4.1 shows the classification used here. Up to 150 causes of chorea have been described (Padberg and Bruyn 1986).

In a personal series (EF-A), as in the literature (Klawans and Brandaburg 1993), there was a predominance of females (1.5:1). The mean age of onset in 18 cases was 5.36 years and did not differ with sex. The main aetiology was rheumatic chorea (10 patients) Other causes included: benign familial chorea, trauma, vascular disease (four cases), glutaric aciduria, and 'delayed onset' dyskinesia in patients with cerebral palsy. No cause was found for three patients (Fernández-Alvarez 1996). Interestingly, despite the name, all our cases of Huntington chorea showed rigid–hypokinetic syndrome with no chorea.

This chapter will also briefly refer to ballismus and the symptomatic treatment of chorea and ballismus. Huntington chorea has been discussed in Chapter 2.

RHEUMATIC CHOREA (SYDENHAM CHOREA)

Thomas Sydenham masterly described this disease in a book published in 1686 (three years before his death). This was the first movement disorder reported in the scientific medical literature. Sydenham chorea has long been known as a manifestation of rheumatic fever, of which it is a major feature, although infection with streptococcus A is sometimes difficult to demonstrate. The maximum incidence is between 7 and 12 years (Nausieda et al. 1980, Cardoso et al. 1997). There is a 2:1 female predominance but only after age 10 years, which suggests an influence of sex steroids (Bédard et al. 1979). A family history of chorea is found in 13–26% of cases (Aron et al. 1965, Nausieda et al. 1980) suggesting a genetic predisposition. After a marked decrease in incidence of rheumatic chorea in industrialized countries (Nausieda et al. 1980) even greater than that of rheumatic fever in general, recrudescence of chorea (and of rheumatic fever) is being observed in the USA, UK and probably other developed countries (Markowitz 1985, Kavey and Kaplan 1989).

TABLE 4.1
Classification of choreas

Primary genetic
Benign hereditary chorea
Familial inverted choreoatethosis
Huntington chorea

Secondary
Infectious
    Borrelia infection
    Echovirus infection (Peters et al. 1979)
    Endocarditis
    Herpes simplex encephalitis (Gascon et al. 1993)
    HIV infection
    Infectious mononucleosis
    Rheumatic fever
Metabolic
    Biopterin-dependent hyperphenylalanin-aemia (type VI) (Al Aqeel et al. 1991)
    Canavan spongy degeneration
    Ceroid-lipofuscinosis (Dal Canto et al. 1974)
    Creatine deficiency (guanidinoacetate methyltransferase deficiency)
    Galactosaemia
    Gangliosidosis
    Glutaric aciduria
    Lesch–Nyhan disease
    Phenylketonuria
    Wilson disease
Systemic diseases
    Behçet disease (Bussone et al. 1982)
    Dentatorubro-pallidoluysian atrophy (Chapter 6)
    Friedreich ataxia (Hanna et al. 1998)
    Lupus erythematosus
    Machado–Joseph disease (Chapter 6)
    Pontocerebellar hypoplasia type 2 (Chapter 6)
Vascular
    Cyanotic heart disease (Edwards et al. 1975)
    Moyamoya disease (Kazuyoshi et al. 1990, Takanashi et al. 1993)
    Polycythaemia vera
    Transient cerebral ischaemia
Intoxication
    Carbon monoxide
    Methyl alcohol
    Manganese
    Toluene
Others
    Anticardiolipin syndrome
    Ataxia-telangiectasia
    Cardiac surgery with pulmonary bypass and deep hypothermia
    Cardiopathy
    Head trauma
    Holoprosencephaly (Louis et al. 1995)
    Hyper/hypoglycaemia
    Hyper/hyponatraemia
    Hyperparathyroidism
    Hypocalcaemia
    Hypomagnesaemia
    Idiopathic hypoparathyroidism (MacKinney 1962)
    Infantile bilateral striatal necrosis (Chapter 5)
    Intracranial haematoma (Adler and Winston 1984, Bae et al. 1980)
    Lupus anticoagulant
    Mastocytosis (Iriarte et al. 1988)
    Nocturnal seizure
    Serpial or crenae spilloptelous (Fowler et al. 1992)
    Strangulation (Hori et al. 1991).
    Thiamine deficiency
    Thyrotoxicosis (Pozzan et al. 1992).
Iatrogenic
    Oestrogen, oral contraceptives
    Levodopa and dopa agonists
    Hydantoin
    Pemoline
    Lithium
    Methylphenidate

CLINICAL FEATURES

The onset of Sydenham chorea is generally progressive with behaviour disturbances (irritability, change of mood), clumsiness and difficulties in writing. Affected children drop objects and appear restless. They appear to 'make faces' and other gestures that frequently provoke punishment. After days or weeks, choreic movements become evident. Abnormal movements are usually generalized and may include oculogyric episodes but not infrequently are asymmetrical and may be unilateral in up to 20% of cases (Nausieda et al. 1980). Less commonly, the onset is acute. In rare cases it is marked by generalized hypotonia with difficulties in initiating voluntary movements giving the appearance of a paralysis, sometimes unilateral, while abnormal movements are rare and subtle or may be absent altogether, the so-called 'chorea mollis'. Dysarthria is present in 15–40% of cases (Nausieda et al. 1980, Cardoso et al. 1997), and chewing and swallowing may be affected in severe cases. Other rare manifestations include convulsions (Chien et al. 1978), cerebellar and pyramidal signs and papilloedema (Chun et al. 1961). Carditis is present in about 75% of cases (Cardoso et al. 1997).

The natural course extends over weeks to months with alternation of improvement and deterioration (Aron et al. 1965). Later, relapses occur in 10–20% of cases (Nausieda et al. 1980) but can be difficult to differentiate from exacerbations (Berrios et al. 1985). The outcome is usually good, although emotional disturbances (Freeman et al. 1965) or minimal neurological symptoms, e.g. clumsiness, may persist for several months (Bird et al. 1976).

Girls with a history of rheumatic chorea have a higher risk of recurrent chorea during pregnancy (chorea gravidarum) or following the use of contraceptives, suggesting an increased central dopaminergic sensitivity (Nausieda et al. 1983)

LABORATORY EXAMINATIONS

Biological signs indicative of streptococcus A infection when present support the diagnosis, but a quarter of patients have a negative serology for streptococcus A (Taranta and Stollerman 1956) and 90% have negative pharyngeal swabs (Goldenberg et al. 1992), This is because the long interval between the streptococcal infection and the neurological disease allows a return to normal of the tests (Diament 1972).

The EEG frequently shows nonspecific abnormalities (Chien et al. 1978). Even though reversible abnormal findings such as hypodense areas on CT scan or enlargement and increased T_2 signal in the caudate nucleus by MRI (uni- or bilateral) have been reported (Kienzle et al. 1991, Traill et al. 1995), in rheumatic chorea neuroimaging is generally not contributory to diagnosis (Ganji et al. 1988), although statistical analysis of rheumatic chorea cases versus normal controls shows increased sizes of the caudate, putamen and globus pallidus (Giedd et al. 1995). PET scanning has shown reversible glucose hypermetabolism in the striatum (Goldman et al. 1993).

DIAGNOSIS

The diagnosis of Sydenham chorea is essentially based on clinical history and identification of the choreic movements. A past history of streptococcal infections is frequent. The presence of other rheumatic manifestations such as heart disease and laboratory evidence supports the diagnosis.

Behavioural disturbances can suggest, erroneously, a primary psychogenic problem. Tics can be mistaken for chorea. Unilateral cases should be differentiated from acquired hemiplegia. Chorea mollis may rarely suggest quadriparesis, but examination shows that the problem is with initiation of movement rather than a true paralysis. Symptomatic and other choreas should be excluded. They will be described below.

PATHOLOGY

A few pathological studies have demonstrated nonspecific, diffuse lesions of neurons and cerebral vessels (Ichikawa et al. 1980) which, unexpectedly, do not necessarily predominate in the striatum (Oppenheimer and Esiri 1992). Antibodies in the serum of children with rheumatoid fever may react against cytoplasmic antigens in the caudate and subthalamic nuclei, supporting the hypothesis of an immunological mechanism (Husby et al. 1976, Swedo et al. 1994).

PATHOGENESIS

Antineural antibodies against caudate and subthalamic nuclei have been found in patients with rheumatic chorea (Husby et al. 1976). These antineural antibodies appear to arise in response to group A β-haemolytic streptococcal infection. A 45 kd component of brain seems to be a target of antineuronal antibodies detected in patients with rheumatic chorea (Frucht et al. 1997). This abnormal immune response to the pathogen seems to be genetically determined because there is a familial predisposition to the development of rheumatic fever following streptococcal infections (Nausieda et al. 1980). Moreover, because of its preponderance in females, female gender must play some role in the development of the chorea. Some tics and other neuropsychiatric disorders may have the same immune mechanism (Swedo et al. 1994). This syndrome has been termed PANDAS (paediatric autoimmune neuropsychiatric disorders associated with streptococcal infection) (see Chapter 9).

LUPIC CHOREA

Chorea is a rare neurological complication of systemic lupus erythematosus (SLE). It occurs mainly in girls (female to male ratio 8:1), and half of the SLE patients with chorea are below 16 years old (Herd et al. 1978). Chorea may be the initial manifestation and may remain an isolated symptom for years (Groothuis et al. 1977, Bruyn and Padberg 1984, Arisaka et al. 1984, Pincemaille et al. 1987).

The clinical features of lupic chorea are indistinguishable from those of rheumatic chorea and it can also be generalized or unilateral (Lusins and Szilagyi 1975). Chorea may last from a few days to several weeks and frequently recurs. The diagnosis is difficult when chorea is the only manifestation of SLE (Arisaka et al. 1984). A later age of onset than in rheumatic chorea, and an elevated sedimentation rate may suggest the diagnosis, but they are not specific. When chorea supervenes in a known case of SLE it should be distinguished from other complications such as drug toxicity. The outcome of SLE with neurological complications tends to be severe. A mortality rate as high as 12% was reported by Yancey et al. (1981).

LABORATORY EXAMINATIONS
Biological abnormalities include anaemia, leukopenia, lymphopenia, thrombocytopenia, and increased sedimentation rate. In the CSF, increased cell count and protein are frequent. Antinuclear antibodies are always present, but may be found in other autoimmune disorders, such as rheumatoid arthritis. Bicatenary antiDNA antibodies seem to be limited to SLE. Antiphospholipid antibodies are often present (Okseter and Sirnes 1988, Seaman et al. 1995). Renal biopsy may be a useful diagnostic tool. CT and MR scans may be abnormal with atrophy, infarcts or haemorrhages (Bilaniuk et al. 1977, Aisen et al. 1985). The results of PET are controversial (Guttman et al. 1987, Hosokawa et al. 1987).

PATHOPHYSIOLOGY
The mechanisms of lupic chorea are uncertain. Vascular lesions have been implicated but a direct action of antineuronal antibodies now seems more probable (Atkins et al. 1972, Pincemaille et al. 1987).

TREATMENT
The treatment de SLE is beyond the scope of this book. For some authors the treatment of lupic chorea is not different from that of SLE in general (Herd et al. 1978). Others add specific treatment of chorea (Heilman et al. 1971).

CHOREA IN THE ANTIPHOSPHOLIPID SYNDROME
Chorea may be a feature of the antiphospholipid syndrome: recurring episodes of arterial or venous thrombosis, thrombocytopenia and increased levels of antiphospholipid antibodies (lupus anticoagulant, false positive VDRL, and/or anticardiolipin antibodies) are features of this autoimmune disorder that differs from SLE by the absence of the characteristic lesions and biological features of SLE. Although observed predominantly in adults (Bouchez et al. 1985, Okseter and Sirnes 1988, Schiff and Ortega 1992, Hughes 1993), an acute choreic syndrome has been also reported in children (Vilches et al. 1992, Broere et al. 1993, Seaman et al. 1995).

GENETICALLY DETERMINED CHOREAS
In addition to Huntington chorea whose hereditary character has long been known, new forms of genetically determined choreas have been described (Table 4.2).

BENIGN HEREDITARY CHOREA
Haerer et al. (1967) and Pincus and Chutorian (1967), independently described a form

TABLE 4.2
Genetically determined choreas

Huntington disease – AD
Benign familial chorea – AD or AR
Dentatorubro-pallidoluysian atrophy – AD (see Chapter 6)
Familial inverted choreoathetosis – AD
Neuroacanthocytosis – AD or AR
Pontocerebellar hypoplasia type 2 – AR

AD = autosomal dominant; AR = autosomal recessive.

of benign chorea inherited as an autosomal dominant character. Autosomal recessive (Nutting et al. 1969; family C of Chun et al. 1973; Damasio et al. 1977) and X-linked inheritance (Landrieu et al. 1984) have also been reported. The existence of this disease is questioned. A review of reported cases (Schrag et al 2000) has shown that features unusual for chorea were present in a majority of the families, so that in several of them the diagnosis had to be changed at follow-up to that of myoclonic dystonia, Huntington disease, torsion dystonia or atypical ataxia–telangiectasia.

The disorder can become apparent at any age in childhood, commonly around 1 year but sometimes in late childhood or early adolescence (Chun et al. 1973, Harper 1978, Schady and Meara 1988, Wheeler et al. 1993). In early cases, infants are referred for developmental delay. Walking generally begins late (Sadjadpour and Amato 1973, Robinson and Thornett 1985) (18 months to 3 years in the cases of Deonna and Voumard 1979). Gait is awkward with frequent falls. Later, 'unrest' and writing difficulties are the main complaints.

Choreic movements involve any part of the body, mainly the trunk, neck and proximal limbs. Their frequency and intensity vary considerably even within the same family (Haerer et al. 1967); they increase with stress and excitation and disappear during sleep.

The disorder is neither paroxysmal nor progressive. It is not incapacitating – a member of the family reported by Burns et al. (1976) was an aviation pilot – and can regress spontaneously – the father of the patients described by Deonna and Voumard (1979) improved spontaneously at 21 years of age to the point that at 35 years he showed only mild and intermittent sudden hand movements. Intelligence is usually not impaired, although in a few families low–average IQ scores were noted (Haerer et al. 1967, Chun et al. 1973, Sadjadpour and Amato 1973).

Fisher et al. (1979) described as 'inverted chorea' a type in which chorea began in the first months of life and predominated in the lower limbs. Pyramidal tract signs were also present and the disorder was slowly progressive. It was transmitted as an autosomal dominant trait. Propranolol appeared to be effective. Serendipitously, Robinson and Thornett (1985) found a case responsive to steroids.

Diagnostic studies

Neurophysiological (Stapert et al. 1985) and neuroimaging studies (Rice and Terrence 1979) including PET (Kuwert et al. 1990) are normal.

Differential diagnosis

Some investigators (Quinn et al 1988) think that most cases of BHC share many features with essential myoclonus and myoclonic dystonia and may be different expressions of the same disease. As previously discussed, several cases reported as BHC have been later diagnosed as idiopathic torsion dystonia, myoclonic dystonia or Huntington disease, so testing to exclude these diseases may be indicated.

NEUROACANTHOCYTOSIS

The term neuroacanthocytosis applies to a multisystem disease, recessively inherited, due to a mutant gene located at 3q21 (Rubio et al. 1997). Usually, the disease has its onset in adulthood but cases with onset before age 18 years are on record (Bird et al. 1978, Hardie et al. 1991). Clinical features usually include chorea, hence the original terms of 'familial amyotrophic chorea with acanthocytosis' and 'choreo-acanthocytosis' (Ohnishi et al. 1981, Sakai et al. 1981). However, the terms 'neuroacanthocytosis' (Yamamoto et al. 1982) or Levine–Critchley syndrome (Sakai et al. 1985) have prevailed as chorea is not always present. Other movement disorders are often associated with chorea, e.g. rigid–akinetic syndrome, dystonia or tics. Epileptic seizures, dementia, psychiatric syndromes, lip and tongue mutilation, areflexia and neurogenic amyotrophy are variably associated. A related syndrome features tics, parkinsonism, anterior horn cell disease and elevated creatine kinase with slow progression. Spitz et al. (1985) considered this as a distinct syndrome. In one of these patients the onset was at 13 years of age with weakness of the lower limbs.

Laboratory examinations

Acanthocytosis (>3%) is necessary for the diagnosis. Creatine kinase in serum is elevated (Hardie et al. 1991). Neurophysiological studies frequently show an axonal neuropathy. Neuroimaging may show cerebral atrophy (Serra et al. 1987) and an abnormal signal in the caudate nucleus (Hardie et al. 1991).

Differential diagnosis

Acanthocytes are also present in Bassen–Kornzweig disease, where there is absence of beta-lipoproteins, in McLeod syndrome (benign X-linked myopathy) and in Hallervorden–Spatz syndrome (see Chapter 6). These entities are clearly different clinically from neuroacanthocytosis.

Pathology

The pathology resembles that of Huntington disease with marked neuronal loss and gliosis in the caudate, putamen and pallidum. In some cases, lesions are present in the thalamus and substantia nigra, which may explain the rigid–akinetic syndrome, and in the anterior horn of the spinal cord. Rinne et al. (1994) have suggested that preservation of the subthalamic nuclei, cerebral cortex, pons and cerebellum can help differentiate the two diseases. Nerve biopsy may show a chronic axonal neuropathy (Hardie et al. 1991).

OTHER CHOREAS

Focal lesions of the basal ganglia rarely cause chorea. This was the case in only 8% of patients in the review of Bhatia and Marsden (1994). With unilateral lesions, chorea is almost always contralateral, affecting an arm and leg.

Vascular lesions are not an exceptional cause. *Moyamoya* disease (Suzuki and Takaku 1969) may feature movement disorders such as tremor, ballismus or chorea in up to 21% of cases (Kurokawa et al. 1984). The lesion may be suggested by MRI and sometimes by CT scanning and is confirmed by angiography. It rarely results in episodes of acute hemichorea (Watanabe et al. 1990, Pavlakis et al. 1991, Garaizar et al. 1994). In a personal case (EF-A), hemichorea occurred at the age of 12 years during a second episode of the disease.

The association of moyamoya and Down syndrome has been reported (Schrager et al. 1977, Fukushima et al. 1986), presenting with chorea in one case (Takanashi et al. 1993).

Generalized chorea, mainly involving the limbs, facial musculature and tongue, occurs as a complication of *cardiac surgery* in about 1% of children with pulmonary bypass and deep hypothermia (Brunberg et al. 1974, Robinson et al. 1988, Ferry 1990, De Leon et al. 1990, Curless et al. 1994). Associated neurological manifestations include orofacial dyskinesia, hypotonia, affective changes and pseudobulbar signs (CHAP syndrome: Wical and Tomasi 1990). Symptoms appear between two days and two weeks post-operatively. About 50% of cases have a complete regression of the abnormal movements one to four weeks after onset (Gerpelli et al. 1998) but others can have a severe persistent dysphagia and/or dysarthria. In some patients the neurological dysfunction is transient (Brunberg et al. 1974) but a majority experience persistent difficulties. The response to therapy is usually poor, although Blunt et al. (1994) reported a good response in siblings.

The cause of involvement of the basal ganglia is unclear. MRI shows no lesions. Curless et al. (1994) suggested that chorea results from cerebral vasoconstriction caused by hypocapnia.

Recently two patients harbouring the Friedreich ataxia gene mutation exhibited generalized chorea, starting at 10 and 19 years of age, in the absence of cerebellar signs (Hanna et al. 1998).

Perlman and Volpe (1989) have described, in preterm infants with severe broncho-pulmonary dysplasia, a syndrome of abnormal movements of the extremities, limbs and neck that they regarded as choreiform. All infants had feeding difficulties due to abnormal tongue motions. Moreover, these infants presented an abnormal motor activity similar to akathisia. The onset was around the third month, and symptoms disappeared between 15

and 30 months or remained stationary. Treatment with clonazepan improved the disturbance in three patients. The authors attributed the syndrome to chronic hypoxaemia but
all infants were also receiving digoxin, antidiuretics and theophylline aerosols which may
have contributed to the disorder. A similar case but without abnormal tongue movements
has been reported (Hadders-Algra et al. 1994). The authors suggested for this disorder
the term 'infantile chorea'.

Patients with psychomotor developmental arrest starting in infancy, epilepsy, and
later hemiballistic–dystonic movements due to *creatine/phosphocreatine (guanidinoacetate
methyltransferase) deficiency* in muscle and brain has been reported (Stockler et al. 1994,
Schulze et al. 1997). In a personal case (EF-A) epilepsy started at 7 years of age and a
severe ballistic state at 13 years. MR spectroscopy reveals a strong depletion of creatine
in brain and cerebellum. MRI showed pallidal hypointensities in T_1-weighted images and
hyperintensity in T_2-weighted images (Stockler et al. 1994) or myelination delay of
white matter (at age 3 years, Schulze et al. 1997). Guanidinoacetic acid, the immediate
precursor of creatine, is elevated in urine. Oral administration of creatine monohydrate
resulted in a significant improvement of abnormal movements (Stockler et al. 1996,
Schulze et al. 1997), and of both behaviour and epilepsy in a case without abnormal
movements (Ganesan et al. 1997).

Chorea has also been reported in other situations (see Table 4.1)

BALLISMUS

Ballismus is usually considered as an extreme form of chorea. It is rare in infancy and
childhood. At this age, some cases of rheumatic chorea with ballismus have been reported.
Other cases have an unclear cause (Boukthir et al. 1991). My experience (EF-A) is limited
to two cases: a very severe case of rheumatic chorea in a girl of $2^1/_2$ years; and a syndrome
of diffuse vascular involvement in a patient with hyperlipoproteinaemia. Ballismus can
also be unilateral (hemiballismus) due to vascular lesions, infection (Yoshikawa and Oda
1999), or tumours of the subthalamic body or of the caudate nuclei (Bhatia and Marsden
1994) which is the common lesion in adult cases.

BALLISMUS PRECIPITATED BY FEVER
Febrile illness can be a precipitating factor of severe, long-lasting episodes of intense
chorea or ballismus. Reported cases had pre-existing dyskinetic cerebral palsy often of
undetermined aetiology (Erickson and Chun 1987, Harbord and Kobayashi 1991).
Transaminases, creatine kinase and other enzymes are markedly elevated coinciding with
the maximal ballistic activity, but return to normal range once the movement disorder
improves. EEG does not show paroxysmal activity. The severe prolonged muscular activity
in these patients may be dangerous. Tachycardia, poor peripheral perfusion and dehydra-
tion must be strictly controlled. The marked muscle activity is also responsible for a
further rise in body temperature. These cases have similarities with the status dystonicus
syndrome (Manji et al. 1998) (see Chapter 5).

At the first episode these patients cause diagnostic difficulties. Status epilepticus (in a child with a pre-existing encephalopathy), metabolic disorder (mainly mitochondrial encephalopathy triggered by the increased catabolism produced by the fever), severe rheumatic chorea and encephalitis are the main differential diagnoses. Benzodiazepines, carbamazepine and phenytoin are the most effective drugs.

TREATMENT OF CHOREA AND BALLISMUS

Only a few cases of chorea are due to an aetiologically treatable disease (hyperthyroidism, drugs, infections). In rheumatic chorea, corticosteroids (Green 1978, Robinson and Thornett 1985) and intravenous immunoglobulins have been used. The latter has been recommended by Pranzatelli (1996) early in the course of the disease. Because both chorea and ballismus are considered to be due to increased dopaminergic activity, symptomatic treatment is usually directed at compensating for dopaminergic hyperactivity. Phenothiazines such as chlorpromazine (Pincus and Chutorian 1967, Goetz et al. 1981) or butyrophenones (haloperidol) (Heilman et al. 1971, Loosmore and Wood 1988) are most frequently used. Other drugs such as carbamazepine (Roig et al. 1988, Artigas and Lorente 1989, Roulet and Deonna 1989) and valproate (McLaghlan 1981, Daoud et al. 1990) have also been used. Benefit from reserpine has been reported (Obeso et al. 1978). In chronic medically intractable cases pallidotomy may be useful (Suarez et al. 1997).

REFERENCES

Adler JR, Winston KR (1984) Chorea as a manifestation of epidural hematoma: a case report. *J Neurosurg* 60: 856–7.

Aisen AM, Gabrielsen TO, McCune WJ (1985) MR imaging of systemic lupus erythematosus involving the brain. *AJR Am J Roentgenol* 144: 1027–31.

Al Aqeel A, Ozand P, Gascon GG, et al. (1991) Biopterin dependent hyperphenylalaninemia due to deficiency of 6-pyruvoyl tetrahydropterin synthase. *Neurology* 41: 730–7.

Arisaka O, Obinata K, Sasaki H, et al. (1984) Chorea as an initial manifestation of systemic lupus erythematosus. *Clin Pediatr* 23: 298–300.

Aron AM, Freeman JM, Carter S (1965) The natural history of Sydenham's chorea. *Am J Med* 38: 83–95.

Artigas J, Lorente I (1989) Utilización de la carbamazepina en la coreoatetosis paroxística y en corea de Sydenham. *An Esp Pediatr* 30: 41–4.

Atkins CJ, Kondon JJ, Quismorio FP, Friou GJ (1972) The choroid plexus in systemic lupus erythematosus. *Ann Intern Med* 76: 65–72.

Bae SH, Vates TS, Kenton EJ (1980) Generalized chorea associated with chronic subdural hematoma. *Ann Neurol* 8: 449–50.

Bédard PJ, Langelier P, Dancova J, et al. (1979) Estrogens, progesterone and the extrapyramidal system. In: Poirier LJ, Sourkes TL, Bédard P (eds) *Advances in Neurology, Vol. 24. The Extrapyramidal System and its Disorders.* New York: Raven Press, pp. 411–22.

Berrios X, Quesney F, Morales A, et al. (1985) Are all recurrences of 'pure' Sydenham's chorea true recurrences of acute rheumatic fever? *J Pediatr* 107: 867–72.

Bhatia KP, Marsden CD (1994) The behavioural and motor consequences of focal lesions of the basal ganglia in man. *Brain* 117: 859–76.

Bilaniuk LT, Patel S, Zimmerman RA (1977) Computed tomography of systemic lupus erythematosus. *Radiology* 124: 119–21.

Bird TD, Cederbaum S, Valpey RW, Stahl WL (1978) Familial degeneration of the basal ganglia with acanthocytosis: A clinical, neuropathological and neurochemical study. *Ann Neurol* 3: 253–8.

Bird M, Palkes H, Prensky AL (1976) A follow-up study of Sydenham's chorea. *Neurology* 26: 601–6.

Blunt SB, Brooks DJ, Kennard C (1994) Steroid-responsive chorea in childhood following cardiac transplantation. *Mov Disord* 9: 112–4.

Bouchez B, Arnott G, Hatron PY, et al. (1985) Chorée et lupus erithémateux disseminé avec anticoagulant circulant. *Rev Neurol* 142: 570–6.

Boukthir S, Trabelsi M, Sammoud S, et al. (1991) Paraballisme. Description d'un cas clinique chez l'enfant. *Ann Pédiatr* 38: 358–63.

Broere CAJ, Gabreëls FJM, van der Grond J, et al. (1993) Anti-cardiolipin syndrome and chorea, a non-ischemic connection. A magnetic resonance case study. *Neuropediatrics* 24: 176 (abstract).

Brunberg JA, Doty DB, Reilly EL (1974) Choreoathetosis in infants following cardiac surgery with deep hypothermia and circulatory arrest. *J Pediatrics* 84: 232–5.

Bruyn GW, Padberg G (1984) Chorea and systemic lupus erythematosus: a critical review. *Eur Neurol* 23, 26–33.

Burns J, Neuhauser G, Tomasi L (1976) Benign hereditary nonprogressive chorea of early onset. Clinical genetics of the syndrome and report of a new family. *Neuropädiatrie* 7, 431–8.

Bussone LA, Mantia L, Boiardi A, Giovannini P (1982) Chorea in Behçet syndrome. *J Neurol* 227: 89–92.

Cardoso F, Eduardo C, Silva AP, Mota CCC (1997) Chorea in fifty consecutive patients with rheumatic fever. *Mov Disord* 12: 701–3.

Chien LT, Economides AN, Lemmi H (1978) Sydenham's chorea and seizures. *Arch Neurol* 35: 382–5.

Chun RW, Smith NJ, Forster FM (1961) Papilledema in Sydenham's chorea. *Am J Dis Child* 101: 641–4.

— Daly RF, Mansheim BJ Wolcott GJ (1973) Benign familial chorea with onset in childhood. *JAMA* 225: 1603–7.

Curless RG, Katz DA, Perryman RA, et al. (1994) Choreoathetosis after surgery for congenital heart disease. *J Pediatr* 124: 737–9.

Dal Canto MC, Rapin I, Suzuki K (1974) Neuronal storage disorder with chorea and curvilinear bodies. *Neurology* 24: 1026–32.

Damasio H, Antunes L, Damasio AR (1977) Familial nonprogressive involuntary movements of childhood. *Ann Neurol* 1: 602–3.

Daoud AS, Zaki M, Shakir R, Al-Saleh Q (1990) Effectiveness of sodium valproate in the treatment of Sydenham's chorea. *Neurology* 40: 1140–1.

De Leon S, Ilbawi M, Archilla R, et al. (1990) Choreoathetosis after deep hypothermia without circulatory arrest. *Ann Thorac Surg* 50: 714–9.

Deonna T, Voumard C (1979) Benign hereditary (dominant) chorea of early onset. *Helv Paediatr Acta* 34: 77–83.

Diament AJ (1972) Valor de alguns exames complementares na coréia de Sydenham. *Arq Neuro-psiquiatr* 30: 187–214.

Edwards PD, Prosser R, Wells CEC (1975) Chorea, polycythaemia and cyanotic heart disease. *J Neurol Neurosurg Psychiatry* 38: 729–39.

Erickson GR, Chun RWM (1987) Acquired paroxysmal movement disorders *Pediatr Neurol* 3: 226–9.

Fernández-Alvarez E (1996) Chorea in children. *Acta Neuropediatr* 2: 116–25.

Ferry PC (1990) Neurologic sequelae of open-heart surgery in children. An 'irritating question'. *Am J Dis Child* 144: 369–73.

Fisher M, Sargent M, Drachman D (1979) Familial inverted choreathetosis. *Neurology* 29: 1627–31.

Fowler WE, Kriel RL, Krach LE (1992) Movement disorders after status epilepticus and other brain injuries. *Pediatr Neurol* 8: 281–4.

Freeman J, Aron A, Collard J, et al. (1965) The emotional correlates of Sydenham's chorea. *Pediatrics* 35: 42–9.

Frucht J, Zabriskie J, Trifiletti R (1997) Immunoblot characterization of antineuronal antibodies targets in Sydenham's chorea. *Ann Neurol* 42: 5333 (abstract).

Fukushima Y, Kondo Y, Kuroki Y, et al. (1986) Are Down syndrome patients predisposed to moyamoya disease? *Eur J Pediatr* 144: 516–7.

Ganesan V, Johnson A, Connelly A, et al. (1997) Guanidinoacetate methyltransferase deficiency: New clinical features. *Pediatr Neurol* 17: 155–7.

Ganji S, Duncan C, Frazier E (1988) Sydenham's chorea: Clinical, EEG, CT scan and evoked potential studies. *Clin Electroencephalogr* 19: 114–22.

Garaizar C, Prats JM, Zuazo E, et al. (1994) Chorea of acute onset due to moyamoya disease. *Acta Neuropediatr* 1: 58–63.

Gascon GG, Jarallah A, Okamoto E, et al. (1993) Chorea as a presentation of herpes simplex encephalitis relapse. *Brain Dev* 15: 178–81.

Gerpelli JLD, Azaka E, Riso A, et al. (1998) Choreoathetosis after cardiac surgery with hypothermia and extracorporeal circulation. *Pediatr Neurol* 19: 113–8.

Giedd JN, Rapoport JL, Kruesi MJ, et al. (1995) Sydenham's chorea: Magnetic resonance imaging of the basal ganglia. *Neurology* 45: 2199–202.

Goetz CG, Weiner WJ, Klawans HL (1981) Treatment of choreas. In: Barbeau A (ed) *Disorders of Movement*. Lancaster: MTP Press, pp. 29–41.

Goldenberg J, Ferraz M, Fonseca A, et al. (1992) Sydenham's chorea: clinical and laboratory findings. Analysis of 187 cases. *Rev Paul Med* 110: 152–7.

Goldman S, Amrom D, Szliwowski HB, et al. (1993) Reversible striatal hypermetabolism in a case of Sydenham's chorea. *Mov Disord* 8: 355–8.

Green LN (1978) Corticosteroids in the treatment of Sydenham's chorea. *Arch Neurol* 35, 53.

Groothuis JR, Groothuis DR, Mukhopadhyay D, et al. (1977) Lupus-associated chorea in childhood. *Am J Dis Child* 131: 1131–4.

Guttman M, Lang AE, Garnett ES, et al. (1987) Regional cerebral glucose metabolism in SLE chorea: Further evidence that striatal hypometabolism is not a correlate of chorea. *Mov Disord* 2: 201–10.

Hadders-Algra M, Bos AF, Martijn A, Prechtl HFR (1994) Infantile chorea in an infant with severe bronchopulmonary dysplasia: an EMG study. *Dev Med Child Neurol* 36: 173–82.

Haerer AF, Currier RD, Jackson JF (1967) Hereditary nonprogresive chorea of early onset. *N Engl J Med* 276: 1220–4.

Hanna MG, Davis MB, Sweeney MG, et al. (1998) Generalized chorea in two patients harboring the Friedreich's ataxia gene trinucleotid repeat expansions. *Mov Disord* 13: 339–40.

Harbord MG, Kobayashi JS (1991) Fever producing ballismus in patients with choreoathetosis. *J Child Neurol* 6: 49–52.

Hardie RJ, Pullon HWH, Harding AE, et al. (1991) Neuroacanthocytosis. A clinical, haematological and pathological study of 19 cases. *Brain* 104: 13–49.

Harper PS (1978) Benign hereditary chorea. Clinical and genetic aspects. *Clin Genet* 13: 85–95.

Heilman KM, Kohler WC, Lemaster PC (1971) Haloperidol treatment of chorea associated with systemic lupus erythematosus. *Neurology* 21: 963–5.

Herd JK, Medhi M, Uzendoski DM, Saldivar VA (1978) Chorea associated with systemic lupus erythematosus: Report of two cases and review of the literature. *Pediatrics* 61: 308–15.

Hori A, Hirosi G, Kataoka S, et al. (1991) Delayed postanoxic encephalopathy after strangulation: Serial neuroradiological and neurochemical studies. *Arch Neurol* 48: 871–4.

Hosokawa S, Ichiya Y, Kuwabara Y, et al. (1987) Positron emission tomography in cases of chorea with different underlying diseases. *J Neurol Neurosurg Psychiatry* 50: 1284–7.

Hughes GRV (1993) The antiphospholipid syndrome: ten years on. *Lancet* 342: 341–3.

Husby G, van de Rijn I, Zabriskie JB, et al. (1976) Antibodies reacting with cytoplasm of subthalamic and caudate nuclei neurons in chorea and acute rheumatic fever. *J Exp Med* 144: 1094–110.

Ichikawa K, Kim RC, Givelber H, Collins GH (1980) Chorea gravidarum. Report of a fatal case with neuropathological observations. *Arch Neurol* 37: 429–32.

Iriarte JM, Mateu J, Cruz G, Escudero J (1988) Chorea: A new manifestation of mastocytosis. *J Neurol Neurosurg Psychiatry* 51: 1457–63.

Kavey RE, Kaplan EL (1989) Resurgence of acute rheumatic fever. *Pediatrics* 84: 585–6.

Kazuyoshi W, Tamiko N, Mitsuo M, et al. (1990) Moyamoya disease presenting with chorea. *Pediatr Neurol* 6: 40–2.

Kienzle GD, Breger RK, Chun RWM, et al. (1991) Sydenham chorea: MR manifestations in two cases. *AJNR* 12: 73–6.

Klawans HG, Brandaburg MM (1993) Chorea in childhood. *Pediatr Ann* 22: 43–50.

Kurokawa T, Chen YJ, Tomita S, et al. (1984) Cerebral occlusive disease with and without the moyamoya vascular network in children. *Neuropediatrics* 16, 29–32.

Kuwert T, Lange HW, Langen KJ, et al. (1990) Normal striatal glucose consumption in two patients with benign hereditary chorea as measured by positron emission tomography. *J Neurol* 237: 80–4.

Landrieu P, Benchet MI, Tardieu M, Lapresle J (1984) Chorée familiale, nonprogressive, liée au sexe. *Rev Neurol* 140: 432–3.

Loosmore SJ, Wood K (1988) Benign hereditary chorea: a case report. *Br J Psychiatry* 152: 131–4.

Louis DE, Lynch T, Cargan AL, Fahn S (1995) Generalized chorea in an infant with semilobar holoprosencephaly. *Pediatr Neurol* 13: 355–7.

Lusins JO, Szilagyi PA (1975) Clinical features of chorea associated with systemic lupus erythematosus. *Am J Med* 58: 857–61.

MacKinney AS (1962) Idiopathic hypoparathyroidism presenting as chorea. *Neurology* 12: 485–91.

McLaghlan KS (1981) Valproic acid in Sydenham's chorea. *BMJ* 283, 274–5.

Manji II, Howard RS, Miller DH, et al. (1998) Status dystonicus: The syndrome and its management. *Brain* 141: 243–52.

Markowitz M (1985) The decline of rheumatic fever: Role of medical intervention. *J Pediatr* 106: 545–50.

Nausieda PA, Grossman BJ, Koller WC, et al. (1980) Sydenham chorea: An update. *Neurology* 30: 331–4.

— Bieliauskas LA, Bacon LD, et al. (1983) Chronic dopaminergic sensitivity after Sydenham's chorea. *Neurology* 33: 750–4.

Nutting PA, Cole BR, Schimke RN (1969) Benign, recessively inhereted choreoatethosis of early onset. *J Med Genet* 6: 408–10.

Obeso JA, Marti-Masso JF, Astudillo W, et al. (1978) Treatment of hemiballism with reserpine. *Ann Neurol* 4: 581–3.

Ohnishi A, Sato Y, Nagara H, et al. (1981) Neurogenic muscular atrophy and low density of large amyelinated fibers of sural nerve in neuroacanthocytosis. *J Neurol Neurosurg Psychiatry* 44: 645–8.

Okseter K, Sirnes K (1988) Chorea and lupus anticoagulant: a case report. *Acta Neurol Scand* 78: 206–9.

Oppenheimer DR, Esiri MR (1992) Diseases of the basal ganglia, cerebellum and motor neurons. In: Adams JH, Duchen LW (eds) *Greenfield's Neuropathology.* London: Arnold, pp. 988–1045.

Padberg G, Bruyn GW (1986) Chorea: differential diagnosis. In: Vinken PJ, Bruyn GW, Klawans HL (eds) *Handbook of Clinical Neurology, Vol. 5.* Amsterdam: Elsevier, pp. 549–64.

Pavlakis SG, Scheneider S, Black K, Gould RJ (1991) Steroid responsive chorea in moyamoya disease. *Mov Disord* 6: 347–9.

Perlman JM, Volpe JJ (1989) Movement disorder of premature infants with severe bronchopulmonary dysplasia: A new syndrome. *Pediatrics* 84: 215–8.

Peters ACB, Vielvoye GJ, Versteeg J, et al. (1979) ECHO 25 focal encephalitis and subacute hemichorea. *Neurology* 29: 676–80.

Pincemaille O, Jeannoel P, Pouzol P, et al. (1987) Chorée aigue, lupus érythémateux disseminé et anticorps antiphospholipides. A propos d'une observation. *Pediatrie* 42: 157–60.

Pincus JH, Chutorian A (1967) Familial benign chorea with intention tremor: A clinical entity. *J Pediatr* 70: 724–9.

Pozzan GB, Battistella PA, Rigon F, et al. (1992) Hyperthyroid-induced chorea in an adolescent girl. *Brain Dev* 14: 126–7.

Pranzatelli MR (1996) Antidyskinetic drug therapy for pediatric movement disorders. *J Child Neurol* 11: 355–69.

Quinn NP, Rothwell JC, Thompson PD, Marsden CD (1988) Hereditary myoclonic dystonia, hereditary torsion dystonia, and hereditary essential myoclonus: An area of confusion. *Adv Neurol* 50: 391–401.

Rice E, Terrence C (1979) Computerized tomography in hereditary nonprogressive chorea. *Arch Neurol* 36: 249–50.

Rinne JO, Daniel SE, Scaravilli F, et al. (1994) The neuropathological features of neuroacanthocytosis. *Mov Disord* 9: 297–304.

Robinson RO, Thornett CE (1985) Benign hereditary chorea—response to steroids. *Dev Med Child Neurol* 27: 814–6.

— Samuels M, Pohl KRE (1988) Choreic syndrome after cardiac surgery. *Arch Dis Child* 63: 1466–9.

Roig M, Montserrat L, Gallart A (1988) Carbamazepine: An alternative drug fot the treatment of nonhereditary chorea. *Pediatrics* 82: 492–5.

Roulet E, Deonna T (1989) Successful treatment of hereditary dominant chorea with carbamazepine. *Pediatrics* 83: 1077.

Rubio JP, Danek S, Stone C, et al. (1997) Chorea–acanthocytosis: Linkage to chromosome 9q21. *Am J Hum Genet* 61: 899–908.

Sadjadpour K, Amato RS (1973) Hereditary nonprogressive chorea of early onset – a new entity? *Adv Neurol* 1: 79–91.

Sakai T, Mawatari S, Iwashita H, et al. (1981) Neuroacanthocytosis: Clues to clinical diagnosis.

Arch Neurol 38: 335–8.

Sakai T, Iwashita H, Kakugawa M (1985) Neuroacanthocytosis syndrome and choreoacanthocytosis (Levine–Critchley syndrome). *Neurology* 35: 1679.

Schady W, Meara RJ (1988) Hereditary progressive chorea without dementia. *J Neurol Neurosurg Psychiatry* 51, 295–7.

Schiff DE, Ortega JA (1992) Chorea, cosinophilia, and lupus anticoagulant associated with acute lymphoblastic leukemia. *Pediatr Neurol* 8: 466–8.

Schrag A, Quinn NP, Bhatia KP, Marsden CD (2000) Benign hereditary chorea: Entity or syndrome? *Mov Disord* 15: 280–8.

Schrager GO, Solomon JC, Cohen SJ, Vigman MP (1977) Acute hemiplegia and cortical blindness due to moya moya disease: Report of a case in a child with Down's syndrome. *Pediatrics* 60: 33–7.

Schulze A, Hess T, Wevers R, et al. (1997) Creatine deficiency syndrome caused by guanidino-acetate methyltransferase deficiency: Diagnostic tools for a new inborn error of metabolism. *J Pediatr* 131: 626–31.

Seaman DE, Londino AV, Kinoh CK, et al. (1995) Antiphospholipid antibodies in pediatric systemic lupus erythematosus. *Pediatrics* 96: 1040–5.

Serra S, Xerra A, Scribano E, et al. (1987) Computerized tomography in amyotrophic choreo-acanthocytosis. *Neuroradiology* 29: 480–2.

Spitz MC, Jankovic J, Killian JM (1985) Familial tic disorder, parkinsonism, motor neuron disease, and acanthocytosis: a new syndrome. *Neurology* 35: 366–70.

Stapert JLRH, Busard BLSM, Gabreëls FJM, et al. (1985) Benign (nonparoxysmal) familial chorea of early onset: An electroneurophysiological examination of two families. *Brain Dev* 7: 38–42.

Stockler S, Holzbach U, Hanefeld F, et al. (1994) Creatine deficiency in the brain: A new, treatable inborn error of metabolism. *Pediatr Res* 36: 409–13.

Stockler S, Hanefeld F, Frahm J (1996) Creatine replacement therapy in guanidinoacetate methyl-transferase deficiency: a novel inborn error of metabolism. *Lancet* 348: 789–90.

Suarez JI, Verhagen L, Reich SG, et al. (1997) Pallidotomy for hemiballismus: Efficacy and characteristics of neuronal activity. *Ann Neurol* 42: 807–11.

Suzuki J, Takaku A (1969) Cerebrovascular 'moyamoya' disease. A disease showing abnormal net-like vessels in base of brain. *Arch Neurol* 20: 288–99.

Swedo SE, Leonard HL, Kiessling LS (1994) Speculations on antineuronal antibody-mediated neuropsychiatric disorders of childhood. *Pediatrics* 93: 323–6.

Takanashi J, Sugita K, Honda A, Niimi H (1993) Moyamoya syndrome in a patient with Down syndrome presenting with chorea. *Pediatr Neurol* 9: 396–8.

Taranta A, Stollerman GH (1956) The relationship of Sydenham's chorea and infection with group A streptococci. *Am J Med* 20: 110–75.

Traill Z, Pike M, Byrne J (1995) Sydenham's chorea: a case showing reversible striatal abnormalities on CT and MRI. *Dev Med Child Neurol* 37: 270–3.

Vilches RM, Tamayo JA, Minguez A, Foronda J (1992) Corea y síndrome antifosfolípido primario. *Neurologia* 7: 120 (letter).

Watanabe K, Negoro T, Maehara H, et al. (1990) Moyamoya disease presenting with chorea. *Pediatr Neurol* 6: 40–2.

Wheeler PG, Weaver DD, Dobyns WB (1993) Benign hereditary chorea. *Pediatr Neurol* 9: 337–40.

Wical BS, Tomasi LG (1990) A distinctive neurologic syndrome after induced profound hypothermia. *Pediatr Neurol* 6: 202–5.

Yamamoto T, Hirose G, Shimazaki K, et al. (1982) Movement disorders of familial neuroacantho-cytosis syndrome. *Arch Neurol* 39: 298–301.

Yancey CL, Doughty RA, Athereya BHL (1981) Central nervous system involvement in childhood systemic lupus erythematosus. *Arthritis Rheum* 24: 1389–95.

Yoshikawa H, Oda Y (1999) Hemiballismus associated with influenza A infection. *Brain Dev* 21: 132–4.

5

MOVEMENT DISORDERS WITH DYSTONIA OR ATHETOSIS AS MAIN CLINICAL MANIFESTATION

INTRODUCTION AND CLASSIFICATION

The disorders that feature dystonia and athetosis as their main manifestation continue to raise difficult diagnostic and therapeutic problems. Because of the bizarre symptoms, "Until the 1970's most patients with dystonia were referred to psychiatrists in the belief that these curious motor disorders were an expression of an unhappy mind" (Marsden and Quinn 1990). No precise data are available on the incidence and prevalence of dystonia in children, but in our experience it is the most common movement disorder in this age, after tics (see Fig. 1.5, p. 19).

It is generally accepted that dystonia and hypokinetic–rigid syndrome represent an imbalance between neurotransmitters in opposite directions. Dopa transmission would be increased in dystonia and deficient in parkinsonism, although, paradoxically, features of both syndromes may occur in association as in dystonia–parkinsonism and dopa-responsive dystonia. Moreover, dopa may be helpful in the treatment of some forms of dystonia. Some disorders such as dopa-responsive dystonia may manifest with dystonia when the onset is early in life and with hypokinetic–rigid syndrome later. Both syndromes may also occur in succession in the same patient.

Physiological and semiological aspects of dystonia have been dealt with in Chapter 1.

Various classifications of dystonias have been proposed (Fahn et al. 1987, Fahn 1988) but recent advances in molecular genetics and the recognition of new syndromes have led to a revision of these classifications (see below).

Several mutant genes have been found to be associated with dystonic disorders: the *DYT1* gene on chromosome 9q34 for idiopathic torsion dystonia (ITD); the *DYT2* gene for an autosomal recessive dystonia in the ethnic Gypsy population (unlocalized); the *DYT3* gene for X-linked dystonia–parkinsonism, mapped to X13.1 (Haberhausen et al. 1995); the *DYT4* gene for ITD and whispering dysphonia (Ahmad et al. 1993); the *DYT5* gene for dopa-responsive dystonia due to a deficit in GTP cyclohydrolase I (GCH1) on chromosome 14q; the *DYT6* gene for some cases of ITD linked to chromosome 8 (Almasy et al. 1997); and the *DYT7* gene for adult-onset focal dystonia (torticollis, writer's cramp, blepharospasm), mapped, in a few families, to chromosome 18p (Leube et al. 1996, 1997). Our classification is shown in Tables 5.1 and 5.2.

TABLE 5.1
Classification of dystonias and athetosis according to evolution and topography

Acute	Chronic
Iatrogenic	Generalized
Vascular	Multifocal
Others	Hemidystonia
	Segmental
Transient	Focal
Of the newborn	Blepharospasm
Transient dystonia of infants	Oromandibular dystonia
	Spasmodic dysphonia
Paroxysmal	Spasmodic torticollis
Paroxysmal dyskinesia	Writer's cramp
Due to antiepileptic drugs	Meige syndrome (blepharospasm and
Paroxysmal transient dystonia of infants	oromandibular dystonia)
Benign paroxysmal torticollis of infants	

TABLE 5.2
Classification of dystonias and athetosis according to aetiology

Primary (idiopathic) (when there is not identifiable cause and movement disorder is the only feature)
  Pure (when dystonia is the only abnormal feature)
    Idiopathic torsion dystonia
    Transient idiopathic dystonia of infants
    Paroxysmal idiopathic dystonias (including paroxysmal torticollis)
  Associated (when dystonia is associated to other movement disorder)
    Dopa-responsive dystonia
    Hereditary myoclonic dystonia (autosomal dominant with response to alcohol) (Chapter 8)
    Rapid-onset dystonia–parkinsonism
    Philippine dystonia–parkinsonism
    Juvenile parkinsonism (Chapter 2)
Secondary
  To metabolic disorders
  To heredodegenerative diseases
  To other causes

GENERALIZED IDIOPATHIC (PRIMARY) DYSTONIAS
IDIOPATHIC TORSION DYSTONIA (ITD)

Although cases of this disorder were reported earlier, in 1911 H Oppenheim coined the term 'dystonia' and drew attention to the progressive course and the absence of muscle atrophy, weakness, cerebellar or sensory anomalies. He postulated an organic origin and proposed the names of 'dystonia musculorum deformans' and 'progressiva dysbasia

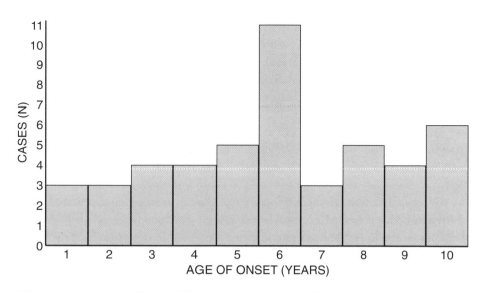

Fig. 5.1. Age at onset in 48 cases of idiopathic torsion dystonia (combined series of Angelini et al. 1989; and personal, EF-A).

lordotica'. However, the general medical belief in a psychogenic origin of the condition persisted until Herz (1944a,b,c) showed its familial basis.

The prevalence of ITD is difficult to assess. About half the patients are not correctly diagnosed (Fletcher et al. 1990, Risch et al. 1995). A prevalence of 1/10,000, with DYT1 frequency between 1/6000 and 1/2000 appears to be a reasonable estimate (Risch et al. 1995). The incidence is five times higher in Ashkenazi Jews than in Caucasians.

The diagnostic criteria for ITD include:
- presence of dystonic postures and/or movements
- normal perinatal and developmental history
- absence of cognitive, pyramidal, cerebellar or sensory anomalies
- exclusion of known cause (e.g. drugs, other known disorders producing dystonia)
- normal results of laboratory and imaging investigations.

Clinical features
Onset is before 15 years in 80% of cases (Marsden and Harrison 1974), and in all of 48 cases in the two series combined in Figure 5.1 (Angelini et al. 1989; and personal, EF-A) it occurred at or before age 10 years. In children the disturbance commonly begins in one limb (arm and leg about equally). ITD linked to chromosome 9q34 usually begins in a limb, whereas, in most non-linked kindreds, onset of dystonia is in the cervical region. Onset with blepharospasm or dysphonia is rare. Inversion of one foot during gait is quite common. Initially, the dystonia appears only for some specific postures

TABLE 5.4
Clinical features in dopa-responsive dystonia*

Onset in early childhood (5.25 ± 2.5 years)
Predominantly postural dystonia with onset in an extremity, usually one lower limb
No torsion of trunk or torticollis
Tremor only in patients older than 10 years, postural in type, with a frequency of
    8–10 Hz
Asymmetry throughout the course (preferential involvement of left side, 2.5 : 1)
Progressive aggravation in awake state
Marked and prolonged effect of L-dopa

*Reproduced by permission from Segawa et al. (1988).

cases (Nygaard et al. 1993a), and cases of unchanging dystonia have been reported in families in which members had typical fluctuating courses (Rondot and Ziegler 1983, Deonna et al. 1986, Nygaard et al. 1991). Sporadic cases without daily variation (Rajput 1973, Willemse et al. 1984), cases with focal dystonia (Deonna and Ferreira 1985, Micheli et al. 1991), with subtle signs sometimes induced only by writing (Steinberger et al. 1998), without progression (Deonna et al. 1997), or needing higher doses of L-dopa for control (Kaiser and Ziegler 1992) may belong to the same disease. Cases with a slower response to L-dopa treatment in which symptoms decreased after several weeks have been reported (Rondot and Ziegler 1983). In one family (Nygaard et al. 1990) various members had DRD and others developed parkinsonism after age 50 years with an excellent and sustained response to L-dopa. In the latter patients, PET showed the typical image seen in DRD (see below) thus suggesting a single disease process with marked clinical heterogeneity depending on age of onset.

Two unrelated patients (previously reported as having 'severely affected DRD' – Hyland et al. 1997) exhibited severe progressive dystonia that improved with combined tetrahydrobiopterin and L-dopa treatment. One had increased plasma levels of phenyl alanine. Both were compound heterozygotes for two different GTP cyclohydrolase mutations (Furukawa et al. 1998).

Laboratory investigations
Routine tests including CSF protein and cells are normal. Levels of homovanillic acid in CSF were low in a majority of studied cases (Gorke and Bartholomew 1990) and became normal on L-dopa therapy (Willemse et al. 1984). All patients studied had much lower CSF levels of tetrahydrobiopterin (a tyrosine hydroxylase cofactor) and of its metabolite neopterin than those with ITD (Lewitt et al. 1986, Fink et al. 1988).

Fluorodopa PET scans are normal (Sawle et al. 1991) in contrast with the reduced fixation of fluorodopa in basal ganglia in patients with childhood or juvenile parkinsonism (Snow et al. 1993; see Chapter 12).

TABLE 5.5

Differential diagnosis of dopa-responsive dystonia (DRD), childhood-onset idiopathic torsion dystonia (ITD) and childhood-onset Parkinson disease (PD)

	DRD	Childhood-onset ITD	Childhood-onset PD
Age at onset	Infancy 12y	Less common <6y	Rarely <8y
Initial signs	Arm or leg dystonia	Foot dystonia, gait disorder	Bradykinesia and rigidity, rest tremor
Foot dystonia	Usually at onset	Onset in 40%, eventually in all	Frequently
Axial dystonia	Rarely	Rarely, onset in 15%	65%
Rest tremor	Late in course	Rarely	May be initial or early sign
Hyperreflexia	Common	No	No
Levodopa	Marked low doses	Rarely mild	Small to moderate doses
Anticholinergic	Marked	May be marked	Yes

Differential diagnosis (Table 5.5)

Diagnostic errors are frequent because knowledge of the disease is still limited and because there are many atypical presentations in which the clinical signs are widely different from those expected from the first reports (Costeff et al. 1987, Steinberger et al. 1998). Many errors could be avoided by the systematic use of the dopa test in all dystonic syndromes.

One of the most common misdiagnoses is that of spastic paraparesis, paraplegia or diplegia because of hyperreflexia, extensor toes, and localization of disturbances in the lower limbs (Boyd and Patterson 1989). The absence of a past history of familial disorder or preterm birth, the presence of mild dystonic/rigid features and of diurnal worsening should suggest the diagnosis. In case of any doubt a therapeutic test is in order. Dystonic–dyskinetic forms of cerebral palsy should be diagnosed only with caution when there is no prenatal or perinatal history of hypoxia, no MRI abnormalities, or where there is any suggestion of fluctuation. Again a dopa test is indicated at the slightest doubt.

The circadian variation of signs may erroneously imply psychogenic motor disturbances. Equinovarus observed in focal cases can be misdiagnosed as an orthopaedic disorder (Steinberger et al. 1998). The differential diagnosis with ITD is easy as an L-dopa test must be systematically performed in such cases, and the same applies to the rare cases of juvenile parkinsonism. The two brothers described in 1971 by Fenichel et al. as having 'hereditary dystonia with muscle abnormalities' were later shown to have DRD (Charles et al. 1995).

Genetics

Cases reported as DRD as well as 'hereditary progressive dystonia with marked diurnal fluctuation' are associated with mutations of the *DYT5* gene (Nygaard et al. 1993b, Tanaka et al. 1995a) at the locus coding for GTP-cyclohydrolase I (GTPCH) gene (*GCH1*) (Ichinose et al. 1994). Usually mutations in GCH1 are dominant, but its penetrance is low (Segawa et al. 1988) and sex-related, more commonly expressed in females. This female preponderance could be explained by a base level of GTP-cyclohydrolase activity lower in females than in males (Ichinoise et al. 1994). Proved carriers of the mutant gene can remain unaffected. For instance, penetrance was 31% in a family reported by Nygaard et al. (1990), but higher penetrance is found if relatives with subtle signs are recognized (Steinberger et al. 1998). Variable levels of mutant mRNA could explain the phenotypic variability among cases with the same mutation (Hirano et al. 1996). Relatives and parents of affected children may present with mild forms of the condition (Steinberger et al. 1998) or with a pure parkinsonian syndrome (Nygaard et al. 1992). In a personal case (EF-A) the father of an affected girl had presented, between the ages of 15 and 40 years, an isolated postural tremor of the hands appearing only at the end of the day.

At least two other metabolic defects have been found to produce the same clinical picture: deficit of tyrosine hydroxylase, a rare, autosomal recessive genetic disorder (Knappskog et al. 1995, Lüdecke et al. 1995, Braütigam et al. 1998, van den Heuvel et al. 1998, Rondot and Wevers 1999); and deficit of L-amino acid decarboxylase, responsible for rare cases also with an autosomal recessive inheritance. In the latter disorder, the syndrome is associated with oculogyric crises (Hyland et al. 1992).

Pathology
In a verified case (Rajput et al. 1994) no abnormalities were found either in the substantia nigra or in the striatum, despite a reduction in the melanin content of the substantia nigra and of the tyrosine hydroxylase protein and dopamine in the striatum.

Pathophysiology
De Jong et al. (1989) studied plasma and urine levels of catecholamine metabolites in three patients after administration of a load of tagged tyrosine and compared these with those in a single control. The results suggested a decreased half-life of brain dopamine due to a storage defect. These data are consistent with a deficit of dopamine due to defective synthesis.

DRD is the consequence of a functional defect in the synthesis of dopamine as a result of a reduced synthesis of tetrahydrobiopterin, a cofactor of tyrosine hydroxylase, as suggested by the excellent and persistent response to L-dopa, the decrease in dopamine metabolites in CSF, the normality or slight decrease of fluorodopa uptake in the striatum as shown by PET and SPECT (Sawle et al. 1991, Snow et al. 1993, Naumann et al. 1997) and neuropathological data (Rajput et al. 1994). Cases of early onset manifest as dystonia, those of late onset as parkinsonism. The metabolism of phenylalanine and other amino acids dependent on tetrahydrobiopterin is not affected enough to produce clinical

disturbances unless the DYT5 mutation inherited from both parents results in a homozygous genotype. In this situation atypical hyperphenylalaninaemia is produced (Niederwieser et al. 1984, Ichinose et al. 1996). As mentioned, compound heterozygotes for
different GTP-cyclohydrolase mutations exhibits an intermediate phenotype with both
DRD and hyperphenylalaninaemia.

Treatment
Administration of small doses (5–30 mg/kg/d) of L-dopa, often combined with an
inhibitor of peripheral decarboxylation, usually produces a rapid response which is
independent of the delay in initiating treatment. A 51-year-old patient who had been
unable to walk for 36 years resumed a normal life after three days of L-dopa (600 mg/d)
(Segawa et al. 1990). Rare cases with slow response to higher doses of L-dopa have been
reported (Kaiser and Ziegler 1992).

The tolerance of treatment is good. The secondary problems that inevitably occur
during L-dopa treatment of parkinsonism such as the 'on–off' phenomenon are never
observed in DSD, and the efficacy of the drug does not decrease even after many years
of therapy. When the dose is excessive, choreic movements can occur but disappear with
reduction of the dose. As treatment is lifelong the lowest effective dose should be used.
When the dose is too low there may be mild stiffness of the limbs or a tremor at the end
of the day. Treatment during pregnancy does not seem to have noxious effect on the fetus
(Cook and Klawans 1985, Ball and Sagar 1995).

Some patients also respond to anticholinergic agents (trihexyphenidyl, benztropine),
carbamazepine or bromocriptine (Nomura et al. 1984), although rarely as completely as
to L-dopa (Nygaard et al. 1991). Tetrahydrobiopterin has been given a trial (Fink et al.
1989) but the results were no better than with L-dopa.

MYOCLONIC DYSTONIA
Clinical features
Myoclonic dystonia is an autosomal dominant disorder with variable expressivity and
high, but incomplete, penetrance (Kyllerman et al. 1990, Fahn and Sjaastad 1991). Age
of onset is before 10 years. Symptoms of myoclonic dystonia include proximal, action-
induced bilateral myoclonic jerks usually involving extremities. Dystonia is often mild,
starting usually in the upper extremities and neck (Quinn and Marsden 1984). Stimulus
sensitivity to sudden noise or tactile stimuli has been described (Kurlan et al. 1988). The
response to alcohol (both dystonia and myoclonus) (Quinn and Marsden 1984) and
sometimes to sodium valproate (for the myoclonus) and trihexyphenidyl (for the dystonia) (Pueschel et al. 1992) is an important diagnostic clue. The disease runs a relatively
benign course.

Differential diagnosis
The association of myoclonus and dystonia may occur in several disorders other than

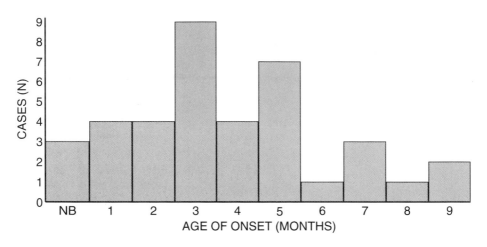

Fig. 5.2. Age at onset in 38 cases of transient idiopathic dystonia of infancy (combined series of Willemse 1986; Deonna et al. 1991; and personal, EF-A). NB = newborn.

myoclonic dystonia, such as idiopathic torsion dystonia (Obeso et al. 1983), essential myoclonus and benign hereditary chorea. Differentiating these entities may be difficult (Quinn et al. 1988). They are all autosomal dominant disorders and, with the exception of ITD, are relatively benign. Some members of the family reported by Kyllerman et al. (1990) had been previously reported as cases of hereditary essential myoclonus (Lundemo and Persson 1985). Confusion may be increased by the relative frequency of dystonic features in some cases of 'hereditary essential myoclonus' and because in myoclonic dystonia, both dystonia and myoclonus could present either independently or in association in different family members (Kurlan et al. 1988). The course of myoclonic dystonia is different from that of ITD with myoclonus. Furthermore, myoclonic jerks are briefer and more 'shock-like' than in ITD (Kurlan et al. 1988, Quinn et al. 1988).

OTHER IDIOPATHIC GENERALIZED DYSTONIAS
A few families with the X-linked dystonia–deafness syndrome (also named Mohr–Tranebjaerg syndrome) have been reported (Scribanu and Kennedy 1976, Tranebjaerg et al. 1995, Hayes et al. 1998). The disease is characterized by early onset sensorineural deafness and severe generalized dystonia starting around 7 years of age. Mental retardation and corticospinal tract involvement are associated features. A candidate gene for this disorder, called *DDP* (deafness/dystonia peptide) has been identified (Jin et al. 1996).

IDIOPATHIC HEMIDYSTONIA; SEGMENTAL AND FOCAL DYSTONIAS
TRANSIENT IDIOPATHIC DYSTONIA OF INFANCY
Willemse (1986) first described this syndrome in four infants who presented between 5 months and 1 year of age with segmental dystonia that disappeared without sequelae. He

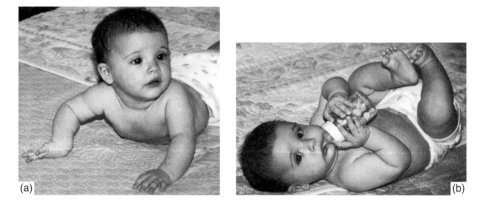

Fig. 5.3. Dystonic posture of the right arm (a) in a patient aged 5 months with transient dystonia of infancy. Note that the dystonic posture disappears during voluntary activity (b).

coined the term 'benign idiopathic dystonia'. Deonna et al. (1991) later reported eight new cases.

The disorder is usually detected before 5 months of age (Fig. 5.2). Affected infants present with abnormal posture, usually limited to one upper limb, although it may occasionally involve the trunk (Deonna et al. 1991), both arms or one side of the body (Figs. 5.3, 5.4). The arm is abducted and the forearm hyperpronated with flexion at the wrist when the infant is at rest. In the prone position, the infant often maintains forced pronation, using the back of the hand as support. The feet may be held in equinovarus. In some infants the abnormal posture is almost permanent even though attenuated during sleep. In others, it is only noticeable during relaxation or in certain positions. An important diagnostic clue is that the dystonic postures disappear when the infant carries out purposive movements with the affected extremity.

The rest of the neurological examination is normal and development proceeds normally, although in one case (Willemse 1986) a mild tremor of the head, arms and tongue was present. It spontaneously disappears around the first birthday, although in one patient (Willemse 1986) it persisted to 3 years of age. The duration of the disorder tends to be longer in cases of early onset (Fig. 5.5). Mild forms may not come to medical attention. Familial cases are known (Willemse 1986; personal observations by EF-A).

Under the term 'transient paroxysmal dystonia of infancy', Angelini et al. (1988) reported nine cases of 'paroxysmal' dystonia with onset between 1 and 5 months of age. The episodes consisted of opisthotonus and symmetrical or asymmetrical dystonia of the upper limbs. The episodes lasted from a few minutes to two hours and were frequent (up to several attacks daily). Their duration tended to increase and the frequency to diminish until disappearance between 8 and 22 months of age in seven children. Affected infants showed no neurological or developmental abnormalities. No other report of this disorder

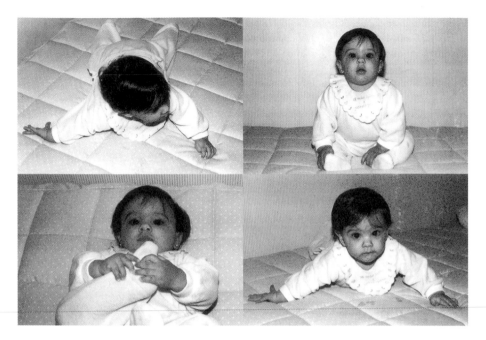

Fig. 5.4. Transient dystonia of infancy. Note that the dystonic posture of the right arm and hand disappear during voluntary activity. (Family photographs.)

has been published, but Patient 1 of the study by Beltran and Coker (1995) concerning infants with a history of intrauterine cocaine exposure might be a similar case. Such 'paroxysmal' cases could be an intermittent form of transient idiopathic dystonia.

Differential diagnosis
Lack of knowledge of the condition due to the rarity of publications on the theme is the main cause of diagnostic errors. Exclusion of orthopaedic problems, brachial obstetric paralysis, cerebral palsy (mainly congenital hemiplegia) and onset of progressive dystonia is usually easy because of the absence of other neurological signs, especially abnormalities of reflexes or tone. A very important key to the diagnosis is that dystonia disappears when the infant performs propositive movements with the affected extremity (Fig. 5.5). Normal manipulation and variation of the dystonia with posture help to exclude hemiplegia. When the clinical signs are typical no complementary studies (neuroimaging, laboratory examinations) are necessary.

Aetiology
The aetiology is unknown. Familial cases suggest a genetic basis. Mild forms may be frequent, and only the most marked cases may come to medical attention.

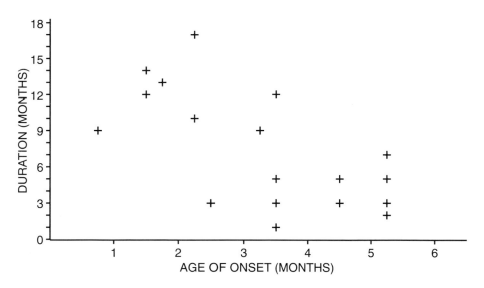

Fig. 5.5. Duration of the dystonia in 18 personal (EF-A) cases of transient dystonia of infancy related to age at onset.

Treatment
Treatment is unnecessary, and aggressive measures such as surgery are to be avoided.

FOCAL, SEGMENTAL AND OTHER LOCALIZED IDIOPHATIC DYSTONIAS
Focal or segmentary dystonia can be the first step of a later generalized idiopathic dystonia. Usually in cases with ITD caused by DYT1 deletion, dystonia begins in a limb, later progressing, sometimes after years, to involve other limbs. The same occurred in the families reported by Almasy et al. (1997), with dystonia linked to chromosome 8. But familial writer's cramp of juvenile onset with proved DYT1 mutation without progress to a generalized dystonia has been reported (Gasser et al. 1998). As mentioned before, cases of focal dystonia in dopa-responsive dystonia have been reported (Deonna and Ferreira 1985, Micheli et al. 1991, Steinberger et al. 1998). In two personal cases (EF-A), with segmentary dystonia of a lower limb without generalization, the onset was at 2.5 and 6 years. In one of these patients the disturbance remitted slowly with carbamazepine treatment to complete recovery.

SECONDARY DYSTONIAS
Dystonia is often a symptom, sometimes the first of a long list of diseases, and is then called secondary dystonia. Such cases have an underlying, demonstrable pathological substrate. Secondary dystonias can be classified into structural, metabolic, degenerative and miscellaneous subgroups that include infantile bilateral striatal or thalamic necrosis.

DYSTONIAS DUE TO STRUCTURAL BRAIN DAMAGE

The most frequent cause of hemidystonia is acute vascular occlusion especially affecting the striatum and/or the caudate (Demierre and Rondot 1983, Pettigrew and Jankovic 1985, Dusser et al. 1986). The first manifestation is generally an acute hemiparesis. Hemidystonia predominates in the upper limb and is very often associated with pyramidal tract signs. The dystonia may appear at the time hemiparesis recovers, but frequently it becomes evident only after several months (Grimes et al. 1982) or even years (Factor et al. 1988). Such late cases are one type of delayed onset dystonia (Midgard et al. 1989; see Chapter 11). In cases of vascular cause, neuroimaging (CT or MRI) (Burton et al. 1984, Perlmutter and Raiche 1984) shows limited lesions that mainly involve the striatum and specially the caudate nucleus.

Hemidystonia has been reported with a variety of other lesions of the basal ganglia. These include infections, especially tuberculous meningitis (Udani et al. 1971), postinfectious encephalitis (Cusmai et al. 1994), tumours (Narbona et al. 1984), arteriovenous malformations (Friedman et al. 1986), AIDS (Nath et al. 1987), porencephalic cysts (Jankovic and Fahn 1988), glutaric aciduria (Awaad et al. 1996), and closed head trauma (Maki et al. 1980, Brett et al. 1981, Pettigrew and Jankovic 1985).

Hemidystonia is an especially common form of secondary dystonia in children. Fourteen of the 19 cases of Demierre and Rondot (1983) had their onset before age 11 years. Bhatia and Marsden (1994) in a review of 240 patients of all ages with focal lesions of the basal ganglia found that 50 of 187 with unilateral lesions presented with hemidystonia, always contralateral to the lesion.

Haar and Dyken (1977) described a family in which four members had left-sided congenital hemiplegia that evolved into hemiathetosis. The abnormal movements first appeared at 8 years. Inheritance was autosomal dominant with incomplete penetrance. Neuroimaging demonstrated right-sided cerebral atrophy. Such patients are reminiscent of those of the hemiparkinsonism–hemiatrophy syndrome (Klawans 1981, Leenders et al. 1986, Giladi et al. 1990). This syndrome is considered a disorder of adults but Lang (1995) has reported a patient with cortical atrophy who presented contralateral hemidystonia after prolonged exercise at age 12 years, and hemiparkinsonism at age 15. Hemiparkinsonism–hemiatrophy patients usually respond well to low doses of L-dopa without significant dopa-induced side-effects.

Focal and segmentary secondary dystonias are uncommon in childhood. The most common focal dystonias include blepharospasm, consisting of repetitive and sustained involuntary contractions of the orbicularis oculi muscle (Grandas et al. 1988), spasmodic dysphonia (Aminoff et al. 1978), spasmodic torticollis and writer's cramp which are generally regarded as mild forms of ITD of adult onset although, for instance, occasional cases of blepharospasm have been observed as early as 11 years of age (Grandas et al. 1988). Writer's cramp has been reported in association with rolandic epilepsy and paroxysmal induced dyskinesia (Guerrini et al. 1999).

Torticollis can be caused by a spinal lesion (Kiwack et al. 1983). In a few cases, dystonia follows a peripheral trauma or surgical operation (Jankovic and van der Linden 1988).

Pathology
In hemidystonia, extensive lesions are usually found in the striatum, in particular the head of the caudate nucleus, the putamen and to a lesser extent the striopallidal fibres, the descending motor pathways and the thalamus (Dooling and Adams 1975, Marsden et al. 1985). Small lesions of the putamen, the head of the caudate or the pallidum have also been reported (Obeso and Gimenez-Roldan 1988).

DYSTONIAS IN METABOLIC DISORDERS
Dystonia is a frequent symptom in the course of many genetic disorders resulting from identified or probable inborn errors of metabolism (Table 5.6). In some, movement disorder is an essential part of the clinical picture, in others only a late or inconstant symptom. 'Degenerative dystonias' are listed in Table 5.7.

Glutaric aciduria and other organic acidaemias with movement disorders
Glutaric aciduria type I (GAI; also termed glutaric acidaemia, L-glutaric aciduria and glutarylCoA dehydrogenase deficiency) is an autosomal recessive disease due to severe reduction or total absence of glutarylCoA dehydrogenase activity (Christensen and Brandt 1978), a mitochondrial enzyme that catalyses dehydrogenation and decarboxylation of glutarylCoA to crotonyl-CoA and probably also decarboxylation of glutaconylCoA. The major precursors of glutarylCoA are the amino acids lysine, hydroxylysine and tryptophan. The GAI gene has been cloned and mapped to the short arm of chromosome 19 (Greenberg et al. 1994, Goodman et al. 1995) thus permitting secure prenatal diagnosis (Busquets et al. 1998). The frequency of GAI is estimated to be 1 in 30,000 neonates (Kyllerman and Steen 1980).

Clinical manifestations generally appear at between 5 and 14 months but mild symptoms such as slight motor delay and hypotonia can be observed at earlier ages. Macrocephaly at birth or developed some time later in infancy is present in about 70% of cases (Iafolla and Kahler 1989, Hoffmann et al. 1996). In two-thirds of cases the disease starts abruptly, on average at 12 months of age, with focal seizures or generalized convulsions, vomiting and obtundation or lethargy, usually following an acute infectious illness. Psychomotor regression and dystonic or choreoathetotic movements then appear (Fig. 5.6). Spasticity may also be evident. Anarthria is common. Comprehension of language is much better than expression, suggesting that cognition is relatively preserved. In the other third of cases the onset is insidious with slowly developing psychomotor delay, hypotonia and dystonic postures (Gregersen et al. 1977, Kyllerman and Steen 1977, Floret et al. 1979, Leibel et al. 1980). Atypical cases, for instance with normality until 8 years of age, have been reported (Haworth et al. 1991). In a personal case with DNA mutation, typical biochemical abnormalities and bilateral putaminal lesion at MRI, the

TABLE 5.6
Metabolic dystonias

2-oxyglutaric aciduria (Kohlschütter et al. 1982, Al Aqeel et al. 1994b)

3-methylglutaconic aciduria

4-hydroxybutyric aciduria

Ethylmalonic aciduria (Burlina et al. 1994, Al-Essa et al. 1999)

Biotinidase deficiency (Gascon et al. 1994)

Creatine deficiency syndrome (guanidinoacetate methyltransferase deficiency) (Stockler et al. 1994; see Chapter 4)

D-glyceric acidaemia (Hagberg et al. 1979)

D-2-hydroxyglutaric aciduria (see p. 101)

L-2-hydroxyglutaric aciduria (see p. 100)

Dystonic lipidosis (see p. 105)

Fucosidosis (Gordon et al. 1995)

Galactosaemia

Glutaric aciduria type I (see p. 95)

Hartnup disease (Darras and Gilmore 1985)

Homocystinuria (see p. 103)

Hyperphenylalaninaemia type VI

Idiopathic hypoparathyroidism

Infantile Gaucher disease

Juvenile GM2 and GM1 gangliosidosis (see p. 104)

Juvenile metachromatic leukodystrophy (see p. 105)

Keratan sulphaturia (Maroteaux 1973)

Krabbe leukodystrophy

Lactosuric oligosaccharidosis

Leber hereditary optic neuropathy plus dystonia (mtDNA) (see p. 106)

Leigh syndrome (see p. 105)

Lesch–Nyhan disease (see p. 101)

MELAS

Methylmalonic acidaemia

Mucopolysaccharidoses

Niemann–Pick disease

Propionic acidaemia (Hagberg et al. 1979, Ozand et al. 1994, Haas et al. 1995, Perez-Cerda et al. 1998)

Pyruvate dehydrogenase deficiency

Sulphite-oxidase deficiency

Tyrosinosis

Triose phosphate isomerase deficiency

Wilson disease (Chapter 6)

TABLE 5.7
Degenerative dystonias

Ataxia–oculomotor apraxia
Ataxia–telangiectasia (see p. 107)
Benign familial chorea (Chapter 4)
Ceroid-lipofuscinosis (Greenwood and Nelson 1978)
Dentato-pallidoluysian atrophy (Chapter 6)
Dystonia and sensorineural deafness
Familial dystonic–amyotrophic paraplegia
Hallervorden–Spatz disease (Chapter 6)
Hereditary non-progressive athetoid hemiplegia
Huntington disease (Chapter 2)
Intranuclear neuronal inclusion disease (Chapter 6)
Machado–Joseph disease (striatonigral autosomal dominant degeneration)
Myoclonic hereditary dystonia with nasal malformations
Neuroaxonal dystrophy
Olivocerebellar atrophy
Paraplegia–dystonia–ophthalmoplegia syndrome (adults)
Pelizaeus–Merzbacher disease
Progressive calcification of the basal ganglia (see p. 144)
Progressive pallidal degeneration
Rett syndrome (see p. 110)
Vitamin E deficiency

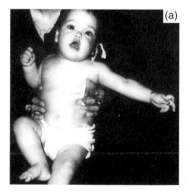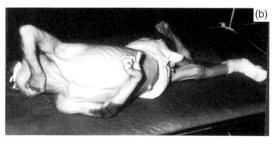

Fig. 5.6. Glutaric aciduria. (a) Left arm dystonia at age 10 months. This girl had an older brother diagnosed with glutaric aciduria and she was presymptomatically diagnosed. In spite of diet and vitaminic treatment she developed the clinical disease. (b) Generalized dystonia in a 5-year-old girl with glutaric aciduria.

only clinical manifestation at 16 years of age was hand tremor (Fernández-Alvarez et al. 1999).

The course of the disorder is variable. Patients in whom treatment was begun before the onset of symptoms have developed normally (Iafolla and Kahler 1989, Hoffmann et al. 1996). In most untreated cases, the disease continues to progress in a stepwise manner with a succession of acute episodes precipitated by febrile illness and infections. In others it remains stationary with severe motor and language sequelae. About half of the untreated patients die before age 4 years during intercurrent illnesses. Some patients remain alive into adolescence (Brandt et al. 1979).

• *Laboratory investigations.* Organic acids in urine are usually abnormal with high, although variable, quantities of glutaric, betahydroxyglutaric (smaller amounts) and occasionally glutaconic acids. In a few patients urine glutaric acid is normal or only slightly elevated. Glutaric acid is also increased in blood and CSF. Serum L-carnitine is usually reduced. During acute episodes a severe acidosis, hypoglycaemia (Floret et al. 1979, Bennett et al. 1986), hyperammonaemia (Leibel et al. 1980) and hypocholesterolaemia may be present. Hyperproteinorrachia is found in a quarter of cases.

Glutaryl CoA dehydrogenase assay in fibroblasts and/or genetic studies should be performed when the condition is strongly suspected on clinical or neuroimaging grounds even in the presence of normal levels of glutaric acid (Campistol et al. 1992, Christensen et al. 1997, Pineda et al. 1998).

In some cases (Goodman et al. 1977) no enzymatic activity is detectable, the levels of glutaric acid are relatively high and the course is progressive, whereas in others (Brandt et al. 1979) there is some residual enzymatic activity and a less severe course without intellectual involvement. Although such differences might suggest different mutations, the correlation between enzymatic activity and clinical severity is far from constant and forms of markedly different severity have been reported in the same sibship despite similar levels of enzymatic deficit.

• *Neuroimaging.* Early signs on CT and MR scans usually include an increase of the subarachnoid spaces with frontotemporal atrophy (Fig. 5.7), subependymal pseudocysts and delayed myelination (Goodman and Noremberg 1983, Iafolla and Kahler 1989). The frontotemporal atrophy may be so marked as to suggest the diagnosis of bilateral sylvian arachnoid cysts (Hald et al. 1991). The caudate and putamen often show decreased density on CT and high signal on T_2 MRI. These lesions may be transient (Aicardi et al. 1985) or improve with therapy (Cho et al. 1995). Chronic subdural effusions and subdural haematomas have been found in some cases (Leibel et al. 1980, Artigas et al. 1993), even as the initial manifestation of the disease (Osaka et al. 1993).

• *Differential diagnosis.* Because beneficial effect of treatment in presymptomatic cases has been reported (Hoffmann et al. 1996), diagnosis at this stage is important. A high

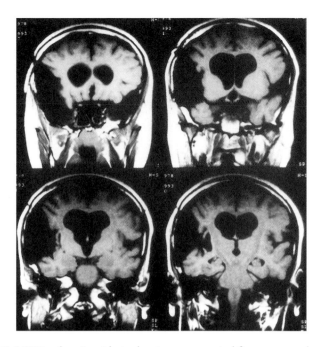

Fig. 5.7. MRI in glutaric aciduria showing asymmetrical frontotemporal atrophy.

level of suspicion in infants with macrocephaly, mild hypotonia and motor delay together with neuroimaging features should lead to a search for organic aciduria.

Increased urine glutaric acid may also be found in glutaric acidaemia type II, glutaryl-CoA oxidase deficiency and alpha-aminoadipic acidaemia (Goodman and Frerman 1995), but the clinical signs are different from GAI. When betahydroxyglutaric acid is found the diagnosis of GAI is almost certain.

On clinical or neuroimaging grounds, the differential diagnosis includes acute encephalitis, Leigh syndrome (Stutchfield et al. 1985), sequelae of hypoxic–ischaemic encephalopathy, other cases of dystonic tetraparesis and the degenerative disorders already mentioned. Because of subdural effusions, child abuse may be erroneously considered.

• *Pathology.* Autopsy studies have shown minimal changes in severely affected patients who died at 1 year of age (loss of neurons and increased astrocytes in the putamen, and to a lesser extent in the caudate nuclei) (Bennett et al. 1986) but changes much more marked in patients who died at more than 2 years of age (Goodman et al. 1977, Leibel et al. 1980, Chow et al. 1988). These findings are remarkably similar to those in the so-called 'familial holotopistic striatal necrosis' or 'familial striatal degeneration' described by Miyoshi et al. (1969) and by Roessman and Schwartz (1973). These cases may have been unrecognized forms of glutaric aciduria.

• *Pathogenesisis.* This is unclear. Goodman et al. (1977) suggested that increased levels of glutaric acid may interfere with the metabolism of glutamic acid (thus resulting in low GABA levels) or that glutaric acid acts as a false neurotransmitter in the place of glutamate.

Glutaric acid concentrations may be increased not only in the brain but in all tissues (Goodman et al. 1977, Leibel et al. 1980, Bennett et al. 1986). The GABA content of putamen, caudate and substantia nigra is markedly decreased.

• *Treatment.* Ideally, treatment should start before onset of clinical symptoms. In such cases, as in symptomatic patients, carnitine administration (Bergman et al. 1989, Hoffmann et al. 1996) and aggressive treatment of acute febrile episodes, including fever control and glucose infusions, can prevent in many cases the development of clinical signs or decrease their severity. A diet low in protein, supplemented with lysine- and tryptophan-free amino acid mixtures have been advised (Goodman et al. 1977, Brandt et al. 1979), but its potential benefit is unclear (Hoffmann et al. 1996) and it can be responsible for serious side-effects.

Treatment should be maintained for years, although after 3–4 years deterioration is rare (Kyllerman et al. 1994). Efforts to stimulate residual enzymatic activity of glutaryl-CoA dehydrogenase have been made, although the lack of correlation between plasmatic and urinary levels of glutaric acid and clinical effects renders this technique of dubious clinical value. Riboflavin is theoretically an active stimulator of glutaryl-CoA dehydrogenase. Therefore, most patients (Brandt et al. 1979, Bennett et al. 1986) receive such treatment but efficacy is hard to assess. Baclofen, an inhibitor of GABA B receptors, is useful in reducing muscle spasms (Brandt et al. 1979, Bennett et al. 1986, Bergman et al. 1989, Awaad et al. 1996, Hoffmann et al. 1996).

Treatment of epileptic seizures – frequently observed during acute episodes – with valproic acid should be avoided because this may promote disturbances in the mitochondrial acetyl-CoA/CoA ratio (Hoffmann et al. 1991). Hoffmann et al. (1996) consider that neurosurgical interventions on subdural effusions or haematomas should be avoided because they do not result in expansion of brain.

There are two diseases with elevated excretion of 2-hydroxyglutaric acid with very different phenotypes and neuroimaging. L-2-Hydroxyglutaric aciduria (Barth et al. 1992) is probably an autosomal recessive disease and features mental deficiency (or mental deterioration), seizures and progressive cerebellar dysfunction. Dystonia is present in about a third of the patients (Barth et al. 1993). Usually the first signs are delay in unsupported walking, abnormal gait, speech delay or severe febrile crisis, but patients without abnormalities until learning difficulties in the first school year have been reported (Barth et al. 1993). Macrocephaly is frequent and can be the presenting feature (Diogo et al. 1996). Intrafamilial clinical heterogeneity has been reported (De Klerk et al. 1997). On neuroimaging all patients show a highly characteristic and consistent pattern of severe progressive loss of myelin most marked in the arcuate fibres, cerebellar vermis atrophy, and intense T_2 signal in both dentate nuclei and often in the caudate nucleus and globus pallidus (van der Knaap and Valk 1995). In addition to L-2-hydroxyglutarate, other organic acids (glycolic, glyceric and others) have an abnormally high concentration in CSF (Hoffmann et al. 1995). D-2-hydroxyglutaric aciduria has a variable clinical symptomatology of early-infantile onset. Some patients show chorea or dystonia. Subependymal cysts over the head or corpus of the caudate nucleus are present when neuroimaging is performed within the first few months of life (van der Knaap et al. 1999).

Methylmalonic aciduria (Stokke et al. 1967) includes a group of biochemically and clinically distinct disorders due to an inborn error in the conversion of methylmalonyl-CoA to succinyl-CoA or defects of cobalamin metabolism. Several cases of acute dystonic syndrome (Korf et al. 1986, Heindereich et al. 1988) have been reported during episodes of metabolic decompensation. Hypodense lesions of the pallidum on CT and/or a high signal in T_2-weighted MRI sequences can be seen. These are different from the putaminal and caudate lesions of glutaric aciduria (De Sousa et al. 1989, Roodhooft et al. 1990, Mirowitz et al. 1991). Familial cases of progressive encephalopathy with dystonia, microcephaly, mental retardation, spasticity and cataracts with an elevated excretion of methylmalonic acid (but less than in typical cases of methylmalonic aciduria) have been reported (Stromme et al. 1995). MRI in one of these patients showed low signal intensity in the globus pallidus, substantia nigra and red nucleus.

3-methylglutaconic aciduria is the landmark of a heterogeneous group of metabolic disorders (Greter et al. 1978, Costeff et al. 1993, Gibson et al. 1993, Gascon et al. 1994). At least four different phenotypes have been described (Al Aqeel et al. 1994a). Type III begins around the age of 1 year as a progressive encephalopathy with rigidity and choreic movements (Gibson et al. 1988, 1991; Gascon et al. 1994). A subclass of type III (Costeff et al. 1989) resembles Behr syndrome (optic atrophy, ataxia, spastic paraparesis or pyramidal tract signs) but 'choreiform movements' (Elpeleg et al. 1994) are often present.

4-hydroxybutyric aciduria is an autosomal recessive disorder caused by the deficiency of succinic semialdehyde dehydrogenase. Urinary 4-hydroxybutyric acid is 300–1000 times that of normal. It is a rare progressive encephalopathy with variable clinical manifestations. Cases with onset in early infancy and choreoathetosis, severe dystonia or myoclonus have been reported (Rahbeeni et al. 1994).

Lesch–Nyhan disease

Lesch–Nyhan disease is an X-linked disorder of purine metabolism resulting from deficiency of hypoxanthine-guanine phosphoribosyltransferase (HGPRT). The disease usually has its onset between 6 and 18 months of age, with delayed psychomotor development, hypotonia or spasticity. Abnormal movements begin as fine athetoid movements of the hands and feet. They are predominantly dystonic (Fig. 5.8) but may include chorea and tremor. A remarkable feature is an aggressive behaviour (85% of cases) directed both to the self and to surrounding persons. Automutilation, particularly affecting the lips and fingers, usually begins with tooth eruption but may begin as late as 16 years. Dysarthria

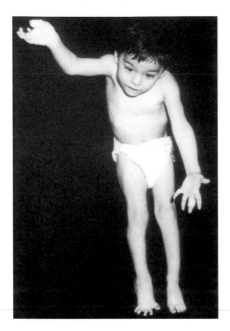

Fig. 5.8. Lesch–Nyhan disease. Generalized dystonia at 2 years 9 months of age. This boy, the only child of healthy parents, showed developmental delay. At age 16 months automutilation started. Biological and enzymatic studies showed typical results of Lesch–Nyhan disease.

is also a frequent symptom. Affected children also present extraneurological symptoms such as haematuria, crystalluria and signs of hyperuricaemia such as renal stones, gouty arthritis and tophi (Christie et al. 1982). An early sign may be the appearance of an orange-coloured crystalline material in the nappies. Other features include vomiting, anaemia, reduced growth and delayed bone age.

A few patients with involuntary movements, spasticity but normal cognitive function and behaviour (no self-mutilation) considered as an atypical neurological variant have been reported (Bakay et al. 1979, Gottlieb et al. 1982, Mitchell and McInnes 1984, Adler and Wrabetz 1996).

The HPRT gene has been localized to Xq26–q27 (Pai et al. 1980). Prenatal diagnosis is possible by enzyme assay (Alford et al. 1995) or DNA analysis by fibroblast cultures or chorionic villus obtained by amniocentesis.

• *Laboratory examination.* Levels of uric acid in urine are increased three- to four-fold. Patients excrete 3–4 mg of uric acid per mg of creatinine (normal <1 mg). Hyperuricaemia is frequent.

• *Differential diagnosis.* The differential diagnosis is mainly with dyskinetic cerebral palsy and other forms of secondary dystonia. Automutilation is a useful feature but can be absent (Gottlieb et al. 1982) or start as late as the mid-teens (Mitchell and McInnes 1984) in rare atypical cases. Moreover, automutilation can also be observed in cases of

TABLE 5.8
Observations of homocystinuria with dystonia

Reference	Type	Sex	Onset (years)	Localization	Evolution
Hagberg et al. (1970)	?	M	14	Torticollis	Progressive
Kempster et al. (1988)	CSD	M	18	Cerv→Trunk→UE	Died 22y
	CSD	M	10	Cerv→Trunk→LE	Alive at 19y
	CSD	F	9	Generalized	Alive at 26y
Davous and Rondot (1983)	?	M	21	Torticollis	NR
Personal case (EF-A) (Fig. 5.9)	CSD	M	9	Left hemidystonia	Alive at 19y

CSD = cystathionine synthetase deficiency; UE = upper extremities; LE = lower extremities; NR = not reported.

severe mental retardation of various causes, in autism, and in some types of sensory neuropathy.

• *Pathogenesis.* The neurological disease does not result from the excess production of uric acid. Allopurinol treatment can prevent systemic complications of hyperuricaemia but does not alleviate neurological signs even when administered from birth. Automutilation has been thought to be due to hypersensitivity of dopamine receptors D1 to a normal amount of dopamine (Golstein et al. 1985).

Pathological studies have not shown any structural changes (Watts et al. 1982). Marked reduction of homovanillic acid has been reported in the striatum and limbic area (Lloyd et al. 1981) and in CSF (Silverstein et al. 1985).

• *Treatment.* Allopurinol is indicated for renal and gouty manifestations. Unfortunately, allopurinol has no effect on the neurological symptoms. For self-mutilation, 5-hydroxy-L-tryptophan (Mizuno et al. 1975) and naltrexone (Anderson and Ernst 1994) may be useful, and behavioural therapy seems to be moderately effective (McGreevy and Arthur 1987).

Homocystinuria
A few cases of homocystinuria (Carson et al. 1963, Dunn et al. 1966) with onset of dystonia after the diagnosis of homocystinuria had been established have been reported (Table 5.8). In these cases dystonia was slowly progressive and reached a plateau. Pathological lesions included arterial and venous thrombosis of the cerebral cortex and basal ganglia (Gibson et al. 1964).

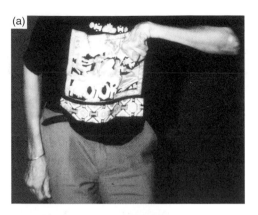

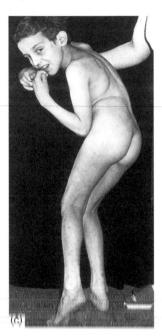

Fig. 5.9. Dystonia in homocystinuria.

(a, b) This patient was diagnosed with homocystinuria at age 5 years. At 9 years left arm dystonia started, evolving to left hemidystonia.

(c) Another unrelated case showing trunk and left hemidystonia (photo courtesy Dr Jaime Campos, Madrid).

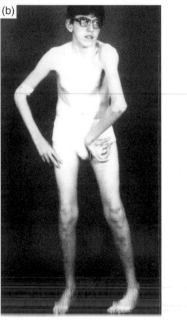

The cause of the movement disorder is obscure. Vascular disease is probable, but in case 1 of Kempster et al. (1988) autopsy showed no pathology in the vessels of the basal ganglia.

Dystonias due to other metabolic disorders
• *GM1 and GM2 gangliosidosis.* Focal or generalized movement disorders with dystonia, athetosis, tremor or rigidity, usually as late manifestations, were present in a third of the patients with GM2 gangliosidosis reported by Meek et al. (1984) and Oates et al. (1986) and in all 16 patients of a Japanese series of GM1 gangliosidosis (Yoshida et al. 1992). In

both diseases, cases in which dystonia was the main manifestation in association with hypokinetic–rigid syndrome were reported (Goldman et al. 1981; Meek et al. 1984; Guazzi et al. 1988; Nardocci et al. 1992, 1993). Oromandibular dyskinesia, bradykinesia and rest tremor can be also observed (Rapin et al. 1976, Nardocci et al. 1993). Cases with progressive dystonia as the main sign are on record (Hardie et al. 1988). Intellectual deterioration is always present, usually associated with ataxia and spasticity, seizures and myoclonus.

Neuroimaging can be normal or show nonspecific features such as cerebral atrophy predominantly in the frontal lobe, areas of demyelination and atrophy in the corpus callosum (see Fig. 5.7). Symmetrical hyperintensity in the putamen (Inui et al. 1990, Uyama et al. 1992) on T_2-weighted MRI has been reported in adult patients with GM1 gangliosidosis. In the case of an 11-year-old child with GM1 there was hypointensity in the putamen and globus pallidus similar to that found in Hallervorden–Spatz syndrome (Tanaka et al. 1995b).

The diagnosis is based on enzymatic studies. In GM1 gangliosidosis, levels of beta-galactosidase in leukocytes or fibroblasts are low or undetectable. In GM2 gangliosidosis, betahexosaminidase A in serum, leukocytes and fibroblasts is reduced but enzymatic diagnosis can be missed if the enzymatic activity is tested only with conventional synthetic substrates. Tests for the presence of the activator protein or use of sulphated substrates are sometimes necessary.

The dominant movement disorders in these patients are probably due to predom-inant basal ganglia intraneuronal storage of gangliosides in the late-onset form of ganglio-sidosis (Kobayashi and Suzuki 1981), whereas in the early-onset form the neuronal storage is ubiquitous (Yoshida et al. 1992). In all forms, however, the ganglion cells in the submucosal enteric plexus contain the characteristic inclusions, a useful complementary diagnostic feature.

• *Juvenile dystonic lipidosis* (Karpati et al. 1977). This term has been applied to a small group of patients with progressive dystonia and evidence of lipid storage disorder. Most such cases probably belong to type C Niemann–Pick disease (Karpati et al. 1977) and feature vertical supranuclear gaze palsy, especially on looking downward (Neville et al. 1973). Clinical manifestations at onset usually include intellectual regression and gait disorder. Movement disorder can predominate and consists mainly (Fig. 5.10) of dys-tonia. Cerebellar and pyramidal signs then appear, and splenomegaly is common (but not constant).

Dystonia may be a manifestation of advanced stages of *metachromatic leukodystrophy* (Fig. 5.11). Lang et al. (1985) reported a juvenile form manifested purely by dystonia and severe intellectual deficit with a protracted course. Nerve biopsy showed metachromasia and Schwann cell laminar inclusions despite normal conduction velocities.

In *subacute necrotizing encephalomyelopathy* (Leigh syndrome) movement disorder of any type including hypokinetic–rigid syndrome, chorea, myoclonus or dystonia may be

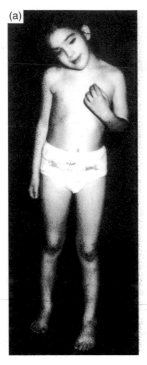

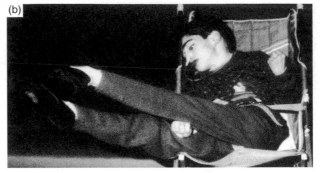

Fig. 5.10. Dystonic lipoidosis. Onset in this girl was at age 4 years with learning difficulties and clumsiness. On examination at 6 years the only neurological abnormality was light conjugate vertical ocular paresis. Three months later quite suddenly she developed a right laterocollis (a). Medullar puncture showed Niemann–Pick cells. Three years later (b) the dystonia was generalized with dystonic spasms. She died at 14 years. (This patient never developed visceromegaly.)

the presenting and the most obvious clinical features (Rondot et al. 1982, Campistol et al. 1986, Gallego et al. 1986, Lera et al. 1994). In many cases, dystonia is only one of the complex manifestations of this syndrome as reported in 19 of the 34 patients reviewed by Macaya et al. (1993).

Symmetrical lucencies affecting mainly the putamina have been described on CT scans (Campistol et al. 1984), and high signal is usually present on T_2-weighted MRI sequences. Similar anomalies are sometimes visible also in the midbrain, periaqueductal grey matter, the onate nucleus and cerebral cortex (Koch et al. 1986, Davis et al. 1987) Such images are common to several mitochondrial diseases.

• *Leber hereditary optic neuropathy (LHON)* (De Vivo and Di Mauro 1990). In several families, LHON and/or dystonia (Novotny et al. 1986) were associated with a heteroplasmic G-to-A point mutation in the *ND6* gene of the mitochondrial DNA, causing a defect in oxidative phosphorylation. In childhood-onset cases, manifestations ranged from pure dystonia with normal cognition to severe generalized dystonia associated with variable degrees of dementia, bulbar and corticospinal tract dysfunction, and short stature (Shofner et al. 1995). The mildest manifestations were observed in adolescent-onset LHON. Frequently these patients exhibited on MRI unilateral or bilateral basal ganglia lesions, sometimes silent.

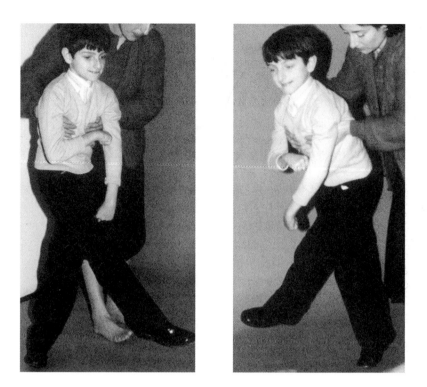

Fig. 5.11. Juvenile metachromatic leukodystrophy. The disease in this boy started at age 4 years with change of mood and difficulties at school. Diagnosed at 6 years. Dystonia started at 10 years in the hands and spreads to the legs. Notice the peculiar dystonic disturbance of the gait. He died at 15 years.

Several families with optic atrophy, dystonia and hypodensities of the basal ganglia are on record. In a patient of Nigro et al. (1990), muscle biopsy showed ragged red fibres and subsarcolemmal mitochondrial aggregates. A partial deficiency of cytochrome B was demonstrated.

DYSTONIAS DUE TO 'DEGENERATIVE' DISORDERS

Dystonia or chorea are present in 50% of cases of *ataxia–telangiectasia* (AT), an autosomal recessive disease. Dystonia in AT is usually a late sign (Fig. 5. 12) and its frequency can increase to 90% in late cases (Woods and Taylor 1992), but in some patients dystonia, athetosis or hypokinetic–rigid syndrome may be a prominent and initial sign (Koep et al. 1994). Chorea is often the first manifestation. Atypical cases may begin with resting tremor (Hiel et al. 1994). Bodensteiner et al. (1980) reported the case of a 9-year-old girl in whom the disorder began with dystonia that increased over the years. Multiple telangiectasias suggested the diagnosis. Lesions in the lenticular nucleus have been described (Demaerel et al. 1992).

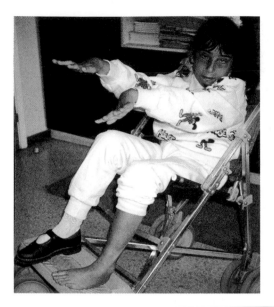

Fig. 5.12. Ataxia–telangiectasia in a girl aged 12 years, demonstrating dystonia of the hands and left foot. The dystonia was noticed at age 9 years.

The cause of dystonia in AT is unclear. In pathological study of 17 cases of AT with movement disorder, abnormalities of the basal ganglia were found in 10. Lesions were found only in long-standing cases. In two of these (Agamanolis and Greenstein 1979), Lewy bodies similar to those found in Parkinson disease were present. In four there was only neuronal loss and gliosis in the striatum.

Patients with the syndrome of *ataxia–ocular motor apraxia* (Aicardi et al. 1988) may also exhibit dystonic features.

A limited number of families (Dick and Stevenson, 1953) with *spastic paraplegia, amyotrophy and dystonia*, the so-called 'familial amyotrophic dystonic paraplegia' have been reported. Other features may include tremor, nystagmus and mental retardation. In the family described by Gilman and Horenstein (1964) the disease was transmitted as an autosomal dominant trait.

INFANTILE BILATERAL STRIATAL OR THALAMIC NECROSIS

Following the initial description in 1924 by D Paterson and EA Carmichael, Friede (1989) proposed the term 'infantile bilateral striatal necrosis' (IBSN) to designate a neuropathological syndrome featuring bilateral symmetrical spongy degeneration of both putamina and caudate nuclei and occasionally of the thalami. The number of cases has increased with the change from a neuropathological to a neuroimaging syndrome. A follow-up of the neuroimaging has been published by Fujita et al. (1994). The lesions can now been recognized in living patients by CT that shows hypodense images in the involved areas and, better, by MRI that shows an increased T_2 signal in the same zones (Leuzzi et al. 1988).

Recent progress in the knowledge of mitochondrial disorders and organic acidurias shows that symmetrical striatal lesions are common in these diseases (Goodman and Noremberg 1983, Campistol et al. 1987), and suggests that many of the cases reported as IBSN may have been due to metabolic disorders decompensated by an acute infection, e.g. glutaric aciduria. Gascon et al. (1994) think that "those cases in which no organic aciduria was identified and lactic acidosis was not documented, are unproven mitochondrial disorders". However, evidence for an inflammatory condition has been brought forward in a number of cases (Brandel et al. 1996).

Typical cases of acute IBSN are characterized by an acute onset of rigidity, dystonia, chorea, ballismus (Yamamoto et al. 1997), and a stereotyped response to stimuli whether pleasant or painful, with monotonous crying, grimacing and hyperextension of the neck. Epilepsy is rare. Some patients develop symptoms soon after a variety of infections, including respiratory tract infections, mumps or *Mycoplasma pneumoniae* infection (Brandel et al. 1996). On imaging, there is often extensive oedema of the white matter in addition to symmetrical hypodensities of the striatum. MRI lesions can disappear after a period of time or persist (Roig et al. 1990, Fujita et al. 1994). Some patients may die shortly after the acute phase, but usually a gradual improvement occurs, in some cases even after several months, although sequelae such as dystonia (Goutières and Aicardi 1982) or hemiparesis (Fujita et al. 1994) can result. The clinical picture is distinctive and different from that of the chronic forms (Mito et al. 1986) in which hypodensities are less extensive and limited to the striatum.

Although some familial cases are on record (Broessmann and Schwartz 1973, Craver et al. 1996) most cases of IBSN are sporadic. Goutières and Aicardi (1982) proposed to group the cases into three categories: (1) definite or probable subacute necrotizing encephalopathy (Leigh syndrome) (see above); (2) familial cases of insidious onset and slowly progressive course; and (3) cases presenting with abrupt neurologic dysfunction following an acute systemic infectious disease. This last category has been named Goutières–Aicardi syndrome (Brandel et al. 1996), a confusing eponym because there exists another condition with a similar name, and the term 'acute encephalopathy with bilateral striatal necrosis' (Rosemberg et al. 1991) seems more appropriate.

The pathogenesis remains unknown but a parainfectious mechanism is probable.

Cases of *acute necrosis of both thalami* ('acute necrotizing encephalopathy of children' – Mizuguchi et al. 1995) following an acute viral infection have been reported initially from Japan where this condition seems mostly to occur (Wang et al. 1994, Mizuguchi 1997), although it has also been reported in Caucasians (Eicke et al. 1992, Pedro et al. 1995, Campistol et al. 1998). Half the cases started acutely between 6 and 18 months of age (Mizuguchi 1997). Hyperthermia, coma and decerebrate or decorticate postures are very common in the acute stage. The course is severe, leading to death in a quarter of the cases or to severe residual impairment with quadriplegia, microcephaly, dystonia and mental retardation. Early in the course bilateral hyperechogenic thalamic lesions may be observed by ultrasound; CT or MRI also shows lesions in the pons, mesencephalon,

TABLE 5.9
Secondary dystonias, not metabolic or degenerative (or unknown metabolic abnormalities)

Alternating hemiplegia of childhood
Brain tumours (Narbona et al. 1984)
Basal ganglia infarction (Giroud and Dumas 1988)
Chromosome 18p (or 18q) deletion (Gordon et al. 1995, Awaad et al. 1999)
HIV infection (Nath et al. 1987)
Meningitis/encephalitis (Gollomp and Fahn 1987, Silverstein and Brunberg 1995, Hargrave and
     Webb 1998)
Moyamoya disease
Neuroacanthocytosis
Neuroaxonal dystrophy (Aicardi and Castelein 1969)
Ophthalmoplegia–paraplegia dystonia (adults)
Pelizaeus–Merzbacher disease (Boulloche and Aicardi 1986)
Pontocerebellar hypoplasia type 2 (Chapter 6)
Rett syndrome (Al Mateen et al. 1986, Fitzgerald et al. 1990, Narbona and Poch-Olive 1985)
Vascular malformation (Friedman et al. 1986)

cerebellum and white matter. Hyperproteinorrachia can be present. Causal or associated viral infections have been demonstrated in several cases (Ochi et al. 1986, Protheroe and Mellor 1991, Oki et al. 1995). These cases show some similarities to those of IBSN, so the term 'infantile thalamic bilateral necrosis' has been suggested (Campistol et al. 1998).

OTHER SECONDARY DYSTONIAS
As seen in Tables 5.6 and 5.7, generalized dystonia can be a major or accessory feature of many disorders. In addition, a long list of other disorders can cause acute dystonia (Table 5.9).

In alternating hemiplegia of childhood, tonic and dystonic episodes, often unilateral, are present in 90% of cases (Aicardi et al. 1995) and are often the first manifestation. The movement disorder, initially paroxysmal, tends to become permanent, and generalized choreoathetosis is almost constant in the late stages although dystonia may also be present (Aicardi et al. 1995, Sakuragawa 1995). Flunarizine is partially effective in about half of the patients (Casaer 1987).

CONDITIONS THAT SIMULATE DYSTONIA (PSEUDODYSTONIAS)
Essential Setting-Sun Sign
A few cases of infants with self-limited setting-sun sign as the only neurological abnormality and normal neuroimaging have been reported (Cernerud 1945, Biglan 1984). Associated downward nystagmus has been occasionally noted (Biglan 1984). Usually the sign is observed shortly following birth and may last for several months (Miller and Packard 1998). Development is normal.

Downward deviation of both eyes in the neonatal period without eyelid retraction and with normal oculocephalic response has been observed in five of 242 prospectively examined healthy newborn infants (Hoyt et al. 1980)

SANDIFER SYNDROME

Kinsbourne (1964) published the first cases of this syndrome that had been recognized by Paul Sandifer (see Murphy and Gellis 1977). The syndrome may appear in the neonatal period or up to 3 years of age. It is characterized by intermittent postures of hyperextension of the head often associated with rotation or tilting that may also involve the trunk. Abnormal movements may increase during or immediately after feeding and disappear during sleep (Gellis and Feingold 1971).

The syndrome occurs in children with gastro-oesophageal reflux, often associated with hiatus hernia (Werlin et al. 1980). Symptoms of reflux may be absent. In young infants, cyanosis, apnoea and paroxysmal stiffness may be prominent (Werlin et al. 1980).

The diagnosis may be difficult: benign paroxysmal torticollis and psychiatric syndromes can be suspected (Bray et al. 1977), and reflux is frequent in children with cerebral palsy, especially dyskinetic forms (Stephenson 1990). Moreover, metoclopramide often used to treat reflux can induce dystonia. Cases are often misdiagnosed as epileptic seizures. The pathogenesis of Sandifer syndrome is unclear. It does not depend of the degree of reflux (Mandel et al. 1989), and the dystonic attitudes may, in fact, increase reflux.

Mechanical or postural treatment of reflux or correction of hiatus hernia results in rapid resolution of symptoms. Surgery may be necessary in some cases.

SYMPTOMATIC TREATMENT OF DYSTONIA

Although a large number of pharmaceuticals and other therapeutic methods have been used in the treatment of dystonia, both idiopathic and symptomatic, only a few controlled studies are available. The response to therapy is unpredictable and the mechanisms of action unknown.

This section is concerned only with the treatment of generalized or focal dystonias, excluding dopa-responsive dystonia (see p. 89).

The agents commonly used include dopaminergic, anticholinergic and antidopaminergic drugs, benzodiazepines and baclofen. In focal or segmental dystonias, botulinum toxin may be useful. Finally, various surgical therapies have been tried.

A trial of L-dopa is indicated in all cases of idiopathic dystonia because (1) patients diagnosed with ITD may in fact have DRD without fluctuation; (2) it is sometimes effective in ITD (Willemse et al. 1984, De Yebenes et al. 1988); and (3) even some secondary dystonias may respond to the drug (Fletcher et al. 1993). Small doses are used (62.5–100 mg, 2–3 times daily) in association with a carboxylase inhibitor (carbidopa, benzerazide) (Marsden and Quinn 1990, Nygaard et al. 1991). Such a dose, given over a few days, is usually sufficient to assess the efficacy and may be secondarily adjusted.

However, cases with a lesser sensitivity may require higher dosages and prolonged therapy. Marsden (1981) advises a trial of three months.

In the most common situation when there is no response to L-dopa, various agents can be tested in a trial-and-error process. Each expert has their own strategy. Fahn (1983) and Marsden et al. (1984) recommend very high doses of benzhexol (trihexyphenidyl, Artane) whose effect was demonstrated by a double-blind trial (Burke et al. 1986b). The proposed initial dose is 4–5 mg/d; the dose is then increased slowly (2.5 mg/d every other week) to reach doses as high as 80 mg/d in children. Side-effects (dryness of mouth, constipation, blurred vision, urinary hesitancy, anorexia, chorea, confusion and psychosis) can be avoided in many cases if the dose progression is slow enough. Pilocarpine eye drops or oral physostigmine can also prevent side-effects (Greene 1995). Benefit can be observed at low dose but may not appear for many weeks. A dramatic effect after some weeks or months of therapy is reportedly obtained in 62% of cases (Greene et al. 1988). The treatment seems to be more effective in early treated patients. Our experience with the use of high doses in children has been less favourable. One of my patients (EF-A) aged 19 years presented a psychotic process while taking 49 mg/d of benzhexol.

When benzhexol fails, Marsden et al. (1984) advise the use of a combination of benzhexol, tetrabenazine (75 mg/d), and pimozide (6–12 mg/d), a potent antagonist of dopamine. Weiner and Lang (1989) add to benzhexol, progressively increasing doses of benzodiazepines (diazepam or clonazepam). Greene and Fahn (1992) advise the use of baclofen as the third drug to be tried after L-dopa and anticholinergics. Doses range from 40 to 180 mg/d. The main side-effects are lethargy, dry mouth and dizziness. Rapid decrease in the dose of baclofen may produce seizures or psychosis (Greene 1995).

Fourteen per cent of patients with adult or childhood onset get some benefit from clonazepam (Greene 1995). Diazepam in high dosage (100 mg/d) produced dramatic improvement in one case (Ziegler 1981). Carbamazepine is recommended in moderate doses (Marsden et al. 1984, Greene et al. 1988). In three personal cases (EF-A) of early-onset segmental dystonia, carbamazepine was very useful. Haloperidol, pimozide, phenothiazines, amantadine, cyproheptadine, tricyclic antidepressants (Greene et al. 1988) and even lithium have been tried. Tetrabenazine, a dopamine antagonist, has given variable results (Asher and Aminoff 1981, Jankovic 1982). Lang and Marsden (1982) found a high incidence of side-effects with this drug.

The role of continuous infusion of intrathecal baclofen, a method used in the treatment of severe spasticity, remains uncertain in dystonia (Ford et al. 1996).

The beneficial effects on chronic dystonia of pharmacological agents are often limited and transient. It may be wiser to accept the persistence of some dystonia rather than to use massive doses, as the effect of drugs on higher cognitive functions is poorly known.

Severe episodes of generalized dystonia in patients with primary or secondary dystonia can occur. The terms 'status dystonicus' (Manji et al. 1998) or 'dystonic storms' (Vaamonde et al. 1994) have been used. Treatment of this situation is difficult. Because bulbar and respiratory complications are frequent, management in an intensive care setting is necessary.

Surgical treatment by stereoataxic thalamotomy was extensively used by Cooper et al. (1976) who claimed significant benefit in 70% of cases. Andrew et al. (1983), however, reported less favourable results. A major problem is that a bilateral operation is required for the common generalized cases, with a high risk of pseudobulbar paralysis with dysphagia and dysarthria. The best results have been in cases of hemidystonia (Andrew et al. 1983). The risk has been estimated to be 11% in unilateral operation and up to 56% in bilateral cases (Andrew et al. 1983). In addition, recurrence of symptoms is frequent following an initial improvement.

The efficacy of other surgical techniques such as cerebellar or cervical cord stimulation (Waltz 1981) is not demonstrated (Goetz et al. 1988). A beneficial effect on dystonia of chronic high frequency stimulation of the thalamic ventrolateral nucleus, pallidum and subthalamic nucleus has been reported (Blond et al. 1992, Sellal et al. 1993). These techniques appear promising and are being intensively studied (Volkman et al. 1998, Benabid et al. 2000).

In dysphonia spasmodica, tracheotomy (Corbin et al. 1987), resection of a vocal cord or section of the recurrent nerve (Levine et al. 1979) have been used, but botulinum toxin is now the treatment of choice (Miller 1987, Ludlow et al. 1988).

Botulinum toxin is now mainly used for the treatment of focal dystonias. Local injection in the region of motor plates produces in a few hours reduction of dystonia of the injected muscles which is maximal after a few days. After about 12 weeks motor power returns which may be due to the development of new synapses. Repeat injection is equally effective except in rare cases in which antibodies to the toxin develop (Brin et al. 1987, Jankovic and Schwartz 1991). Serotypes A and, recently, F (when resistance to A has developed) are used.

Selection of muscles to be treated is based on clinical examination, sometimes helped by EMG (Ostergaard et al. 1994). The dose used varies with the muscle mass and the degree of contracture and is usually of 40–100 units per muscle, distributed in three to five injections. Maximum total dose is 300 units. The toxin is diluted with saline (50 U/ml) We use the scale of Tsui et al. (1986) for grading the therapeutic effect. The area affected is dose-dependent (Borodic et al. 1994), and unwanted effects may result when other muscles are reached (Borodic et al. 1990).

Physiotherapy is useful for preventing or treating muscle retractions. Psychotherapeutic support is obviously necessary in a chronic disabling disease with preservation of intellectual function.

In summary, treatment of generalized dystonia in children requires consistency and common sense on the part of the family, patient and physician. The physician must keep in mind that benefit of treatment is seldom complete and stable, and advise the patient and family accordingly.

There are few reliable rules for determining the order of medication trials. There is

TABLE 5.10
Proposed treatment in generalized dystonia

Levodopa/carbidopa
↓
High-dose anticholinergics
↓
Other drugs: baclofen, carbamazepine, clonazepam, tetrabenazine
↓
Mixed therapy: anticholinergic + pimozide, and/or tetrabenazine and/or haloperidol
↓
Continuous infusion of intrathecal baclofen or chronic high-frequency basal nucleus stimulation

a consensus for the initial trial of L-dopa followed by anticholinergics. In case of failure, the ensuing steps are less secure. A proposed scheme is shown in Table 5.10.

REFERENCES

Adler CH, Wrabetz L (1996) Lesch–Nyhan variant: Dystonia, ataxia, near-normal intelligence, and no self-mutilation. *Mov Disord* 11: 583–4.

Agamanolis DP, Greenstein JI (1979) Ataxia–telangiectasia – A report of a case with Lewy bodies and vascular abnormalities within cerebral tissue. *J Neuropath Exp Neurol* 38: 475–89.

Ahmad F, Davis MB, Waddy HM, et al. (1993) Evidence for locus heterogeneity in autosomal dominant torsion dystonia. *Genomics* 15: 9–12.

Aicardi J, Barbosa C, Andermann E, et al. (1988) Ataxia–ocular motor apraxia: A syndrome mimicking ataxia–telangiectasia. *Ann Neurol* 24: 407–502.

— Bourgeois M, Goutières F (1995) Alternating hemiplegia in childhood: Clinical findings and diagnostic criteria. In: Andermann F, Aicardi J, Vigevano F (eds) *Alternating Hemiplegia in Childhood.* New York: Raven Press, pp. 3–18.

— Castelein P (1969) Infantile neuroaxonal dystrophy. *Brain* 102: 727–48,

Goutières F, Saudubray JM, Oyier H (1985) CT scans of infants with glutaric aciduria. *Dev Med Child Neurol* 27: 403–6.

Al Aqeel A, Rashed PT, Ozand J, et al. (1994a) Methylglutaconic aciduria. Ten new cases with a possible new phenotype. *Brain Dev* 16 (suppl): 23–32.

— — — et al. (1994b) A new patient with α-ketoglutaric aciduria and progressive extrapyramidal tract disease. *Brain Dev* 16 (suppl): 33–7.

Al-Essa MA, Al-Shamsan LA, Ozand PT (1999) Clinical and brain 18-fluoro-2-deoxyglucose positron emission tomographic findings in ethylmalonic aciduria, a progressive metabolic disease. *Eur J Ped Neurol* 3: 125–7.

Alford RL, Bedman JB, O'Brien WE et al. (1995) Lesch–Nyhan syndrome: Carrier and prenatal diagnosis. *Prenat Diagn* 15: 329–37.

Almasy L, Bressman SB, Raymond D, et al. (1997) Idiopathic torsion dystonia linked to chromosome 8 in two Mennonite families. *Ann Neurol* 42: 670–3.

Al Mateen M, Philipart M, Shields WD (1986) Rett syndrome: A commonly overlooked progressive encephalopathy in girls. *Am J Dis Child* 140, 761–76.

Aminoff MJ, Dedo HH, Izdebski K (1978) Clinical aspects of spasmodic dysphonia. *J Neurol Neurosurg Psychiatry* 41: 361–5.

Anderson LT, Ernst M (1994) Self-injury in Lesch–Nyhan disease. *J Autism Dev Disord* 24: 67–81.

Andrew J, Fowler CL, Harrison MJG (1983) Stereoataxic thalamotomy in 55 cases of dystonia. *Brain* 106: 981–100.

Angelini L, Rumi V, Nardocci N (1987) Idiopathic and symptomatic dystonias. In: Angelini L, et al. (eds) *Extrapyramidal Disorders in Childhood*. Amsterdam: Elsevier, pp. 81–98.

— Lamperti E, Nardocci N (1988) Transient paroxysmal dystonia in infancy. *Neuropediatrics* 19: 171–4.

— Nardocci N, Rumi V, Lampertie (1989) Idiopathic dystonia with onset in childhood. *J Neurol* 236: 319–21.

Artigas J, Ribes A, Rovira A, et al. (1993) Aciduria glutarica tipo I con quistes aracnoideos. *Rev Neurol* 23: 153–6.

Asher SW, Aminoff MJ (1981) Tetrabenazine and movement disorders. *Neurology* 31: 1051–4.

Awaad Y, Shamato H, Chugani H (1996) Hemidystonia improved by baclofen and PET scan findings in a patient with glutaric aciduria type I. *J Child Neurol* 11: 167–9.

Awaad Y, Munoz S, Nigro M (1999) Progressive dystonia in a child with chromosome 18p deletion, treated with intrathecal baclofen. *J Child Neurol* 14: 75–7.

Bakay B, Nissinen E, Sweetman L, et al. (1979) Utilization of purines by an HPRT variant in an intelligent, nonmutilative patient with features of the Lesch–Nyhan syndrome. *Pediatr Res* 13: 1365–70.

Ball MC, Sagar HJ (1995) Levodopa in pregnancy. *Mov Disord* 10: 115.

Barth PG, Hoffmann GF, Jaeken J, et al. (1992) L-2-Hydroxyglutaric acidemia: A novel inherited neurometabolic disease. *Ann Neurol* 32: 66–71.

— — — et al. (1993) L-2-Hydroxyglutaric acidaemia: Clinical and biochemical findings in 12 patients and preliminary report on L-2-hydroxyacid dehydrogenase. *J Inherited Metab Dis* 16: 753–61.

Batshaw ML, Wachtel RC, Deckel AW, et al. (1985) Munchausen's syndrome simulating torsion dystonia. *N Engl J Med* 312: 1437–9.

Beltran RS, Coker SB (1995) Transient dystonia of infancy, a result of intrauterine cocaine exposure? *Ped Neurol* 12: 354–6.

Benabid AL, Benazzouz A, Limousin P, et al. (2000) Dyskinesias and the subthalamic nucleus. *Ann Neurol* 47 (suppl. 1): S189–S192.

Benecke R, Strümper P, Weiss H (1992) Electron transfer complex I defect in idiopathic dystonia. *Ann Neurol* 32: 683–6.

Bennett MJ, Marlow N, Pollitt RJ, Wales JKH (1986) Glutaric aciduria type I: Biochemical investigations and postmortem findings. *Eur J Pediatr* 145: 403–5.

Bergman I, Finegold D, Gatner JC, et al. (1989) Acute profound dystonia in infants with glutaric acidemia. *Pediatrics* 83: 228–34.

Bhatia KP, Marsden CD (1994) The behavioural and motor consequences of focal lesions of the basal ganglia in man. *Brain* 117: 859–76.

Biglan AW (1984) Setting sun sign in infants. *Am Orthoptic J* 34: 114–6.

Blond S, Caparros-Lefebvre D, Parker F, et al. (1992) Control of tremor and involuntary movement disorders by chronic stereotactic stimulation of the ventral intermediate thalamic nucleus. *J Neurosurg* 77: 62–

Bodensteiner JB, Goldblum RM, Goldman AS (1980) Progressive dystonia masking ataxia in ataxia–telangiectasia. *Arch Neurol* 37: 464–5.

Borodic GE, Ferrante R, Pearce B, Smith K (1994) Histological assessment of dose-related diffusion and muscle fiber response after therapeutic botulinum A toxin injections. *Mov Disord* 9: 31–9.

Borodic GE, Joseph M, Fay L, et al. (1990) Botulinum A toxin for the treatment of spasmodic torticollis: Dysphagia and regional toxin spread. *Head Neck* 12: 382–98.

Boulloche J, Aicardi J (1986) Pelizaeus–Merzbacher disease: Clinical and nosological study. *J Child Neurol* 1: 233–9.

Boyd K, Patterson V (1989) Dopa responsive dystonia: a treatable condition misdiagnosed as cerebral palsy. *BMJ* 298: 1019–20.

Brandel J-P, Vidailhet M, Noseda G, et al. (1996) *Mycoplasma pneumoniae* postinfectious encephalomyelitis with bilateral striatal necrosis. *Mov Disord* 11: 333–5.

Brandt NJ, Gregersen N, Christensen E, et al. (1979) Treatment of glutaryl-CoA dehydrogenase deficiency (glutaric aciduria). *J Pediatr* 94: 669–73.

Braütigam C, Wevers RA, Jansen RJT, et al. (1998) Biochemical hallmarks of tyrosine hydroxylase deficiency. *Clin Chem* 44: 1897–904.

Bray PF, Herbst JJ, Johnson DG, et al. (1977) Childhood gastro-oesophageal reflux. Neurologic and psychiatric syndromes mimicked. *JAMA* 237: 1342–5.

Bressman SB, De Leon D, Brin MF, et al. (1989) Idiopathic dystonia among Ashkenazi Jews: Evidence for autosomal dominant inheritance. *Ann Neurol* 26: 612–20.

— De Leon D, Kramer PL, et al. (1994a) Dystonia in Ashkenazi Jews: Clinical characterization of a founder mutation. *Ann Neurol* 36: 771–7.

— Hunt AL, Heiman GA, et al. (1994b) Exclusion of the DYT1 locus in a non-Jewish family with early-onset dystonia. *Mov Disord* 9: 626–32.

— Warner TT, Almasy L, et al. (1996) Exclusion of the DYT1 locus in familial torticollis. *Ann Neurol* 40: 681–4.

Brett EM, Hoare RD, Sheehy MP, Marsden CD (1981) Progressive hemidystonia due to focal basal ganglia lesion after mild head trauma. *J Neurol Neurosurg Psychiatry* 44: 460.

Brin MF, Fahn S, Moskowitz C, et al. (1987) Localized injections of botulinum toxin for the treatment of focal dystonia and hemifacial spasm. *Mov Disord* 2: 237–54.

Broessmann U, Schwartz JF (1973) Familial striatal degeneration. *Arch Neurol* 29: 314–7.

Bundey S, Harrison MJG, Marsden CD (1975) A genetic study of torsion dystonia. *J Med Genet* 12: 12–19.

Burke RE, Brin MF, Fahn S, et al. (1986a) Analysis of the clinical course of non-Jewish autosomal dominant torsion dystonia. *Mov Disord* 1: 163–78.

Fahn S, Marsden CD (1986b) Torsion dystonia: A double blind prospective trial of high dosage trihexyphenidyl. *Neurology* 36: 160–4.

Burlina AB, Dionisi-Vici C, Bennett MJ, et al. (1994) A new syndrome with ethylmalonic aciduria and fatty acid oxidation in fibroblasts. *J Pediatr* 124: 74–86.

Burton K, Farrell K, Li D, Calne DB (1984) Lesions of the putamen and dystonia: CT and magnetic resonance imaging. *Neurology* 34: 962–5.

Busquets C, Coll MJ, Christensen E, et al. (1998) Feasibility of molecular prenatal diagnosis of glutaric aciduria type I in chorionic villi. *J Inherited Metab Dis* 21: 243–6.

Campistol J, Fernandez-Alvarez E, Cusi V (1984) CT scan appearance in subacute necrotising encephalomyelopathy. *Dev Med Child Neurol* 26: 519–22.

— Cusi V, Vernet A, Fernández-Alvarez E (1986) Dystonia as a presenting sign of subacute necrotizing encephalomyelopathy in infancy. *Eur J Pediatr* 144: 589–91.

— Fernández-Alvarez E, Ruscalleda J (1987) CT appearance of low attenuation areas in basal ganglia in childhood: Report of 23 cases. *Computerized Radiol* 11: 229–35.

— Ribes A, Alvarez L, et al. (1992) Glutaric aciduria type I: Unusual biochemical presentation. *J Pediatr* 121: 83–6.

Carson NAJ, Cusworth DC, Dent CE, et al. (1963) Homocystinuria: A new inborn error of metabolism associated with mental deficiency. Arch Dis Child 38: 425–36.

Casaer P (1987) Flunarizine in alternating hemiplegia in childhood. An international study of 12 children. *Neuropediatrics* 18: 191–5.

Cernerud L (1945) The setting sun sign eye phenomenon in infancy. *Dev Med Child Neurol* 17: 447–55.

Charles PD, Davis TL, Robertson D, FenicheL GM (1995) Dystonia and unique muscle features. A 23-year follow-up and correction of diagnosis in two brothers. *Arch Neurol* 52: 825–6.

Cho CH, Mamourian AC, Filiano J, Nordgren RE (1995) Glutaric aciduria: Improvement MR appearance after aggressive therapy. *Pediatr Radiol* 25: 484–5.

Chow CW, Haan EA, Goodman SI, et al. (1988) Neuropathology in glutaric acidemia type I. *Acta Neuropathol* 76: 590–4.

Christensen E, Brandt NJ (1978) Studies on glutaryl-CoA dehydrogenase on leukocytes, fibroblasts and amniotic fluid cells. The normal enzyme and the mutant form in patients with glutaric aciduria. *Clin Chem Acta* 88: 267.

— Ribes A, Busquets C, et al. (1997) Compound heterozygotes with S227P mutation on one allele in the glutaryl-CoA dehydrogenase gene is associated with no or very low glutarate excretion. *J Inherited Metab Dis* 20: 383–6.

Christie R, Bay C, Kaufman A, et al. (1982) Lesch–Nyhan disease: clinical experience with nineteen patients. *Dev Med Child Neurol* 24: 293–306.

Cook DG, Klawans HL (1985) Levodopa during pregnancy. *Clin Neuropharmacol* 8: 93–5.

Cooper IS, Cullinan T, Riklan, M (1976) The natural history of dystonia. In: Eldridge R, Fahn S (eds) *Advances in Neurology. Vol. 14. Dystonia.* New York: Raven Press, pp. 157–69.

Corbin D, Williams A, Johnson AP (1987) Dystonia complicated with respiratory obstruction. *J Neurol Neurosurg Psychiatry* 50: 1707.

Costeff H, Gadoth N, Mendelson L, et al. (1987) Fluctuating dystonia responsive to levodopa. *Arch Dis Childh* 62: 801–4.

— — Apter N, et al. (1989) A familial syndrome of infantile optic atrophy, movement disorder, and spastic paraplegia. *Neurology* 39: 595–7.

— Elpeleg O, Apter N, et al. (1993) 3-Methylglutaconic aciduria in "optic atrophy plus". *Ann Neurol* 33: 103–4.

Craver RD, Duncan MC, Nelson JS (1996) Familial dystonia and choreoathetosis in three generations associated with bilateral striatal necrosis. *J Child Neurol* 11: 185–8.

Cusmai R, Bertini E, Di Capua M, et al. (1994) Bilateral, reversible, selective thalamic involvement demonstrated by brain RM and acute severe neurological dysfunction with favourable outcome. *Neuropediatrics* 25: 44–7.

Darras BT, Gilmore HE (1985) Focal intermittent dystonia in Hartnup disease. *Ann Neurol* 18: 397–8.

Davis PC, Hoffman JC, Braun IF, et al. (1987) MR of Leigh's disease (subacute necrotizing encephalomyelopathy). *Am J Neuroradiol* 8: 71–5.

De Jong APJM, Haan EA, Manson JI, et al. (1989) Kinetic study of catecholamine metabolism in hereditary progressive dystonia. *Neuropediatrics* 20: 3-11.

De Klerk JBC, Huijmans JGM, Stroink H, et al. (1997) L-2-Hydroxyglutaric aciduria: Clinical heterogeneity versus biochemical homogeneity in a sibship. *Neuropediatrics* 28: 314–7.

Demaerel P, Kendall BE, Kingsley D (1992) Cranial CT and RMI in diseases with DNA repair defects. *Neuroradiology* 34: 117–21.

Demierre B, Rondot P (1983) Dystonia caused by putamino-capsulo-caudate lesions. *J Neurol Neurosurg Psychiatry* 46: 404–9.

Deonna T, Ferreira A (1985) Idiopathic fluctuating dystonia: a case of foot dystonia and writer's cramp responsive to L-dopa. *Dev Med Child Neurol* 27: 814–21.

— Fernández E, Gardner-Medwin D, et al. (1986) Dopa-sensitive progressive dystonia of child-hood with fluctuations of symptoms. Segawa's syndrome and possible variants. Results of a collaborative study of the European Federation of Child Neurology Societies. *Neuropediatrics* 17: 86–93.

— Ziegler AL, Nielsen J (1991) Transient idiophatic dystonia in infancy. *Neuropediatrics* 22: 220–4.

— Roulet E, Ghika J, Esiger P (1997) Dopa-responsive childhood dystonia: a forme fruste with writer's cramp, triggered by exercise. *Dev Med Child Neurol* 39: 49–53.

De Sousa C, Piesowicz AT, Brett EM, Leonard JV (1989) Focal changes in the globi pallidi asso-ciated with neurological dysfunction in methylmalonic acidaemia. *Neuropediatrics* 20: 199–201.

De Vivo DC, Di Mauro S (1990) Mitochondrial encephalomyopathies. *Int Pediatr* 5: 112–20.

De Yebenes JG, Moskowitz C, Fahn S, Saint-Hilaire MH (1988) Long-term treatment with levo-dopa in a family with autosomal dominant torsion dystonia. In: Fahn S, Marsden CD, Calne DF (eds) *Advances in Neurology. Vol. 50. Dystonia 2.* New York: Raven Press, pp. 101–11.

Dick AP, Stevenson CJ (1953) Hereditary spastic paraplegia. Report of a family with associated extrapyramidal signs. *Lancet* 1, 21.

Diogo L, Fineza I, Canha J, et al. (1996) Macrocephaly as the presenting feature of L-2-hydroxy-glutaric aciduria in a 5-months-old boy. *J Inherited Metab Dis* 19: 369–70.

Dooling EC, Adams RD (1975) The pathological anatomy of posthemiplegic athetosis. *Brain* 98: 29–48.

Dunn HG, Perry TL, Dolman CL (1966) Homocystinuria. A recently discovered cause of mental defect and cerebrovascular thrombosis. *Neurology* 16: 407–20.

Dusser A, Goutières F, Aicardi J (1986) Ischemic strokes in children. *J Child Neurol* 1: 131–6.

Eicke M, Briner J, Willi U, et al. (1992) Symmetrical thalamic lesions in infants. *Arch Dis Childh* 62: 15–19.

Elpeleg ON, Costeff H, Joseph A, et al. (1994) 3-Methylglutaconic aciduria in the Iraqi–Jewish 'optic atrophy plus' (Costeff) syndrome. *Dev Med Child Neurol* 36: 167–72.

Eldridge R (1970) The torsion dystonias: Literature review on genetic and clinical studies. *Neurology* 20 (suppl): 78.

Gottlieb R (1976) The primary hereditary dystonias: Genetic classification of 768 families and revised estimate of gene frequency, autosomal recessive form and related bibliography. *Adv Neurol* 14: 457–74.

— Harla A, Cooper IS, Riklan M (1970) Superior intelligence in recessively inherited torsion dystonia. *Lancet* 1: 64.

Factor SA, Sanchez-Ramos J, Weiner WJ (1988) Delayed onset dystonia associated with cortico-spinal tract dysfunction. *Mov Disord* 3: 201–10.

Fahn S (1983) High dosage anticholinergic therapy in dystonia. *Neurology* 33: 1255–61.

— (1988) Concept and classification of dystonia. *Adv Neurol* 50: 1–8.

— Sjaastad O (1991) Hereditary essential myoclonus in a large Norwegian family. *Mov Disord* 6: 237–47.

— Williams DW (1988) Psychogenic dystonia. *Adv Neurol* 50: 431.

— Marsden CD, Calne DB (1987) Classification and investigations of dystonia. *Mov Disord* 2: 332–58.

Fenichel GM, Olson WH, Kilrov AW (1971) Hereditary dystonia associated with unique features in skeletal muscle. *Arch Neurol* 25: 552–9.

Fernández-Alvarez E, Peña J, Lorente I (1980) Distonía muscular deformante. In: Fernández-Alvarez E, Fejerman N, Campos J (eds) *Actualidades en Neuropediatria.* Barcelona: Edicion Medica y Técnica, pp. 179–203.

— Ribes A, Vilaseca MA (1999) Forme atypique d'acidurie glutarique. *Rev Neurol* 155: 980 (abstract).

Fink JK, Barton N, Cohen W, et al. (1988) Dystonia with marked diurnal variation associated with biopterin deficiency. *Neurology* 38: 707–11.

— Ravin P, Argoff CE, et al. (1989) Tetrahydrobiopterin administration in biopterin deficient progressive dystonia with marked diurnal fluctuation. *Neurology* 39: 1393–5.

Fitzgerald PM, Jankovic J, Glaze DG, et al. (1990) Extrapyramidal involvement in Rett's syndrome. *Neurology* 40: 293–5.

Fletcher NA, Harding AE, Marsden CD (1990) Genetic study of idiopathic torsion dystonia in the United Kingdom. *Brain* 113: 380–94.

— Thompson PD, Scadding JW, Marsden CD (1993) Successful treatment of childhood onset symptomatic dystonia with levodopa. *J Neurol Neurosurg Psychiatry* 56: 865–7.

Floret D, Divry P, Dingeon N, Monnet P (1979) Acidurie glutarique: Une nouvelle observation. *Arch Fr Pédiatr* 36: 462–70.

Ford B, Greene P, Louis DE, et al. (1996) Use of intrathecal baclofen in the treatment of patients with dystonia. *Arch Neurol* 53: 1241–6.

Friede RL (1989) *Developmental Neuropathology.* Vienna: Springer.

Friedman DI, Jankovic J, Rolak LA (1986) Arteriovenous malformation presenting as hemidystonia. *Neurology* 36: 1590–3.

Furukawa Y, Kish SJ, Bebin M, et al. (1998) Dystonia with motor delay in compound heterozygotes for GPT-cyclohydrolase I gene mutations. *Ann Neurol* 44: 10–16.

Fujita K, Takeuchi Y, Nishimura A, et al. (1994) Serial MRI in infantile bilateral striatal necrosis. *Pediatr Neurol* 10: 157–60.

Gallego J, Obeso JA, Delgado G, Villanueva JA (1986) Enfermedad de Leigh con distonia de torsión como única manifestación clínica. *Arch Neurobiol* 49: 73–8.

Gascon GG, Ozand PT, Brismar J (1994) Movement disorders in childhood organic acidurias. Clinical, neuroimaging, and biochemical correlations. *Brain Dev* 16 (suppl): 94–103.

Gasser T, Windgassen K, Bereznai B, et al. (1998) Phenotypic expression of the DYT1 mutation: A family with writer's cramp of juvenile onset. *Ann Neurol* 44: 126–8.

Gellis SS, Feingold M (1971) Syndrome of hiatus hernia with torsion spasms and abnormal posturing. *Am J Dis Child* 121: 53–4.

Gibson JB, Carson NAJ, Neill DW (1964) Pathological findings in homocystinuria. *J Clin Path* 17: 427–37.

Gibson KM, Nyhan WL, Sweetman L, et al. (1988) 3-Methylglutaconic aciduria: a phenotype in which activity of 3-methylglutaconyl-coenzyme A hydrolase is normal. *Eur J Pediatr* 148: 76–82.

— Sherwood WG, Hoffmann GF, et al. (1991) Phenotypic heterogeneity in the syndromes of 3-methylglutaconic aciduria. *J Pediatr* 118: 885–90.

— Elpeleg ON, Jalobs C, et al. (1993) Multiple syndromes of 3-methylglutaconic aciduria. *Pediatr Neurol* 9: 120–3.

Giladi N, Burke RE, Kostic V, et al. (1990) Hemiparkinsonism–hemiatrophy syndrome: Clinical and neuroradiological features. *Neurology* 40: 1731–4.

Gilman S, Horenstein S (1964) Familial amyotrophic dystonic paraplegia. *Brain* 87: 51–66.

— Junck L, Young AB, et al. (1988) Cerebral metabolic activity in idiopathic dystonia studied with positron emission tomography. In: Fahn S, Marsden CD, Calne DF (eds) *Advances in Neurology. Vol. 50. Dystonia 2.* New York: Raven Press, pp. 231–6.

Giroud M, Dumas R (1988) Dystonie secondaire à un infarctus putamino-capsulo-caudé chez l'enfant. *Rev Neurol* 144: 375–7.

Goetz CG, Penn RD, Tanner CM (1988) Efficacy of cervical cord stimulation in dystonia. *Adv Neurol* 50: 645–9.

Goldman JE, Katz D, Rapin I, et al. (1981) Chronic GM1 gangliosidosis presenting as dystonia. I. Clinical and pathological features. *Ann Neurol* 9: 465–75.

Gollomp SM, Fahn S (1987) Transient dystonia as a complication of varicella. *J Neurol Neurosurg Psychiatry* 50: 1228–9.

Golstein M, Anderson LT, Reuben R, Dancis J (1985) Self-mutilation in Lesch–Nyhan disease is caused by dopaminergic denervation. *Lancet* 1: 338–9.

Goodman SI, Frerman FE (1995) Organic acidemias due to defects in lysine oxidation: 2-keto-adipic acidemia and glutaric acidemia. In: Scriver CR, Beaudet AL, Sly WS, Valle D (eds) *The Metabolic Basis of Inherited Disease.* New York: McGraw-Hill, pp. 1451–60.

— Noremberg MD (1983) Glutaric acidemia as a cause of striatal necrosis in childhood. *Ann Neurol* 13: 582–3.

— — Shikes RH, et al. (1977) Glutaric aciduria: Biochemical and morphologic considerations. *J Pediatr* 90: 746–50.

— Kratz LE, Di Giulio KA, et al. (1995) Cloning of glutaryl-CoA dehydrogenase cDNA, and expression of wild type and mutant enzymes in *Escherichia coli. Hum Mol Genet* 4: 1493–8.

Gordon BA, Gordon KE, Seo HC, et al. (1995) Fucosidosis and dystonia. *Neuropediatrics* 26: 325–7.

Gordon MF, Bressman S, Brin MF, et al. (1995) Dystonia in a patient with deletion of 18q. *Mov Disord* 10: 496–9.

Gorke W, Bartholomew K (1990) Biochemical and neurophysiological investigations in two forms of Segawa's disease. *Neuropediatrics* 21: 3–8.

Gottlieb RP, Koppel MM, Nyhan WL, et al. (1982) Hyperuricaemia and choreoathetosis in a child without mental retardation or self-mutilation – a new HPRT variant. *J Inherited Metab Dis* 5: 183–6.

Goutières F, Aicardi J (1982) Acute neurological dysfunction associated with destructive lesions of the basal ganglia in children. *Ann Neurol* 12, 328–32.

Grandas F, Elston J, Quinn N, Marsden CD (1988) Blepharospasm: A review of 264 patients. *J Neurol Neurosurg Psychiatry* 51, 767–72.

Greenberg CR, Duncan AMV, Gragory CA, et al. (1994) Assignment of human glutaryl-CoA dehydrogenase gene (*GCDH*) to the short arm of chromosome 19 (19p13.2) by in situ hybridization and somatic cell hybrid analysis. *Genomics* 21: 289–90.

Greene P (1995) Medical and surgical therapy of idiopathic torsion dystonia. In: Kurlan R (ed) *Treatment of Movement Disorders.* Philadelphia: JB Lippincott, pp. 153–81.

— Fahn S (1992) Baclofen in the treatment of idiopathic dystonia in children. *Mov Disord* 7: 48–52.

— Shale H, Fahn S (1988) Analysis of open-label trials in torsion dystonia using high dosages of anticholinergics and other drugs. *Mov Disord* 3: 46–60.

— Kang UJ, Fahn S (1995) Spread of symptoms in idiopathic torsion dystonia. *Mov Disord* 10: 143–52.

Greenwood S, Nelson JS (1978) Atypical neuronal ceroid-lipofuscinosis. *Neurology* 28: 710–7.

Gregersen N, Brandt NJ, Christensen E, et al. (1977) Glutaric aciduria: Clinical and laboratory findings in two brothers. *J Pediatr* 90: 740.

Greter J, Hagberg B, Stern G, Soderhjelm U (1978) 3-Methylglutaconic aciduria: a report on a sibship with infantile progressive encephalopathy. *Eur J Paediatr* 29: 231–8.

Grimes JD, Hassan MN, Quarrington AM, d'Alton J (1982) Delayed onset post-hemiplegic dystonia: CT demonstration of basal ganglia pathology. *Neurology* 32: 1033.

Guazzi GC, d'Amore I, van Hoof F, et al. (1988) Type 3 (chronic) GM1 gangliosidosis presenting as infanto-choreo athetotic dementia, without epilepsy, in three children. *Neurology* 38: 1124–7.

Guerrini R, Bonanni P, Nardocci N, et al. (1999) Autosomal recessive rolandic epilepsy with paroxysmal exercise-induced dystonia and writer's cramp: Delineation of the syndrome and gene mapping to chromosome 16p12–11.2. *Ann Neurol* 45: 344–52.

Haar F, Dyken P (1977) Hereditary nonprogressive athetosis hemiplegia. A new syndrome. *Neurology* 27: 849–54.

Haas RH, Marsden CD, Capistrano-Strada S, et al. (1995) Acute basal ganglia infarction in propionic acidemia. *J Child Neurol* 10: 18–22.

Haberhausen G, Schmit Y, Kohler A, et al. (1995) Assignment of the dystonia/parkinsonism syndrome locus, DYT3 to a small region within a 1-8-Mb YAC contig of Xq13.1. *Am J Hum Genet* 57: 644–50.

Hagberg B, Kyllerman M, Steen G (1979) Dyskinesia and dystonia in neurometabolic disorders. *Neuropädiatrie* 10: 305–20.

Hald JK, Nakstad PH, Skjeldal OH, Stromme P (1991) Bilateral arachnoid cysts of the temporal fossa in four children with glutaric aciduria type I, *AJNR* 12: 407–9.

Hardie RJ, Young EP, Morgan-Hughes JA (1988) Hexosaminidase A deficiency presenting as juvenile progressive dystonia. *J Neurol Neurosurg Psychiatry* 51: 446–59.

Hargrave DR, Webb DW (1998) Movement disorders in association with herpes simplex virus encephalitis in children: a review. *Dev Med Child Neurol* 40: 640–2.

Haworth JC, Booth FA, Chudley AE, et al. (1991) Phenotypic variability in glutaric aciduria type I: Report of fourteen cases in five Canadian Indian kindreds. *J Pediatr* 118: 52–8.

Hayes MW, Ouvrier RA, Evans W, et al. (1998) X-linked dystonia–deafness syndrome. *Mov Disord* 13: 303–8.

Heindereich R, Natowitcz M, Hainline BE, et al. (1988) Acute extrapyramidal syndrome in methylmalonic acidemia: "metabolic stroke" involving the globus pallidus. *J Pediatr* 113: 1022–7.

Herz E (1944a) Dystonia. Historical review: Analysis of dystonic symptoms and physiologic mechanism involved. *Arch Neurol Psychiatry* 51: 305–18.

— (1944b) Dystonia. II. Clinical classification. *Arch Neurol Psychiatry* 51: 319–55.

— (1944c) Dystonia. III. Pathology and conclusions. *Arch Neurol Psychiatry* 52: 20–6.

Hiel JAP, Weemaes CMR, Sweets DFMC, et al. (1994) Late-onset ataxia–telangiectasia in two brothers presenting with juvenile resting tremor. *Mov Disord* 9: 460–2.

Hirano M, Tamaru Y, Ito H, et al. (1996) Mutant GTP cyclohydrolase I levels contribute to dopa-responsive dystonia onset. *Ann Neurol* 40: 796–8.

Hoffmann GF, Trefz FK, Barth P, et al. (1991) Glutaryl-CoA dehydrogenase deficiency. A distinct encephalopathy. *Pediatrics* 88: 1194–203.

— Jakobs C, Holmes B, et al. (1995) Organic acids in cerebrospinal fluid and plasma of patients with L-2-hydroxyglutaric aciduria. *J Inherited Metab Dis* 18: 189–93.

— Athanassopoulos S, Burlina AB, et al. (1996) Clinical course, early diagnosis, treatment, and prevention of disease in glutaryl-CoA dehydrogenase deficiency. *Neuropediatrics* 27: 115–23.

Hornykiewicz O, Kish SJ, Becker LE, et al. (1986) Brain neurotransmitters in dystonia musculo-rum deformans. *N Engl J Med* 315: 347–53.

Hoyt CS, Mousel DK, Weber AA (1980) Transient supranuclear disturbances of gaze in healthy neonates. *Am J Ophthalmol* 89: 708–13.

Hyland K, Surtees RAH, Rodeck C (1992) Aromatic L-aminoacid decarboxylase deficiency: Clinical features, diagnosis and treatment of a new inborn error of neurotransmitter amine synthesis. *Neurology* 42: 1980–8.

Hyland K, Fryburg JS, Wilson WG, et al. (1997) Oral phenylalanine loading in dopa-responsive dystonia: A possible diagnostic test. *Neurology* 48: 1290–7.

Iafolla AK, Kahler SG (1989) Megaloencephaly in the neonatal period as the initial manifestation of glutaric aciduria type I. *J Pediatr* 114:1004–6.

Ichinose H, Ohye T, Takahashi E, et al. (1994) Hereditary progressive dystonia with marked diur-nal fluctuation caused by mutations in the GTP cyclohydrolase 1 gene. *Nature Genet* 8: 236–42.

— — Matsuda Y, et al. (1996) Characterization of mouse and human GTP cyclohydrolase I genes. *J Biol Chem* 270: 1062–71.

Inui K, Namba R, Ihara Y, et al. (1990) A case of chronic GM1 gangliosidosis presenting as dystonia: Clinical and biochemical studies. *J Neurol* 237: 491–3.

Jankovic J (1982) Treatment of hyperkinetic movement disorders with tetrabenazine: A double-blind crossover study. *Ann Neurol* 11: 41–7.

— Fahn S (1988) Dystonic syndromes. In: Jankovic J, Tolosa E (eds) *Parkinson's Disease and Movement Disorders.* Baltimore/Munich: Urban & Schwartzenberg, pp. 283–314.

— Penn AS (1982) Severe dystonia and myoglobinuria. *Neurology* 32: 1195–7.

— Schwartz K (1991) Clinical correlates of response to botulinum toxin injections. *Arch Neurol* 48: 1253–6.

— van der Linden (1988) Dystonia and tremor induced by peripheral trauma. Predisposing factors. *J Neurol Neurosurg Psychiatry* 51: 1512–9.

Jin H, May M, Tranebjaerg L, et al. (1996) A novel X-linked gene, *DDP*, shows mutations in families with deafness (DFN-1), dystonia, mental deficiency and blindness. *Nature Genet* 14: 177–89.

Kaiser R, Ziegler G (1992) Hereditary progressive dystonia with diurnal fluctuation (Segawa's syndrome) – An unusual case. *Neuropediatrics* 23: 268–71.

Karpati G, Carpenter S, Wolfe LS, Andermann F (1977) Juvenile dystonic lipidosis: An unusual form of neurovisceral storage disease. *Neurology* 27: 32–42.

Kemspter PAK, Brenton DP, Gale AN, Stern GM (1990) Dystonia in homocystinuria. *J Neurol Neurosurg Psychiatry* 51: 859–62.

Kinsbourne M (1964) Hiatus hernia with contortions of the neck. *Lancet* 1: 1058–61.

Kiwack KJ, Deray MJ, Shields WD (1983) Torticollis in three children with syringomyelia and spinal cord tumour. *Neurology* 33: 946–8.

Klawans HL (1981) Hemiparkinsonism as a late complication of hemiatrophy: A new syndrome. *Neurology* 31: 625–8.

Knappskog PM, Flatmark T, Mallet J, et al. (1995) Recessively inherited L-dopa-responsive dystonia caused by a point mutation (Q381K) in the tyrosine hydroxylase gene. *Hum Mol Genet* 4: 1209–12.

Kobayashi T, Suzuki K (1981) Chronic GM1 gangliosidosis presenting as dystonia: II. Biochemical studies. *Ann Neurol* 19: 476–83.

Koch TK, Yee MH, Hutchinson HT, Berg BO (1986) Magnetic resonance imaging in subacute necrotizing encephalomyelopathy (Leigh's disease). *Ann Neurol* 19: 605–7.

Kohlschütter A, Behbehani A, Langenbeck U, et al. (1982) A familial progressive neurodegenerative disease with 2-oxyglutaric aciduria. *Eur J Pediatr* 138: 32–7.

Koep M, Schelosky L, Cordes I, et al. (1994) Dystonia in ataxia telangiectasia: Report of a case with putaminal lesions and decreased striatal [123-I]iodobenzamide binding. *Mov Disord* 9: 455–9.

Korf B, Wallman JK, Levy HL (1986) Bilateral lucency of the globus pallidus complicating methyl-malonic acidemia. *Ann Neurol* 20: 364–6.

Kramer PL, De Leon D, Ozelius L, et al. (1990) Dystonia gene in Ashkenazi Jewish population is located on chromosome 9q32–34. *Ann Neurol* 27: 114–20.

Kurlan R, Behr J, Medved L, Shoulson Y (1988) Myoclonus and dystonia: A family study. *Adv Neurol* 50: 385–9.

Kyllerman M, Steen G (1977) Intermittently progressive dyskinetic syndrome in glutaric aciduria. *Neuropädiatrie* 8: 397–404.

— Steen G (1980) Glutaric aciduria. A 'common' metabolic disorder? *Arch Fr Pédiatr* 37: 279 (letter).

— Forsgren L, Sanner G, et al. (1990) Alcohol-responsive myoclonic dystonia in a large family: Dominant inheritance and phenotypic variation. *Mov Disord* 5: 270–9.

— Skjeldal OH, Lundberg M, et al. (1994) Dystonia and dyskinesia in glutaric aciduria type I: Clinical heterogeneity and therapeutical considerations. *Mov Disord* 9: 22–30.

Lang AE (1995) Hemiatrophy, juvenile-onset exertional alternating leg paresis, hypotonia, and hemidystonia and adult-onset parkinsonism: The spectrum of hemiparkinsonism–hemiatrophy syndrome. *Mov Disord* 10: 489–95.

— Marsden CD (1982) Alphamethylparatyrosine and tetrabenazine in movement disorders. *Clin Neuropharmacol* 5: 375–87.

— Clarke JTR, Resch L, et al. (1985) Progressive long-standing "pure" dystonia: A new phenotype of juvenile metachromatic leukodystrophy (MLD). *Neurology* 35 (suppl 1): 194.

Ledoux MS, Lorden JL, Ervin JM (1993) Cerebellotomy eliminates the motor syndrome of the genetically dystonic rat. *Exp Neurol* 120: 302–10.

— Rutledge SL, Mountz JM, Darji JT (1995) SPECT abnormalities in generalized dystonia. *Pediatr Neurol* 13: 5–10.

Leenders KL, Frackowiak RSJ, Quinn N, et al. (1986) Ipsilateral blepharospasm and contralateral hemidystonia and parkinsonism in a patient with a unilateral rostral brainstem–thalamic lesion: Structural and functional abnormalities studied with CT, MRI, and PET scanning. *Mov Disord* 1: 51–8.

Leibel RL, Shih VE, Goodman SI, et al. (1980) Glutaric acidemia: A metabolic disorder causing progressive choreoathetosis. *Neurology* 30: 1163–8.

Lera G, Bhatia K, Marsden CD (1994) Dystonia as the major manifestation of Leigh's syndrome. *Mov Disord* 9: 642–9.

Leube B, Rudnicki D, Ratzlaff T, et al. (1996) Idiopathic dystonia – Assignment of a gene to chromosome 18p in a German family with adult onset, autosomal dominant inheritance and purely focal distribution. *Hum Mol Genet* 5: 1673–7.

— Hendgen T, Kessler KR, et al. (1997) Sporadic focal dystonia in Northwest Germany: Molecular basis on chromosome 18p. *Ann Neurol* 42: 111–4.

Leuzzi V, Favata Y, Seri S (1988) Bilateral striatal necrosis. *Dev Med Child Neurol* 30: 252–7.

Levine HL, Wood BG, Batza E, et al. (1979) Recurrent laryngeal nerve section for spasmodic dysphonia. *Ann Otol Rhinol Laringol* 88: 527–30.

Lewitt PA, Miller LP, Levine RA, et al. (1986) Tetrahydrobiopterin in dystonia: Identification of abnormal metabolism and therapeutic trials. *Neurology* 36: 760–4.

Lloyd KG, Hornykiewicz O, Davidson L, et al. (1981) Biochemical evidence of dysfunction of brain neurotransmitters in the Lesch–Nyhan syndrome. *N Engl J Med* 305: 1106–11.

Lüdecke B, Dworniczak B, Bartholomé K, et al. (1995) A point mutation in the tyrosine hydroxylase gene associated with Segawa syndrome. *Hum Genet* 95: 123–5.

Ludlow CL, Nauton RF, Sedory SE, et al. (1988) Effects of botulinum toxin injections on speech in adductor spasmodic dysphonia. *Neurology* 38: 1220–5.

Lundemo G, Persson HE (1985) Hereditary essential myoclonus. *Acta Neurol Scand* 72: 176–9.

Macaya A, Munell F, Burke RE, De Vivo DC (1993) Disorders of movement in Leigh syndrome. *Neuropediatrics* 24: 60–7.

Maki Y, Akimoto H, Enomoto T (1980) Injuries of basal ganglia following head trauma in children. *Child's Brain* 7: 11–13.

Mandel H, Tirosh E, Berant M (1989) Sandifer syndrome reconsidered. *Acta Pediatr Scand* 78: 797–9.

Manji H, Howard RS, Miller DH, et al. (1998) Status dystonicus: The syndrome and its management. *Brain* 141: 243–52.

Maroteaux P (1973) Un nouveau type de mucopolysacharidose avec athétose et élimination urinaire de keratan sulfate. *Nouv Press Med* 11: 975–9.

Marsden CD (1981) Treatment of torsion dystonia. In: Barbeau A (ed) *Disorders of Movement.* Lancaster: NTP Press, pp. 81–104.

— Harrison MJG (1974) Idiopathic torsion dystonia (dystonia musculorum deformans). A review of forty two patients. *Brain* 97: 793–810.

— Quinn NP (1990) The dystonias. *BMJ* 300: 139–44.

— Harrison JG, Bundey S (1976) Natural history of idiopathic torsion dystonia. *Adv Neurol* 14: 177–87.

— Marion MH, Quinn N (1984) The treatment of severe dystonia in children and adults. *J Neurol Neurosurg Psychiatry* 47: 1166–73.

— Obeso JA, Zarranz JJ, Lang AE (1985) The anatomical basis of symptomatic hemidystonia. *Brain* 108: 463–83.

McGreevy P, Arthur M (1987) Effective behavioral treatment of self-biting by a child with Lesch–Nyhan syndrome. *Dev Med Child Neurol* 29: 529–40.

Meek D, Wolfe LS, Andermann E, Andermann F (1984) Juvenile progressive dystonia: A new phenotype of GM2 gangliosidosis. *Ann Neurol* 15: 348–52.

Micheli F, Fernandez Pardal M, Gatto E, Paradiso G (1991) Dopa responsive dystonia masquerading as idiopathic kyphoscoliosis. *Clin Neuropharmacol* 14: 367–71.

Midgard R, Aarli JA, Julsrud OJ, Odegaard H (1989) Symptomatic hemidystonia of delayed onset. Magnetic resonance demonstration of pathology in the putamen and the caudate nucleus. *Acta Neurol Scand* 79: 27–31.

Miller M (1987) Botulinum toxin injection of the vocal fold for spasmodic dysphonia: A preliminary report. *Arch Otholaryngol Head Neck Surg* 113, 603–5.

Miller VS, Packard AM (1998) Paroxysmal downgaze in term newborn infants. *J Child Neurol* 13: 294–5.

Mirowitz SA, Sartor K, Prensky AJ, et al. (1991) Neurodegenerative diseases in childhood: MR and CT evaluation. *J Comput Assist Tomogr* 15: 210–22.

Mitchell G, McInnes RR (1984) Differential diagnosis of cerebral palsy: Lesch–Nyhan syndrome without self-mutilation. *Can Med Assoc J* 130: 1323–4.

Mito T, Tanaka T, Becker LE, et al. (1986) Infantile bilateral striatal necrosis: Clinicopathological classification. *Arch Neurol* 43: 677–80.

Miyoshi K, Matsuoka T, Mizushima S (1969) Familial holotopistic striatal necrosis. *Acta Neuropathol* 13: 240–9.

Mizuguchi M (1997) Acute necrotizing encephalopathy of childhood: A novel form of acute encephalopathy prevalent in Japan and Taiwan. *Brain Dev* 19: 81–92.

— Abe J, Mikkaichi K, et al. (1995) Acute necrotizing encephalopathy of childhood: A new syndrome presenting with multifocal, symmetric brain lesions. *J Neurol Neurosurg Psychiatry* 58: 555–61.

Mizuno T, Yagari Y (1975) Prophylactic effect of L-5-hydroxytryptophan on self-mutilation in the Lesch–Nyhan syndrome. *Neuropediatrics* 6: 13–23.

Murphy WJ, Gellis SS (1977) Torticollis with hiatus hernia in infancy. Sandifer syndrome. *Am J Dis Child* 311: 564–5.

Mowat AP (1973) Dystonic reactions to drugs. *Dev Med Child Neurol* 15: 654–5.

Narbona J, Obeso JA, Martinez-Lage JM, Marsden CD (1984) Hemi-dystonia secondary to localized basal ganglia tumor. *J Neurol Neurosurg Psychiatry* 47: 704–9.

Narbona J, Poch-Olive MI (1985) Dystonie dans le syndrome de Rett. In: Szcliwowski H, Borman J (eds) *Progress en Neurologie Pédiatrique.* Brussels: Prodim, p. 248.

Nardocci N, Bertagnolio B, Rumi V, Angelini L (1992) Progressive dystonia symptomatic of juvenile GM2 gangliosidosis. *Mov Disord* 7: 66–7.

— — — et al. (1993) Chronic GM1 gangliosidosis presenting as dystonia: Clinical and biochemical studies in a new case. *Neuropediatrics* 24: 164–6.

Nath A, Jankovic J, Pettigrew LC (1987) Movement disorders and AIDS. *Neurology* 37: 37–41.

Naumann M, Pirker W, Reiners K, et al. (1997) [123 I (-CIT single-photon emission tomography in dopa-responsive dystonia. *Mov Disord* 12: 448–51.

Neville BGR, Lake BD, Stephens R, Sanders MD (1973) A neurovisceral storage disease with vertical supranuclear ophthalmoplegia and its relationship to Niemann–Pick disease. *Brain* 96: 97–120.

Niederwieser A, Blau N, Wang M, et al. (1984) GTP cyclohydrolase I deficiency, a new enzyme defect causing hyperphenylalaninemia with neopterin, biopterin, dopamine, and serotonin deficiencies and muscular hypotonia. *Eur J Pediatr* 141: 208–14.

Nigro MA, Martens ME, Awerbuch GI, et al. (1990) Partial cytocrome b deficiency and generalized dystonia. *Pediatr Neurol* 6: 407–10.

Nomura Y, Kase M, Igawa C, et al. (1984) A female case of hereditary progressive dystonia with marked diurnal fluctuation with favorable response to anticholinergic drugs for 25 years. *Clin Neurol* 22: 723.

Novotny EJ, Sing G, Wallace DC, et al. (1986) Leber's disease and dystonia: A mitochondrial disease. *Neurology* 36: 1053–60.

Nygaard TG (1993) Dopa-responsive dystonia: Delineation of the clinical syndrome and clues to pathogenesis. *Adv Neurol* 60: 577–85.

— Marsden CD, Duvoisin RC (1988) Dopa responsive dystonia. *Adv Neurol* 50: 377–84.

— Trugman JM, de Yebenes JG, Fahn S (1990) Dopa responsive dystonia: The spectrum of clinical manifestations in a large North American family. *Neurology* 40: 66–9.

— Marsden CD, Fahn S (1991) Dopa responsive dystonia: Long term treatment response and prognosis. *Neurology* 41: 174–81.

— Takahashi H, Heiman GA, et al. (1992) Long-term treatment response and fluorodopa positron emission tomographic scanning of parkinsonism in a family with dopa-responsive dystonia. *Ann Neurol* 32: 603–8.

— Snow BJ, Fahn S, Calne DB (1993a) Dopa responsive dystonia: Clinical characteristics and definition. In: Segawa M (ed) *Hereditary Responsive Dystonia with Marked Diurnal Fluctuation.* New York: Parthenon, pp. 21–35.

— Wilhelmsen KC, Risch NJ, et al. (1993b) Linkage mapping of dopa-responsive dystonia (DRD) to chromosome 14q. *Nature Genet* 5: 386–91.

Oates CE, Bosch EP, Hart MN (1986) Movement disorders associated with chronic GM2 gangliosidosis: Case report and review of the literature. *Eur Neurol* 25: 154.

Obeso JA, Gimenez-Roldan S (1988) Clinicopathological correlation in symptomatic dystonia. In: Fahn S, Marsden CD, Calne DF (eds) *Advances in Neurology. Vol. 50. Dystonia 2.* New York: Raven Press, pp. 113–32.

— Rothwell LC, Lang AE, Marsden CD (1983) Myoclonic dystonia. *Neurology* 33: 825–30.

Ochi J, Ukomo T, Uenoyama Y, et al. (1986) Symmetrical low density areas in bilateral thalami in an infant with measles encephalitis. *Comput Radiol* 10: 137–9.

Oki J, Yoshida H, Tokumitsu S, et al. (1995) Serial neuroimages of acute necrotizing encephalopathy associated with human herpesvirus 6 infection. *Brain Dev* 17: 356–9.

Osaka H, Kimura S, Nezu A, et al. (1993) Chronic subdural hematoma as an initial manifestation of glutaric aciduria type I. *Brain Dev* 15: 125–7.

Ostergaard L, Fulgsang-Frederiksen A, et al. (1994) Quantitative EMG in botulinum toxin treatment of cervical dystonia. A double-blind, placebo-controlled study. *EEG Clin Neurophysiol* 93: 434–9.

Ozand PT, Rashed M, Gascon GG, et al. (1994) Unusual presentations of propionic acidemia. *Brain Dev* 16 (suppl): 46–57.

Ozelius LO, Kramer PL, Moskowtiz CB, et al. (1989) Human gene for torsion dystonia located on chromosome 9q32–34. *Neuron* 2: 1427–34.

— Hewett JW, Page CE, et al. (1997) The early onset dystonia gene (*DYT1*) encodes an ATP-binding protein. *Nature Genet* 17: 40–8.

Pai GS, Sprenkle JA, Do TT, et al. (1980) Localization of loci for HPRT and glucose-6-phosphate dehydrogenase and biochemical evidence for non-random X-chromosome expression from studies of a human X-autosome translocation. *Proc Nat Acad Sci USA* 77: 2810.

Pedro J, Lobo N, Levy A (1995) Acute infantile thalamic necrosis. *Dev Med Child Neurol* 37: 1006–19.

Perez-Cerda C, Merinero B, Marti M, et al. (1998) An unusual late-onset case of propionic acidaemia: Biochemical investigations, neuroradiological findings and mutation analysis. *Eur J Pediatr* 157: 50–2.

Perlmutter JS, Ralche MR (1984) Pure hemidystonia with basal ganglion abnormalities on positron emission tomography. *Ann Neurol* 15: 228–33.

Pettigrew LC, Jankovic J (1985) Hemidystonia: A report of 22 patients and a review of the literature. *J Neurol Neurosurg Psychiatry* 48: 650–7.

Pineda M, Ribes A, Busquets C, et al. (1998) Glutaric aciduria type I with high residual glutaryl-CoA dehydrogenase activity. *Dev Med Child Neurol* 40: 840–2.

Protheroe SM, Mellor DH (1991) Imaging in influenza A encephalitis. *Arch Dis Childh* 66: 702–5.

Pueschel SM, Friedman JH, Shetty T (1992) Myoclonic dystonia. *Child's Nerv Syst* 8: 61–6.

Quinn NP, Marsden CD (1984) Dominantly inherited myoclonic dystonia with dramatic response to alcohol. *Neurology* 34: 236–7.

— Rothwell JC, Thompson PD, Marsden CD (1988) Hereditary myoclonic dystonia, hereditary torsion dystonia, and hereditary essential myoclonus: An area of confusion. *Adv Neurol* 50: 391–401.

Rahbeeni Z, Ozand PT, Rashed M, et al. (1994) 4-Hydroxybutyric aciduria. *Brain Dev* 16 (suppl): 64–71.

Rajput AH (1973) Levodopa in dystonia musculorum deformans. *Lancet* 24: 432.

— Gibb WRG, Zhong XH, et al. (1994) Dopa-responsive dystonia: Pathological and biochemical observations in a case. *Ann Neurol* 35: 396–402.

Rapin I, Suzuki K, Suzuki K, Valsamis MP (1976) Adult (chronic) GM2 gangliosidosis: Atypical spinocerebellar degeneration in a Jewish sibship. *Arch Neurol* 33: 120–30.

Reichmann H, Naumann M, Hauck S, Janetzky B (1994) Respiratory chain and mitochondrial deoxyribonucleic acid in blood cells from patients with focal and generalized dystonia. *Mov Disord* 9: 597–600.

Risch N, De Leon D, Ozelius L, et al. (1995) Genetic analysis of idiopathic torsion dystonia in Ashkenazi Jews and their recent descent from a small founder population. *Nature Genet* 9: 152–9.

Roessmann U, Schwartz JF (1973) Familial striatal degeneration. *Arch Neurol* 29: 314–7.

Roig M, Macaya A, Munell F, Capdevila A (1990) Acute neurologic dysfunction associated with destructive lesions of the basal ganglia. A benign form of infantile bilateral striatal necrosis. *J Pediatr* 117: 578–81.

Rondot P, Wevers RA (1999) Dystonie dopa-sensible. Forme récessive. Mutation du gène de la tyrosine-hydroxylase. *Bull Acad Nat Med* 183: 639–47.

— Ziegler M (1983) Dystonia L-dopa responsive or juvenile parkinsonism? *J Neural Transm Suppl* 19: 273–81.

— de Recondo J, Davous P, et al. (1982) Rigidité extrapyramidale avec dystonie, atrophie optique et atteinte bilatérale du putamen chez un adolescent. Forme juvénile de la maladie de Leigh. *Rev Neurol* 138: 143–8.

— Aicardi J, Goutières F, Ziegler M (1992) Dopa-sensitive dystonia. *Rev Neurol* 148: 680–8.

Roodhooft AM, Baumgartner ER, Martin JJ, et al. (1990) Symmetrical necrosis of the basal ganglia in methylmalonic acidemia. *Eur J Pediatr* 149: 582–4.

Rosemberg S, Amaral LC, Kliemann SE, Arita FN (1991) Acute encephalopathy with bilateral striatal necrosis. A distinctive clinicopathological condition. *Neuropediatrics* 23: 310–5.

Rothwell JC, Obeso JA (1987) The anatomical and physiological basis of torsion dystonia. *Mov Disord* 2: 313–31.

Rutledge JN, Hilal SK, Silver AJ, et al. (1988) Magnetic resonance imaging of dystonic states. In: Fahn S, Marsden CD, Calne DF (eds) *Advances in Neurology. Vol. 50. Dystonia 2.* New York: Raven Press, pp. 265–75.

Sakuragawa N (1995) Clinical findings in 23 Japanese patients with alternating hemiplegia of child-hood. In: Andermann F, Aicardi J, Vigevano F (eds.) *Alternating Hemiplegia in Childhood.* New York: Raven Press, pp. 43–7.

Sawle GV, Leenders KL, Brooks DJ, et al. (1991) Dopa-responsive dystonia: [18F] dopa positron emission tomography. *Ann Neurol* 30: 24–30.

Scribanu N, Kennedy C (1976) Familial syndrome with dystonia, neural deafness and possible intellectual impairment: Clinical course and pathological findings. In: Eldridge R, Fahn S (eds) *Advances in Neurology. Vol. 14. Dystonia.* New York: Raven Press, pp. 235–43.

Segawa M, Nomura Y (1993) Hereditary progressive dystonia with marked diurnal fluctuation. In: Segawa M (ed) *Hereditary Progressive Dystonia.* New York: Parthenon, pp. 3–19.

— Hosaka A, Miyagawa F, et al. (1976) Hereditary progressive dystonia with marked diurnal fluctuation. In: Fahn S, Eldridge R. (eds) *Advances in Neurology. Vol. 14. Dystonia.* New York: Raven Press, pp. 215–22.

— Nomura Y, Tanaka S, et al. (1988) Hereditary progressive dystonia with marked diurnal fluctuation. Considerations on its pathophysiology on the characteristics of clinical and polysomnographical findings. In: Fahn S, Marsden CD, Calne DF (eds) *Advances in Neurology. Vol. 50. Dystonia 2.* New York: Raven Press, pp. 367–76.

— — Yamashita S, et al. (1990) Long-term effects of L-dopa on hereditary progressive dystonia with marked diurnal fluctuation. In: Berardelli A, Benecke RM, Manfredi M, Marsden CD (eds) *Motor Disturbances II.* London: Academic Press, pp. 305–18.

Sellal F, Hirsch E, Barth P, et al. (1993) A case of symptomatic hemidystonia improved by ventro-posterolateral thalamic electrostimulation. *Mov Disord* 8: 515–8.

Shoffner JM, Brown MD, Stugard C, et al. (1995) Leber's hereditary optic neuropathy plus dystonia is caused by a mitochondrial DNA point mutation. *Ann Neurol* 38: 163–9.

Silverstein FS, Brunberg JA (1995) Postvaricella basal ganglia infarction in children. *AJNR* 16: 449–52.

— Johnston MV, Hutchinson RJ, Edwards NL (1985) Lesch–Nyhan syndrome: CSF neurotransmitter abnormalities. *Neurology* 35, 907–11.

Snow BJ, Nygaard TG, Takahashi H, Calne DB (1993) Positron emission tomographic studies of dopa-responsive dystonia and early onset idiopathic parkinsonism. *Ann Neurol* 34: 733–8.

Steinberger D, Webwe Y, Korinthenberg R, et al. (1998) High penetrance and pronounced variation in expressivity of GCH1 mutations in five families with Dopa-responsive dystonia. *Ann Neurol* 43: 634–9.

Stephenson JBP (1990) *Fits and Faints. Clinics in Developmental Medicine no 109.* London: Mac Keith Press.

Stockler S, Holzbach U, Hanefeld F, et al. (1994) Creatine deficiency in the brain: A new, treatable inborn error of metabolism. *Pediatr Res* 36: 409–13.

Stokke O, Eldjarn L, Norum KR, et al. (1967) Methylmalonic acidemia: A new inborn error of metabolism which may cause fatal acidosis in the neonatal period. *Scand J Clin Lab Invest* 20: 313–28.

Stromme P, Stokke O, Jellum E, et al. (1995) Atypical methylmalonic aciduria with progressive encephalopathy, microcephaly and cataract in two siblings – a new recessive syndrome? *Clin Genet* 48: 1–5.

Stutchfield P, Edwards MA, Gray RGF, et al. (1985) Glutaric aciduria type I misdiagnosed as Leigh's encephalopathy and cerebral palsy. *Dev Med Child Neurol* 27: 514–21.

Tanaka H, Endo K, Tsuji S, et al. (1995a) The gene for hereditary progressive dystonia with marked diurnal fluctuation maps to chromosome 14q. *Ann Neurol* 37: 405–8.

— Momoi T, Yoshida A, et al. (1995b) Type 3 GM1 gangliosidosis: Clinical and neuroradiological findings in an 11-year-old girl. *J Neurol* 242: 299–303.

Trane Bjaerg L, Schwartz C, Eriksen H, et al. (1995) A new X linked recessive deafness syndrome with blindness, dystonia, fractures and mental deficiency is linked to Xq22. *J Med Genet* 32: 257–63.

Tsui JK, Stoessl AJ, Eisen A, et al. (1986) 1986) Double-blind study of botulinum toxin in spasmodic torticollis. *Lancet* 2: 245–7.

Udani PM, Parekh UC, Dastur DK (1971) Neurological and related syndromes in CNS tuberculosis. *J Neurol Sci* 14: 341–57.

Uyama E, Terasaki T, Watanabe S, et al. (1992) Type 3 GM1 gangliosidosis: Characteristic MRI findings correlated with dystonia. *Acta Neurol Scand* 86: 609–15.

Vaamonde J, Narbona J, Weiser R, et al. (1994) Dystonic storms: A practical management problem. *Clin Neuropharmacol* 17: 344–7.

van den Heuvel LPWJ, Luiten B, Smeitink JAM, et al. (1998) A common point mutation in the tyrosine hydroxylase gene in autosomal recessive L-dopa-responsive dystonia in the Dutch population. *Hum Genet* 102: 644–6.

Van der Knaap MS, Valk J (1995) *Magnetic Resonance of Myelin, Myelination, and Myelin Disorders. 2nd edn.* Berlin: Springer-Verlag, pp. 220–2.

— Jakobs C, Hoffmann GF, et al. (1999) D-2-Hydroxyglutaric aciduria: Biochemical marker of clinical disease entity? *Ann Neurol* 45: 111–9.

Waltz JM (1981) Surgical approach to dystonia. In: Marsden CD, Fahn S (eds) *Movement Disorders*. London: Butterworth, pp. 300–7.

Wang HS, Huang SC, Hung PC (1994) Acute encephalopathy with panthalamic plus lesion: A major occurrence in oriental children? *Pediatr Neurol* 11: 135–6.

Watts RWE, Spellacy E, Gibbs DA, et al. (1982) Clinical, postmortem, biochemical and therapeutic observations on the Lesch–Nyhan syndrome with particular reference to the neurological manifestations. *Q J Med* 201: 43–78.

Weiner WJ, Lang AE (1989) *Movement Disorders. A Comprehensive Survey.* Mount Kisko, NY: Futura.

Werlin SL, d'Souza BJ, Hogan WJH, et al. (1980) Sandifer syndrome: an unappreciated clinical entity. *Dev Med Child Neurol* 22: 374–8.

Willemse J (1986) Benign idiopathic dystonia in the first year of life. *Dev Med Child Neurol* 28: 355–63.

— van Nieuwenhuizen O, Gooskens FH, Westenbergh GM (1984) Treatment of nonfluctuating progressive dystonia: A neuropharmacological approach. *Neuropediatrics* 15: 208–10.

Wolfson LI, Shapless NS, Thal LJ, et al. (1983) Decreased ventricular fluid in norepinephrine metabolite in childhood onset dystonia. *Neurology* 33: 369–72.

Woods CG, Taylor AMR (1992) Ataxia–telangiectasia in the British Isles: The clinical and laboratory features of 70 affected individuals. *Q J Med* 298: 169–79.

Yamamoto K, Chiba H, Ishitobi M, et al. (1997) Acute encephalopathy with bilateral striatal necrosis: Favourable response to corticosteroid therapy. *Eur J Paediatr Neurol* 1: 41–5.

Yanagisawa N, Goto A, Narabayashi H (1972) Familial dystonia musculorum deformans and tremor. *J Neurol Sci* 16: 125–36.

Yoshida K, Oshima A, Sakuraba H, et al. (1992) GM1-gangliosidosis in adults: Clinical and molecular analysis of 16 Japanese patients. *Ann Neurol* 31: 328–32.

Zeman W (1970) Pathology of the torsion dystonias (dystonia musculorum deformans). *Neurology* 20: 79–88.

— Dyken (1967) Dystonia musculorum deformans. Clinical, genetic and pathoanatomical studies. *J Psychiat Neurol Neurochir* 70: 77–121.

Ziegler DK (1981) Prolonged relief of dystonic movements with diazepam. *Neurology* 31: 1457–8.

Zweig RM, Hedreen JC, Jankel WR, et al. (1988) Pathology in brainstem regions of individuals with primary dystonia. *Neurology* 38: 702–6.

6
DISEASES WITH SEVERAL TYPES OF MOVEMENT DISORDER

In some disorders, several types of abnormal movements may coexist and none is characteristic so they cannot be dealt with in the chapters dedicated to specific types of abnormal movements. They are considered in this chapter, which covers Wilson disease, Hallervorden–Spatz disease and miscellaneous multisystem diseases.

WILSON DISEASE (WD)
WD (familial progressive hepatolenticular degeneration) is caused by abnormal deposition of copper in the liver, brain, cornea and other tissues. It is a genetically determined disorder with autosomal recessive inheritance. The gene has been mapped to chromosome 13, and cloned (Bull and Cox 1993, Petrukhin et al. 1993). The gene product is a protein very similar (54–76% homologous) to that of Menkes disease gene *MNK* (Petrukhin et al. 1994, Tanzi et al. 1993). The basic defect is of P-type ATPases involved in the cellular transport of copper. At least 100 different mutations have been identified (Thomas et al. 1995). Prevalence is estimated as between 0.5 (Scheinberg and Sternlieb 1999) and 3 per 100,000 (Saito 1981).

CLINICAL FEATURES
The age of onset, presenting symptoms and symptomatology of WD are quite variable. Major features are due to lesions of liver and/or brain. In most cases, clinical presentation depends on the organ most affected so that hepatic and neurological forms can be separated, even though in some cases both categories of symptoms can occur together or in succession and different forms also can occur in the same family (Walshe 1986).

Age of onset and clinical presentation both seem to be related to the characteristics of the mutation but there is no clear or constant correlation between the type of mutation and the clinical phenotype, both because of the large number of mutations detected and because most patients are compound heterozygotes. Mutations that are predicted to completely suppress the function of the gene have a younger average age of onset that missense mutations (Thomas et al. 1995). Factors other than the mutation such as dietary copper intake (copper is more available from meat than it is from vegetable foods) can also influence the phenotypic expression (Thomas et al. 1995).

Neurological manifestations (Table 6.1) usually appear after age 10 years, although onset of neurological symptoms in patients as young as 4 years has been occasionally reported (Walshe 1986, Kudo and Arima 1987). In children, neurological forms generally

TABLE 6.1
Type of first manifestations in Wilson disease
(N = 217)*

Hepatic	94
Neurological	90
Hepatic and neurological	4
Psychiatric	2
Rheumatological	2
Spontaneous mandibular dislocation	1
Presymptomatic diagnosis	24

*Reproduced by permission from Walshe (1986).

begin insidiously with mild tremor, dysarthria (Liao et al. 1991), writing difficulties, ataxic gait or dystonic movements, although rigid–akinetic syndrome, psychiatric disturbances or epilepsy (Stremmel et al. 1991) may be the first manifestation. Even hemiplegia has exceptionally been the initial feature (Lingam et al. 1987).

Four main neurological presentations can be described.

* The *dystonic form* is the most frequent. Focal dystonic postures, becoming generalized, is a quite frequent pattern of evolution in untreated cases. Facio-lingual and pharyngeal involvement is often prominent in these cases.

• The *pseudo-sclerotic form* is marked by dysarthria, intention tremor and asterixis.

• The *rigid–akinetic form* (rare in children) mimics juvenile parkinsonism.

• The *choreic form* is also infrequent in children.

About one-third of patients present for fairly long periods with *mental deterioration* and *psychiatric problems* (Oder et al. 1991).

Tremor frequently begins in an upper extremity and secondarily becomes generalized. Resting tremor with parkinsonian characteristics is most common (Walshe 1986), but postural tremor exacerbated with voluntary movements may also be seen. It can take the form of the so-called 'batwing' tremor when sought for in a patient with abducted shoulders and flexed arms. Action and/or postural dystonia may not differ from that in idiopathic torsion dystonia and tends to generalize rapidly. Gait may be 'staggering' and precipitate torsional movements. Retraction of the upper lip with an apparently fixed 'smile' and drooling is frequent. Facial grimacing is often a very prominent feature of WD. All movements increase with tension, improve with sedation and can disappear with sleep.

The language disorder consists of a peculiar dysarthria with monotonous speech as a consequence of complex abnormal movements of the tongue, lips, soft palate and vocal cords, and may evolve to complete anarthria if no treatment is given. In severe cases dysphagia may be associated (Haggstrom and Hirschowitz 1980).

Psychiatric manifestations and behaviour disorders are of special interest as they can remain isolated for months or years and are often responsible for diagnostic errors. About

25% of patients are first seen by psychiatrists (Scheinberg and Sternlieb 1999). Psychiatric disturbances are variable and may include anxiety neurosis, depression, antisocial behaviour and schizo-affective disease (Medalia et al. 1988).

Ocular abnormalities are usually silent but have a great diagnostic value. The most important is the Kayser–Fleischer ring, a golden coloured or brown–green pigmentation surrounding the corneal limb and representing a granular deposit of copper in Descemet's membrane (Harry and Tripathi 1970). Slit-lamp examination is usually necessary to demonstrate it, although it is sometimes visible with the naked eye. Even though a similar ring can exceptionally be observed with slit-lamp in other hepatic diseases (e.g. primary biliary cirrhosis, chronic active hepatitis or cryptogenetic cirrhosis) (Scheinberg and Sternlieb 1999), it is practically pathognomonic for WD. The Kayser–Fleischer ring almost always precedes the appearance of neurological abnormalities. However, a few undoubted cases of neurological WD with normal slit-lamp examination are on record (Ross et al. 1985, Lingam et al. 1987).

The 'sunflower cataract' is an uncommon manifestation of WD. It consists of a disc-shaped opacity with peripheral extensions towards the borders of the lens (Wiebers et al. 1977). It does not interfere with vision and, like the Kayser–Fleischer ring, disappears with treatment.

Hepatic abnormalities are the first manifestations of the disease in 50% of cases and can coexist with neurological forms in the same sibship. They are proteiform and include acute transient hepatitis, fulminating hepatitis, chronic active hepatitis and cirrhosis. Most patients with hepatic WD develop a Kayser–Fleischer ring but many can remain neurologically normal.

A less usual manifestation of WD is haemolytic anaemia (Werlin et al. 1978) which may also precede the neurological disturbances by months or years and is an important early diagnostic feature. Other blood anomalies (thrombocytopenia, coagulation problems) are probable consequences of liver and spleen involvement.

Skeletal abnormalities are frequent in WD and include articular degeneration, Schmorl nodules and narrowing of the intervertebral spaces. Renal tubular defects with proteinuria, microscopic haematuria and defect of acidification can occasionally produce a Fanconi syndrome. Dermatologic, cardiac and endocrine manifestations are infrequent.

BIOCHEMICAL INVESTIGATIONS

These are generally sufficient to confirm the clinical diagnosis. Plasma ceruloplasmin in WD is decreased to less than 20 mg/dL (normal values: 30–40 mg/dL) in 90–95% of patients (Gibbs and Walshe 1979, Brewer and Yuzbasiyan-Gurkan 1992), but normal blood ceruloplasmin values are more frequent in those patients with the hepatic form. Ceruloplasmin normally combines with copper and plays a role in its transport out of the liver. However, low ceruloplasmin has no primary role in the pathogenesis of WD and is, in fact, a secondary phenomenon. The gene for ceruloplasmin has been mapped to chromosome 3, whereas the WD gene maps to chromosome 13. Ceruloplasmin may also

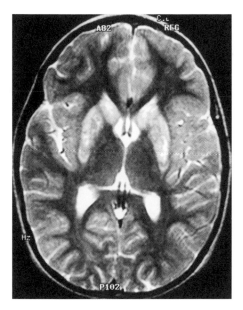

Fig. 6.1. T₂-weighted MRI of a 10-year-old boy with Wilson disease, showing symmetrical hyperintensity of caudate and lenticular nuclei.

be decreased in non-WD neonates (thus making the presymptomatic diagnosis difficult in this age group – Starosta-Rubinstein 1995), and in Menkes disease, the nephrotic syndrome, liver failure, enteropathy with protein loss, and sprue. About 20% of carriers of WD have hypoceruloplasminaemia. Rare cases of familial deficiency of ceruloplasmin are known (Edwards et al. 1979, Miyajima et al. 1987) but it is not related to WD and is not usually associated with clinical symptoms.

Cupraemia is decreased to less than 50 μg/dL while cupruria is augmented to more than 100 μg/dL. The former is a very specific finding because the only situation, other than WD, in which urinary copper may be elevated is obstructive liver disease (Brewer 1995). When in doubt, determination of cupruria following administration of penicillamine is more sensitive. The final test is determination of copper content in biopsied liver. Levels higher than 250 μg/g dry tissue are diagnostic.

NEUROIMAGING

In neurologically symptomatic patients, especially advanced cases, CT scans before treatment usually show areas of hypodensity in the putamen, caudate, dentate, red nucleus and cerebellar cortex. Dilatation of the ventricular system can also be associated (Williams and Walshe 1981). These areas do not take up contrast (Harik and Donovan 1981).

MRI is more sensitive (Fig. 6.1). It usually shows hypointensity on T₁-weighted and hyperintensity on T₂-weighted sequences in the lenticular nuclei, brainstem, claustrum and white matter (Starosta-Rubinstein et al. 1987, Sener 1993a). T₂ hypointensity has also been shown and may be explained by the paramagnetic effect of copper deposition

(Yuh and Flickinger 1988, Brugières et al. 1992), but high T_2 signal is more common. Sometimes cavitation of the basal ganglia can be found (Sener 1993b). CT and MRI also usually show a significant degree of cortical atrophy in the frontal lobes. CT and MRI abnormalities decrease and may disappear following treatment (Rothfus et al. 1977, Lingam et al. 1987).

DIAGNOSIS

Many of the initial clinical symptoms in WD are nonspecific, so a high index of suspicion is in order if detrimental diagnostic delay is to be avoided. Many cases are wrongly considered as 'neuropsychiatric' disorders. In one of my (EF-A) patients, the diagnosis was delayed because of atypical signs of polyneuropathy.

Slit-lamp examination in search of Kayser–Fleischer ring, and determination of serum ceruloplasmin and 24-hour copper excretion provide essential diagnostic clues. MRI and CT are useful and not infrequently suggest a diagnosis that had not been clinically considered.

The finding of low ceruloplasmin levels in apparently normal persons without Kayser–Fleischer ring may pose a diagnostic problem. Once previously quoted causes of low ceruloplasmin have been excluded, one is most likely dealing with a heterozygote for WD. If there is any evidence of copper accumulation by slit-lamp or chemical examination, treatment is indicated. Investigation of copper metabolism in siblings and close relatives should be systematic when WD is diagnosed.

Prenatal diagnosis is sometimes possible, but the large number of mutations makes it impractical in most cases. However, exclusion of the diagnosis may be possible when haplotypes of both affected and non-affected relatives are known. An acquired form of hepatolenticular degeneration has been reported and is obviously important for genetic reasons to be distinguished from WD (Victor et al. 1965).

PATHOLOGY

The characteristic CNS lesion is bilateral degeneration of the putamen with discoloration, softening and even cavitation. In advanced cases, thalamic nuclei, including the red nucleus, and cerebellar nuclei are similarly affected. Involvement of hemispheric white matter is rarely the most pronounced anomaly (Ishino et al. 1972). Cerebellar atrophy with neuronal loss and glial proliferation is frequent (Schulman and Barbeau 1963). Microscopically there is a marked proliferation of Alzheimer type II glia. Capillaries are congested and perivascular spaces are dilated.

PATHOGENESIS

The pathogenesis of the disease is imperfectly understood, although it is clearly due to a positive copper balance caused by an inability to excrete the normal amount of copper in the bile (Frommer 1974). Hypoceruloplasminaemia has no primary role in the pathogenesis of WD. Accumulation of copper is the cause of dysfunction and of damage to affected organs, especially brain and liver. Copper storage occurs first in the liver. When liver is saturated, storage affects the CNS, kidneys and eyes. Excess copper, mainly in ionic state, causes cell injury by harmful effects on mitochondria, peroxisomes and plasma membranes, destabilization of DNA, and inhibition of a large number of enzymes (Scheinberg and Sternlieb 1999). Probably copper exerts its toxic effects through an oxidant-damaging mechanism (Brewer and Yuzbasiyan-Gurkan 1992).

In the brain the putamen, globus pallidus and caudate are unusually sensitive to copper. White matter and cerebral cortex are also sensitive.

TREATMENT

The prognosis of WD has been transformed first by the discovery of the therapeutic efficacy of British anti-lewisite (BAL), then by that of D-penicillamine (dimethylcysteine) (Walshe 1956). The therapeutic goal is to increase the excretion of copper above what is ingested so as to restore a normal balance, or at least to improve it in symptomatic patients, or to prevent the development of the illness in presymptomatic persons (Starosta-Rubinstein 1995). The prognosis is largely dependent on the condition of patients at onset of therapy and on regularity of administration (Arima et al. 1977, Kudo and Arima 1987). Ideally, treatment is best started in the presymptomatic stage.

The drug to be used as initial therapy in neurological WD is controversial (LeWitt 1999). Penicillamine is still the most commonly used. Some authors consider it as the 'first choice' (Walshe 1999), while others write that it "should not be used [for initial therapy], pure and simple" (Brewer 1999). D-Penicillamine increases urinary copper excretion, produces regression of symptoms and improves function of the kidney, liver and brain, although it has no effect on such disturbances as osteoporosis or arthropathies. The daily dose is 20–30 mg/kg in three divided doses. It is best given on an empty stomach to maximize absorption (Bergstrom et al. 1981). Excretion of urinary copper should be verified to adjust the dose if necessary. In many cases, aggravation of the symptoms is observed during the first two months of treatment, so it is recommended to start with a low dose and increase it slowly (Brewer et al. 1987). Neurological deterioration coincident with penicillamine therapy is not rare. The mechanism of neurological worsening in such cases is not known with certainty. In these situations new white matter lesions may appear (Brewer et al. 1987).

The response to treatment can be dramatic in established cases. However, in late treated cases recovery is usually incomplete. Interruption of the treatment may result in fatality (Walshe and Dixon 1986).

About 20% of patients exhibit severe side-effects to the penicillamine which include fever, rashes, lymphadenopathy, leukopenia and thrombocytopenia. Later, arthritis, kidney disease or pancytopenia may occur. Penicillamine also may cause autoimmune conditions such as optic neuritis, IgA deficiency (Proesmans et al. 1976), myasthenia gravis (Masters et al. 1977) or dermatomyositis. Because of its nonspecificity as a chelator, penicillamine can produce zinc deficiency that can be responsible for skin lesions (van Caillie-Bertrand et al. 1985a). Penicillamine being an antagonist of vitamin B_6, pyridoxine (50 mg/d) should be added. Corticosteroids may be useful to attenuate some of the side-effects of penicillamine.

In rare emergency situations, plasma exchange or albumin infusions that increase copper binding capacity can be necessary.

The use of TETA (triethylene tetramine hydrochloride) has been suggested in an effort to avoid the problems of penicillamine therapy. Like D-penicillamine it acts as a chelator and increases copper excretion. The dose is 40–60 mg/kg/d in three divided doses. Unlike with D-penicillamine, toxic reactions are infrequent.

Another method proposed is the use of zinc acetate or zinc sulphate to block the absorption of copper in the intestine (Brewer et al. 1983, van Caillie-Bertrand et al. 1985b). In addition, zinc induces the synthesis of metallothionines that help decrease the absorption of copper. Brewer (1999) considers zinc as the treatment of choice for main-tenance therapy (including presymptomatic patients). Recommended doses of zinc sulphate are 50–100 mg three times daily (one hour before or one hour after meals) for patients under 10 years and 200–300 mg for those over this age. The dose of zinc acetate is 25% lower than zinc sulphate. It is an irritant of the intestinal mucosa, produces diarrhoea and may be rejected by patients Walshe (1986).

Tetrathiomolybdate has been also introduced (Brewer et al. 1991). It prevents copper absorption and also renders plasma copper unavailable for cellular uptake and depletes the copper pool. The recommended dose is 2–3 mg/kg/d.

Decreasing ingestion of copper is an adjuvant to therapy. A strict copper-deficient diet is difficult to observe but patients should be instructed to avoid foods with a high copper content such as liver, chocolate, coffee, shellfish, nuts and mushrooms (Starosta-Rubinstein 1995). Potassium iodide (20 mg four times daily) may also help decrease copper absorption.

In patients with fulminant hepatitis or chronic severe hepatic insufficiency unre-sponsive to medical therapy, liver transplant may be indicated (Schilsky et al. 1994).

HALLERVORDEN–SPATZ DISEASE

Hallervorden–Spatz disease (HSD) is characterized, clinically, by a progressive movement disorder, mainly consisting of dystonia or parkinsonism, usually associated with dementia and pyramidal tract signs. The most specific findings are pathological and include: (1) dysmyelination and deposition of iron-staining pigments in the pallidum and usually the pars reticulata of the substantia nigra (Luckenbach et al. 1983); (2) axonal swelling (spheroid bodies) widely distributed in the cerebral cortex and basal ganglia (Dooling et al. 1974); and (3) increased lipofuscin deposition (Jankovic et al. 1985). In a few cases, Lewy bodies can be found, similar to those in idiopathic Parkinson disease (Antoine et al. 1985). Fifty per cent of reported cases are familial and transmitted as an autosomal recessive trait (Elejalde et al. 1979). The gene has been mapped to chromosome 20 (Taylor et al. 1996).

Whether HSD represents a pathological syndrome of iron deposition in the pallidum of variable cause or a specific disease entity is still an unanswered question. The mere presence of excess iron in the basal nuclei even in association with spheroids is probably nonspecific. It is clear, however, that there exists one (or several) genetic disease(s) with iron deposition *and* characteristic clinical features.

CLINICAL FEATURES

In classical descriptions both clinical signs and age of onset are widely variable. In the review by Dooling et al. (1974), 64 pathologically verified HSD cases were classified on the basis of clinical and pathological signs in three groups: (1) cases of early onset "at a young age generally after earliest childhood", with extrapyramidal signs, dementia, progressive course and pathological abnormalities involving the basal ganglia and substantia nigra; (2) cases with the same clinical signs but with sparing of the substantia nigra; (3) 'miscellaneous' cases with atypical clinical signs. Whether all these cases correspond to a single entity or are only part of a pathological spectrum remains to be determined. Gene studies will probably clarify this issue.

A close relationship between age of onset and type of movement disorder is apparent. Dystonia is the main sign in juvenile onset cases, while developmental delay in walking with a protracted course is the first sign in early onset cases. Hypokinetic–rigid syndrome (parkinsonism) is the predominant clinical manifestation in late onset (adult) cases. This chapter considers only early onset and juvenile forms with a well defined clinical symptomatology (Malmstrom-Groth and Kristensson 1982, Fernández-Alvarez 1993).

Early-onset form

In this form, there is an initial silent period of several months. Motor and language delay and mental retardation then become obvious but early milestones are generally achieved. An unstable gait is the first suggestive sign (Fernández-Alvarez 1993) but sitting is achieved at a normal age so the onset can be placed between 6 and 12 months of age. The disorder initially appears more or less static until regression begins at between 5 and 10 years. Motor and language abilities clearly decline, walking worsens with frequent falls, and episodic outbursts of behavioural disturbance are induced by stress. Dystonia (Fig. 6.2) may be an early manifestation but may not be apparent until one year after onset of regression. Contrary to what obtains in idiopathic torsion dystonia, dystonic features often begin in the upper limbs, the trunk and especially the oromandibular muscles.

From this point onwards, the condition quickly worsens, leading to severe generalized dystonia, fixed abnormal limb postures, and severe impairment of speech but with relatively preserved comprehension. The patients become bedridden over a period of several months to two years. Severe generalized dystonic spasms, axial hyperextension, facial grimacing, mutism and dysautonomic disturbances such as difficult swallowing lead to cachexia and death between the ages of 11 and 15 years.

Retinopathy is frequently present and may be an early manifestation. Difficulties in night vision have been noted as early as 2 years of age (Urechia et al. 1950, Fernández-

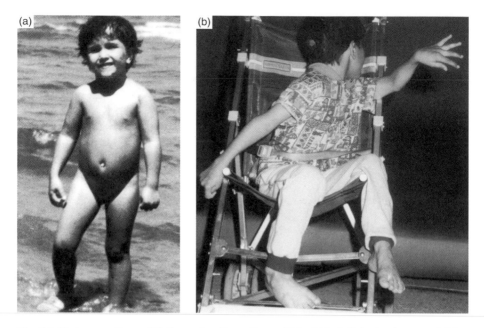

Fig. 6.2. Early-onset form of Hallervorden–Spatz disease. This girl had slight developmental delay. She walked unstably at the age of 3 years. At 2 years her parents had noticed difficulties in night vision. At age 4 a right-sided slightly dystonic posture was noted (a). At 8 years (b) dystonia was generalized.

Alvarez 1993), and retinitis may be a useful clue to early diagnosis. Acanthocytosis is present in many cases.

Variations in the clinical picture may occur within the same sibship.

Juvenile form

This form has its onset between 6 and 14 years of age. The first signs usually include dystonia of the lower limbs or of oromandibular muscles. About one-third of patients then show developmental stagnation or behavioural disorders such as agressivity or impulsivity, followed by intellectual deterioration which preferentially affects short-term verbal memory and mental functions that require conceptual and analogical strategies (Angelini et al. 1992).

The course is progressive and leads to a clinical picture similar to that of the early-onset form with generalized dystonia affecting especially the oromandibular area with 'risus sardonicus', anarthria, dementia, spasticity and abnormal eye movements. Twenty per cent of patients have epileptic seizures. Cerebellar ataxia and amyotrophy are infrequent. Polyneuropathy was present in only one of 11 cases reported by Angelini et al. (1992).

Atypical cases are common but their nosological situation is debatable. Sixteen per cent of the patients reviewed by Dooling et al. (1974) had no cognitive defect. In isolated cases the only extrapyramidal manifestations were postural and intention tremor (Antoine et al. 1985), 'extrapyramidal hypertonicity', and episodes of paroxysmal hemidystonia beginning at age 10.

It has been suggested that acanthocytosis found in some early and juvenile onset cases (Fernández-Alvarez 1993) may define another entity (Luckenbach et al. 1983) for which Higgins et al. (1992) proposed the acronym HARP syndrome (hypobetalipoprotein-aemia, acanthocytosis, retinitis pigmentosa, pallidal degeneration). MR scan showed a typical 'eye of the tiger' image (see below), and except for the disturbance in prebetalipo-protein, the case was typical for HSD. Another case with a milder clinical phenotype has been reported (Orrell et al. 1995). However, Orrel et al. also reported two patients with similar features and normal lipid studies. There is thus little evidence to individualize these cases. A related condition with the presence of sea-blue histiocytes in the bone marrow and cytosomes suggestive of ceroid-lipofuscinosis has been described by Swaiman et al. (1983).

ANCILLARY INVESTIGATIONS
Various CT abnormalities are reported in HSD cases (Boltshauser et al. 1987). Increased density in both pallida is most common and suggestive. However, low or normal density of the pallidum has also been reported. These variations may be related to the stage of evolution of the disorder.

MRI with a 1.5 T machine (Savoiardo et al. 1993) is an essential investigation and is now required for the diagnosis. It shows bilateral areas of increased T_2 signal in the medial part of the pallidum surrounded by a larger zone of markedly low signal (Sethi et al. 1988), the so-called eye of the tiger image (Fig 6.3) (Rutledge et al. 1987). In some cases, only a markedly decreased signal of the pallidum without central hyperdensity is found. The low signal is the result of high iron concentration in both pallida, while the hyperintense area ('the pupil') is due to disintegration of the neuropil with cavitation of the medial part of both nuclei (Schaffert et al. 1989, Savoiardo et al. 1993, Rosemberg et al. 1995). This image has also been reported in cortical–basal ganglionic degeneration, a progressive degenerative disorder of adult onset (Molinuevo et al. 1999). It is not clear at which stage of the disease this image first appears. In the case of Sethi et al. (1988) it was visible one year after onset but in that of Galluchi et al. (1989) there was high signal from the pallidum at 7 years of age, low signal at 8, and at 10 years a typical eye of the tiger image. In the patient of Brouwer et al. (1992) CT and MRI were normal two years after clinical onset and only at 4 years was the typical image present.

Brainstem auditory evoked potentials are normal but visual evoked potentials and ERG are often abnormal and ERG is frequently extinguished.

Zimmerman et al. (1981) reported accumulation of ^{59}Fe transferrin in cultured fibroblasts but this observation has not been confirmed, and the method has not gained clinical acceptance (Vakili et al. 1977).

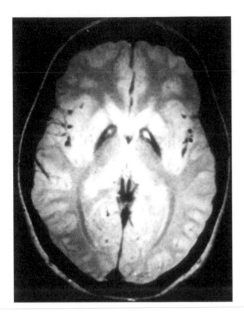

Fig. 6.3. T$_2$-weighted MRI of a patient with Hallervorden–Spatz disease showing the 'eye of the tiger' in the medial part of the pallidum.

DIFFERENTIAL DIAGNOSIS

In early infantile forms, a diagnosis of nonprogressive encephalopathy or cerebral palsy is often erroneously made. The diagnosis of early regression includes a large number of degenerative diseases most of which do not demonstrate prominent extrapyramidal features. Retinopathy and MR images are of obvious diagnostic importance. The diagnosis of *neuroacanthocytosis* should be discarded in cases with acanthocytes. The disease is rare in children and a neuropathy is usually present (see Chapter 4). *Bassen–Korzweig disease* also features acanthocytosis but the clinical picture is mainly ataxic and with peripheral nerve involvement. Late onset idiopathic dystonia can be differentiated in particular by the absence of MR and retinal anomalies.

The presence of spheroids has led to the inclusion of HSD in the spectrum of the neuroaxonal dystrophies together with Seitelberger disease. 'Transitional' forms have been reported (Gilman and Barret 1973, Defendini et al. 1973). It seems likely that the two conditions are different.

PATHOLOGY

The pallidum and substantia nigra normally have a high concentration of iron. In HSD, the accumulation of iron is such that these areas have a characteristic rusty colour. Histologically, iron granules are dispersed in neurons, astrocytes and microglial cells. There is also sometimes extracellular iron surrounding the vessels. The pallidum is demyelinated. 'Pseudocalcic' concretions with a strong affinity for haematoxylin are free in cerebral tissue. Another characteristic finding is the presence of spheroids. These are particularly numerous in the pallidum and substantia nigra but they are also found in the lower brain-stem, white matter and cerebral cortex (Swaiman et al. 1990). These bodies are not specific (Kim et al. 1981). They are present in even greater numbers and with wider distribution in neuroaxonal dystrophy and also in cases of nonspecific, at times congenital encephalopathies.

PATHOPHYSIOLOGY
The mechanisms of HSD are unknown. It is only clear that (1) iron plays an important role in the transport of electrons and the reactions of oxido-reduction, and (2) in ferric form it is toxic to the cell due to its high oxidative potential. Perry et al. (1985) on the basis of an increase in cystein and glutation-cystein, suggested the possibility of a block in the cystein–taurine pathway. Cystein could act as a chelator of iron which would generate free radicals with pseudoperoxidation of neuronal and glial membranes. These authors also found an increase of GABA in the pallidum and the substantia nigra.

TREATMENT
Attempts at treatment by iron chelation with desferroxiamine have been unsuccessful. The increase in lipofuscin and the presence of spheroids have prompted therapy with vitamin E (Luckenbach et al. 1983), with negative results. Symptomatic treatment aims at alleviating the most troublesome clinical anomalies through the administration of L-dopa, bromocriptine or anticholinergic agents, although the tremor usually does not respond to betablockers or primidone. Bilateral thalamotomy has been utilized for control of dystonia but is at best an exceptional indication (Tsukamoto et al. 1992). Treatment of epileptic seizures is obviously indicated.

MULTIPLE SYSTEM ATROPHIES
The term multiple system atrophies (MSAs) designates a group of CNS diseases that share a familial and generally progressive nature and involve simultaneously unrelated structures (brainstem nuclei, cerebellum, inferior olives, substantia nigra, striatum and spinal cord). The lesions have no specific pathological features. The recent demonstration of DNA changes in several of these disorders (dentato-rubro-pallidoluysian atrophy, Steele–Richardson disease, olivopontocerebellar atrophy) will probably clarify their nosology.

MSA can be classified according to their main symptoms into those with mainly extrapyramidal and those with mainly cerebellar symptomatology. Only some of the latter group, which have been reported in children, will be discussed.

MACHADO–JOSEPH DISEASE
Machado–Joseph disease (MJD) (Rosenberg et al. 1978) – also known as Machado disease (Nakado et al. 1972), Azorean disease (Romanul et al. 1977), nigrospinodentate degeneration with nuclear ophthalmoplegia (Woods and Schaumburg 1972) – is an autosomal dominant disorder with variable clinical expression, even in members of

the same family. It was initially described in Portuguese patients from the Azores islands and emigrants therefrom, but has, in fact, a worldwide distribution (Fowler 1984). Although MJD is in some respects similar to the olivopontocerebellar atrophies, its pathology is distinct with always a nigral lesion with neuronal loss and gliosis and variable affectation of subthalamic nucleus, striatum and pallidum. Clinically it is characterized by cerebellar and progressive external ophthalmoplegia, spasticity, and late, peripheral neuropathy.

Type I is characterized by pyramidal and extrapyramidal signs, external ophthalmoplegia and mild ataxia. The onset is usually in adulthood (mean age 41 years) but cases have occurred at 15 years of age (Fowler 1984) and even in the first decade of life (Rosenberg et al. 1978). Dystonia of the extremities and sometimes of the trunk and face is more marked in early onset cases. In some of these cases, both parents were affected so that they were probably homozygous for the condition. Oculomotor anomalies are frequent, with palpebral retraction, nystagmus and defects of conjugate gaze. Intelligence remains normal. The average duration of this type is 15 years (Fowler 1984).

Type II with predominantly extrapyramidal signs and *type III* with additional peripheral amyotrophy are seen only in adults. In fact, recent work showed that the clinical features of MJD may be indistinguishable from those of the other spinocerebellar atrophies (SCAs).

MJD has been shown to be identical with SCA type 3, with the same DNA anomaly (in chromosome 14q, *MJD/SCA3* gene repeat). The symptomatology is highly variable, most forms being indistinguishable from the other SCAs.

PONTOCEREBELLAR HYPOPLASIA TYPE 2

Pontocerebellar hypoplasia type 2 is an autosomal recessive syndrome (Barth et al. 1990) with neurological involvement from birth, myoclonic jerks (Barbot et al. 1997), choreic or dystonic movements starting in the course of the first year (Simonati et al. 1997), acquired microcephaly, severely impaired mental and motor development (lack of visual attention, only reaching unsupported sitting and grasping movements). Epileptic seizures are frequent (Barth et al. 1995).

MRI shows a severe pontocerebellar hypoplasia, involving both the vermis and the cerebellar hemispheres (Fig. 6.4). Supratentorial white matter is generally not involved. (Uhl et al. 1998).

Pathological studies have not been able to explain the chorea in these patients. No biochemical or genetic abnormalities are known.

DENTATO-RUBRO-PALLIDO-LUYSIAN ATROPHY (DRPLA)

DRPLA is an autosomal dominant disease. Although cases were initially reported from Europe and still are observed there (Warner et al. 1994b, 1995), recent cases are overwhelmingly of Japanese origin (Takahashi et al. 1988). The prevalence of the disease in Japan is about 1 per million (Miwa 1994).

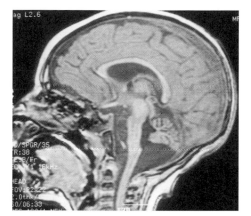

Fig. 6.4. MRI of a 15-month-old girl with pontocerebellar hypoplasia type 2, showing severe pontine and cerebellar hypoplasia. The main sign was severe generalized ballismus.

DRPLA is mostly an adult-onset disease. However, a few infantile cases are on record with onset as early as 1 year (Warner et al. 1995). Anticipation in successive generations has been reported (Warner et al. 1995).

The clinical features vary within the same family and include varying combinations of cerebellar ataxia, epilepsy, dysarthria, pyramidal tract signs, dementia, and abnormal movements including chorea (Warner et al. 1994a), myoclonus, dystonia and parkinsonism. Early onset cases tend to present with a picture of progressive myoclonic epilepsy, whereas abnormal movements may predominate in adults. In children, myoclonic epilepsy and dementia are the most frequent signs (Nielsen et al. 1996) but chorea has been also reported (Becher et al. 1997).

DRPLA is associated with an unstable expansion of a CAG trinucleotide in a cDNA (CTG-B37) on chromosome 12p (Koide et al. 1994, Nagafuchi et al. 1994, Warner et al. 1994b). This repeat in the general population consists of 7–23 trinucleotides and is expanded to 49–75 in DRPLA patients (Koide et al. 1994, Nagafuchi et al. 1994).

Neuroimaging results may be normal or show nonspecific white matter demyelination and atrophy of the cerebellum or brainstem (Warner et al. 1995). Periventricular hyperintensity on T_2-weighted images has been described (Miyazaki et al. 1995).

DRPLA must be differentiated from mitochondrial encephalopathies and cerebellar ataxias, but the clinical features of DRPLA make it difficult to separate, mainly in adults, from Huntington and Machado–Joseph diseases. The most common misdiagnosis is with Huntington disease. As a rule a search of the DRPLA mutation must be considered in families initially diagnosed as having Huntington disease when this has been excluded (Potter et al. 1995, Warner et al. 1995, Nielsen et al. 1996).

Pathologically there is involvement of the dentate nucleus, the external segment of the pallidum and its projections to the subthalamic and, also, the red nucleus. Dentato-rubral involvement is usually more marked and constant than the pallido-luysian lesions (Warner et al. 1994a).

In *progressive pallidal atrophy* (Hunt–van Bogaert disease), neuronal loss is limited to the pallidum. Clinical presentation is that of early onset Parkinson disease or of a progressively generalized dystonia, which in the original two sibs reported by van Bogaert started at age 5–6 years, and in the case of Jellinger (1968) at 14 years. The course was rapid, death occurring after five to ten years.

PALLIDO-PYRAMIDAL ATROPHY

Pallido-pyramidal atrophy (Davison 1954) is a rare condition of probable recessive inheritance characterized at onset by mild cerebellar syndrome and pyramidal features in the lower limbs with secondary development of hypokinetic–rigid syndrome or dystonia. Age of onset is around 10 years. The response to L-dopa is usually excellent and persistent (Horowitz and Greenfield 1975, Tranchant et al. 1991, Nisipeanu et al. 1994). Ancillary examinations are normal. PET studies (Remy et al. 1995) have shown marked dopaminergic denervation of the striatum.

PROGRESSIVE CALCIFICATION OF THE BASAL GANGLIA

Modern neuroimaging techniques, especially CT scanning, have allowed frequent and early identification of basal ganglia calcification. Although in adults 'physiological' calcification of the basal ganglia is seen in about 0.7% of routine CT scans (Harrington et al. 1981, Illum and Dupont 1985), the presence of calcification in children is always abnormal. Encephalopathies with calcification of the basal ganglia are difficult to classify.

Calcification of the basal ganglia is a frequent finding in multiple disorders and represents a heterogeneous syndrome rather than a disease entity. The existence of 'Fahr disease' is much doubted, although the term is often wrongly used for cases of idiopathic basal ganglia calcification.

The main causes of calcification of the basal ganglia (Cohen et al. 1980, Kendall and Cavanagh 1986, Legido et al. 1988, Billard et al. 1989) are shown in Table 6.2.

Familial progressive encephalopathy with calcification of the basal ganglia (Aicardi and Goutières 1984) is an autosomal recessive disorder. Affected patients exhibit dystonia, spasticity, acquired microcephaly and abnormal ocular movements in the first years of life. Neuroimaging shows basal ganglia calcifications, severe and progressive brain atrophy, and hypodensities in the white matter (Bonnemann and Meinecke 1992, Cardenas-Mera et al. 1995, Tolmie et al. 1995, Verrips et al. 1997). In the early years of the disease there is mild CSF lymphocytosis. Elevated levels of interferon alpha are found in CSF and in serum (Lebon et al. 1988). Most patients die within a few years, and those surviving into childhood are severely neurologically impaired (Goutières et al. 1998). Mild cases without deteriorating clinical course have been reported (McEntagart et al. 1998)

Bilateral strio-pallido-dentate calcinosis is an autosomal dominant disorder characterized histologically by calcification of small cerebral vessels which predominates in the basal ganglia but also involves the dentate nuclei and cerebral and cerebellar white matter. Symptoms (mainly mental deterioration, dysarthria and abnormal movements) are only

TABLE 6.2
Conditions associated with calcification of the basal ganglia

Genetic and metabolic disorders	**Tumours**
Down syndrome (Takashima and Becker 1985)	Basal ganglia tumours
	Metastasis
Albright syndrome (renal osteodystrophy)	**Infections**
Cockayne syndrome	Toxoplasmosis
Hallervorden–Spatz disease	Cytomegalovirus
Krabbe leukodystrophy	Cysticercosis
Mitochondrial cytopathies	Viral encephalitis
Tuberous sclerosis	Acquired immunodeficiency syndrome
Carbonic anhydrase II deficiency (Ohlsson et al. 1986; Strisciuglio et al. 1990, 1998; Venta et al. 1991)	Congenital rubella
Lipoid proteinosis (hyalinosis cutis)	**Toxic**
Neurofibromatosis	Carbon monoxide intoxication (Miura et al. 1985)
Phenylketonuria (biopterin reductase deficit)	Lead intoxication
Pyknodysostosis (hydrocephalus, growth retardation)	Chromium intoxication
	Radiation therapy
Microcephaly–intracranial calcification syndrome (congenital microcephaly, basal ganglia calcification, polymicrogyria, autosomal recessive inheritance?) (Burn et al. 1986, Reardon et al. 1994)	Intrathecal methotrexate
	Hypervitaminosis D
	Miscellaneous
	Perinatal hypoxic/ischaemic encephalopathy (Ho et al. 1993)
Endocrinologic disorders	Bilateral striato-pallido-dentate calcinosis (Boller et al. 1977, Ellie et al. 1989)
Primary hypoparathyroidism	Familial idiopathic symmetric basal ganglia calcification
Pseudohypoparathyroidism	Familial progressive encephalopathy with calcification of the basal ganglia (Aicardi and Goutières 1984)
Pseudopseudohypoparathyroidism	
Hyperparathyroidism	
Hypothyroidism	

rarely present before adulthood (Boller et al. 1977, Ellie et al. 1989). About 50% are asymptomatic even at late age.

Calcification of the basal ganglia has also been observed in patients with various neurological symptoms or signs without clear aetiology, as either a familial or a sporadic condition. In the family studied by Larsen et al. (1985) the clinical and X-ray features were variable. Calcifications could also involve subcortical frontal or parietal lobes or cerebellum. Eight of 14 patients with marked clinical symptoms had no calcification on their CT scans, whereas two asymptomatic members showed calcification. Age at disease onset was not uniform. In a patient with onset at 18 months, the predominant features were segmental dystonia, predominating in the upper limbs, lingual dyskinesia and mild cognitive deficit.

REFERENCES

Aicardi J, Goutières F (1984) A progressive familial encephalopathy in infancy with calcifications of the basal ganglia and chronic cerebrospinal fluid lymphocytosis. *Ann Neurol* 15: 49–54.

Angelini L, Nardocci N, Rumi V, et al. (1992) Hallervorden–Spatz disease: Clinical and MRI study of 11 cases diagnosed in life. *J Neurol* 239: 417–25.

Antoine JC, Tommasi M, Chalumeau A, et al. (1985) Maladie de Hallervorden–Spatz avec corps de Lewy. *Rev Neurol* 141: 806–9.

Arima M, Takeshata K, Yoshino K, et al. (1977) Prognosis of Wilson disease in childhood. *Eur J Ped* 126: 147–54.

Barbot C, Carneiro G, Melo J (1997) Pontocerebellar hypoplasia with microcephaly and dyskinesia: Report of two cases. *Dev Med Child Neurol* 39: 554–7.

Barth PG, Vrensen GFJM, Uylings HBM, et al. (1990) Inherited syndrome of microcephaly, dyskinesia and pontocerebellar hypoplasia: A systemic atrophy with early onset. *J Neurol Sci* 97: 25–42.

— Blennow G, Lennard HG, et al. (1995) The syndrome of autosomal recessive pontocerebellar hypoplasia, microcephaly, and extrapyramidal dyskinesia (pontocerebellar hypoplasia type 2). *Neurology* 45: 311–7.

Becher MW, Rubinstein DC, Leggo J, et al. (1997) Dentatorubral and pallidoluysian atrophy (DRPLA). Clinical and neuropathological findings in genetically confirmed North American and European pedigrees. *Mov Disord* 12: 519–30.

Bergstrom RF, Kay DR, Harkcom TM (1981) Penicillamine kinetics in normal subjects. *Clin Pharmacol Ther* 30: 404–13.

Billard C, Dulac O, Boulloche J, et al. (1989) Encephalopathy with calcifications of the basal ganglia in children. A reappraisal of Fahr's syndrome with respect to 14 new cases. *Neuropediatrics* 20: 12–19.

Boller F, Boller M, Gilbert J (1977) Familial idiopathic cerebral calcifications. *J Neurol Neurosurg Psychiatry* 40: 280–5.

Boltshauser E, Lang W, Janzer R, et al. (1987) Computed tomography in Hallervorden–Spatz disease. *Neuropediatrics* 18: 81–3.

Bonnemann CG, Meinecke P (1992) Encephalopathy of infancy with intracerebral calcifications and chronic spinal fluid lymphocytosis: Another case of Aicardi–Goutières syndrome. *Neuropediatrics* 23: 157–61.

Brewer GJ (1995) Practical recommendations and new therapies for Wilson's disease. *Drugs* 50: 240–9.

— (1999) Penicillamine should not be used as initial therapy in Wilson's disease. *Mov Disord* 14: 551–4.

— Yuzbasiyan-Gurkan V (1992) Wilson disease. *Medicine* 71: 139–64.

— Hill GM, Prasad AS, et al. (1983) Oral zinc therapy for Wilson's disease. *Ann Intern Med* 99: 314–9.

— Terry CA, Aisen AM, Gretchen M (1987) Worsening of neurological syndrome in patients with Wilson's disease with initial penicillamine therapy. *Arch Neurol* 44: 490–3.

— Dick RD, Yuzbasiyan-Gurkan V, et al. (1991) Initial therapy of patients with Wilson's disease with tetrathiomolybdate. *Arch Neurol* 48: 42–7.

Brouwer OF, Laboyre PM, Peters ACB, Vielvoye GJ (1992) Follow-up magnetic resonance imaging in Hallervorden–Spatz disease. *Clin Neurol Neurosurg* 94 (suppl): S57–S60.

Brugières P, Combes C, Ricolfi F, et al. (1992) Atypical MR presentation of Wilson disease: A possible consequence of paramagnetic effect of copper? *Neuroradiology* 34: 222–4.

Bull PC, Cox DW (1993) Long range restriction mapping of 13q14.3 focused on the Wilson disease region. *Genomics* 16: 593–8.

Burn J, Wickramasinghe HT, Harding B, Baraitser M (1986) A syndrome with intracranial calcification and microcephaly in two sibs, resembling intrauterine infection. *Clin Genet* 30: 112–6.

Cardenas-Mera N, Campos-Castello J, Ferrando-Lucas MT, Careaga-Maldonado J (1995) Progressive familial encephalopathy in infancy with calcifications of the basal ganglia and cerebrospinal fluid lymphocytosis. *Acta Neuropathol* 1: 207–13.

Cohen CR, Duchesneau PM, Weinstein MA (1980) Calcification of the basal ganglia as visualized by computed tomography. *Radiology* 134: 97–9.

Davison C (1954) Pallido-pyramidal disease. *J Neuropathol Exp Neurol* 13: 50–9.

Defendini R, Markesbery WR, Mastry AR, Duffy PE (1973) Hallervorden–Spatz disease and infantile neuroaxonal dystrophy. Ultrastructural observations, anatomical pathology and nosology. *J Neurol Sci* 20: 7–23.

Dooling EC, Schoene WC, Richardson EP (1974) Hallervorden–Spatz syndrome. *Arch Neurol* 30: 70–83.

Edwards CQ, Williams DM, Cartwright GE (1979) Hereditary hypoceruloplasminemia. *Clin Genet* 4: 311–6.

Elejalde BR, De Elejalde MM, Lopez F (1979) Hallervorden–Spatz disease. *Clin Genet* 16: 1–18.

Ellie E, Julien J, Ferrer X (1989) Familial idiopathic striopallidodentate calcifications. *Neurology* 39: 381–5.

Fernández-Alvarez E (1993) Early infantile type Hallervorden–Spatz's disease. In: Fejerman N, Chamoles NA (eds) *New Trends in Pediatric Neurology.* Amsterdam: Elsevier, pp. 143–8.

Fowler HL (1984) Machado–Joseph–Azorean disease. A ten-year study. *Arch Neurol* 41: 921–5.

Frommer DJ (1974) Defective biliary excretion of copper in Wilson's disease. *Gut* 15: 125–9.

Galluchi M, Cardona F, Arachi M, et al. (1989) Follow-up MR studies in Hallervorden–Spatz disease. *J Comput Assist Tomogr* 14: 118–20.

Gibbs K, Walshe JM (1979) A study of the ceruloplasmin concentrations found in 75 patients with Wilson's disease, their kinships and various control groups. *Q J Med* 48: 447–63.

Gilman S, Barret RE (1973) Hallervorden–Spatz disease and infantile neuroaxonal dystrophy. Clinical characteristics and nosological considerations. *J Neurol Sci* 19: 189–205.

Goutières F, Aicardi J, Barth PG, Lebon P (1998) Aicardi–Goutières syndrome: An update and results of interferon-α studies. *Ann Neurol* 44: 900–7.

Haggstrom G, Hirschowitz BI (1980) Disordered esophageal motility in Wilson's disease. *J Clin Gastroenterol* 2: 273–5.

Harik SI, Donovan J (1981) Computed tomography in Wilson disease. *Neurology* 31: 107–10.

Harrington MG, MacPherson P, McIntosh WB, et al. (1981) The significance of the incidental finding of basal ganglia calcification on computerized tomography. *J Neurol Neurosurg Psychiatry* 44: 1168–70.

Harry J, Tripathi R (1970) Kayser–Fleischer ring: A pathological study. *Br J Ophthalmol* 54: 794–800.

Higgins JJ, Patterson MC, Papadopoulos NM, et al. (1992) Hypoprebetalipoproteinemia, acanthocytosis, retinitis pigmentosa, and pallidal degeneration (HARP syndrome). *Neurology* 42: 194–8.

Ho VB, Fitz CR, Chuang SH, Geyer CA (1993) Bilateral basal ganglia lesions: Pediatric differential considerations. *Radiographics* 133: 269–92.

Horowitz G, Greenfield J (1975) Pallidal–pyramidal syndrome treated with levodopa. *J Neurol Neurosurg Psychiatry* 38: 238–40.

Illum F, Dupont E (1985) Prevalence of CT-detected calcifications in the basal ganglia in idiopathic hypoparathyroidism and pseudohypoparathyroidism. *Neuroradiology* 27: 32–7.

Ishino H, Takashi M, Hayanashi Y, et al. (1972) A case of Wilson's disease with enormous cavity formation of cerebral white matter. *Neurology* 22: 905–9.

Jankovic J, Kirkpatrick JB, Blomquist KA, et al. (1985) Late-onset Hallervorden–Spatz disease presenting as a familial parkinsonism. *Neurology* 35: 227–34.

Jellinger, K (1968) Progressive Pallidumatrophie. *J Neurol Sci* 6: 19–44.

Kendall B, Cavanagh N (1986) Intracranial calcifications in paediatric computed tomography. *Neuroradiology* 28: 234–330.

Kim RC, Ramachandran T, Parisi JE, et al. (1981) Pallidonigral pigmentation and spheroid formation with multiple striatal lacunar infarcts. *Neurology* 31: 774–7.

Koide R, Ikeuchi T, Onodera O, et al. (1994) Unstable expansion of CAG repeat in hereditary dentatorubral–pallidoluysian atrophy (DRPLA). *Nature Genet* 6: 9–13.

Kudo H, Arima M (1987) Factors modifying the prognosis of Wilson's disease in childhood. *J Child Neurol* 2: 57–62.

Larsen TA, Dunn HG, Jan JE, Calne DB (1985) Dystonia and calcification of the basal ganglia. *Neurology* 35: 533–7.

Lebon P, Badoual J, Ponsot G, et al. (1988) Intrathecal synthesis of interferon-alpha in infants with progressive familial encephalopathy. *J Neurol Sci* 84: 201–8.

Legido A, Zimmerman RA, Packer RJ, et al. (1988) Significance of basal ganglia calcification on computed tomography in children. *Pediatr Neurosci* 14: 64–70.

LeWitt P (1999) Penicillamine as a controversial treatment for Wilson's disease. *Mov Disord* 14: 555–6.

Liao KK, Wang SJ, Kwan SY, et al. (1991) Tongue dyskinesia as an early manifestation of Wilson's disease. *Brain Dev* 13: 451–3.

Lingam S, Wilson J, Nazer H, Mowat AP (1987) Neurological abnormalities in Wilson's disease are reversible. *Neuropediatrics* 18: 11–12.

Luckenbach MW, Green WR, Miller NR, et al. (1983) Ocular clinicopathologic correlation of Hallervorden–Spatz syndrome with acanthocytosis and pigmentary retinopathy. *Am J Ophthalmol* 95: 369–82.

Malmstrom-Groth AG, Kristensson K (1982) Neuroaxonal dystrophy in childhood. Report of two cousins with Hallerworden–Spatz [sic] disease and a case of Seitelberger's disease. *Acta Paediatr Scand* 71: 1045–9.

Mantgra CJ, Dawkins JH, Zilko PJ, et al. (1977) Penicillin associated myasthenia gravis, anti acetylcholine receptor and antistriatal antibodies. *Am J Med* 63: 689–94.

McEntagart M, Kamel H, Lebon P, King MD (1998) Aicardi–Goutières syndrome: An expanding phenotype. *Neuropediatrics* 29: 163–7.

Medalia A, Isaacs-Glaberman K, Scheinberg H (1988) Neuropsychological impairment in Wilson's disease. *Arch Neurol* 45: 502–4.

Miura T, Mitomo M, Kawai R, Harada K (1985) CT of the brain in acute carbon monoxide intoxication: Characteristic features and prognosis. *AJNR* 6: 739–42.

Miwa S (1994) Triplet repeats strike again. *Nature Genet* 6: 3–4.

Miyajima H, Nishimura Y, Mizoguchi K, et al. (1987) Familial apoceruloplasmin deficiency associated with blepharospasm and retinal degeneration. *Neurology* 37: 761–7.

Miyazaki M, Kato T, Hashimoto T, et al. (1995) MR of childhood-onset dentatorubral–pallidoluysian atrophy. *AJNR* 16: 1834–6.

Molinuevo JL, Muñoz E, Valdeoriola F, Tolosa E (1999) The eye of the tiger sign in cortical–basal ganglionic degeneration. *Mov Disord* 14: 169–71.

Nagafuchi S, Yanagisawa H, Sato K, et al. (1994) Dentatorubral and pallidoluysian atrophy expansion of an unstable CAG trinucleotide in chromosome 12p. *Nature Genet* 6: 14–18.

Nakado K, Dawson DM, Spence A (1972) Machado disease: A hereditary ataxia in Portuguese immigrants to Massachusetts. *Neurology* 22: 49–55.

Nielsen JE, Sorensen SA, Hasholt L, Norremolle (1996) Dentato-pallidoluysian atrophy. Clinical features of a five-generation Danish family. *Mov Disord* 11: 533–41.

Nisipeanu P, Kuritzky A, Kornczyn AD (1994) Familial levodopa-responsive parkinsonian–pyramidal syndrome. *Mov Disord* 9: 673–5.

Oder W, Grimon G, Kolleger H, et al. (1991) Neurological and neuropsychiatric spectrum of Wilson's disease: A prospective study of 45 cases. *J Neurol* 238: 154–9.

Ohlsson A, Cumming WA, Paul A, Sly WS (1986) Carbonic anhydrase II deficiency syndrome: Recessive osteopetrosis with renal tubular acidosis and cerebral calcification. *Pediatrics* 77: 371–81.

Orrell JA, Harding AE, Marsden CD (1995) Acanthocytosis, retinitis pigmentosa, and pallidal degeneration: A report of three patients, including the second reported case with hypoprebetalipoproteinemia (HARP syndrome). *Neurology* 45: 487–92.

Perry TL, Norman MG, Yong VM, et al. (1985) Hallervorden–Spatz disease: Cysteine accumulation and cysteine dioxygenase deficiency in the globus pallidus. *Ann Neurol* 18: 482–9.

Petrukhin K, Fischer SG, Pirastu M, et al. (1993) Mapping, cloning and genetic characterization of the region containing the Wilson disease gene. *Nature Genet* 3: 338–43.

— Lutsenko S, Chernov I, et al. (1994) Characterization of the Wilson disease gene encoding a P-type copper transporting ATPase: Genomic organization, alternative splicing, and structure/function predictions. *Hum Molec Genet* 3: 1647–56.

Potter NT, Meyer MA, Zimmerman AW, et al. (1995) Molecular and clinical findings in a family with dentatorubral–pallidoluysian atrophy. *Ann Neurol* 37: 273–7.

Proesmans W, Jaeken J, Eeckels R (1976) D-Penicillamine induced IgA deficiency in Wilson's disease. *Lancet* 2: 804–5.

Reardon W, Hockey A, Silberstein P, et al. (1994) Autosomal recessive congenital intrauterine infection-like syndrome of microcephaly, intracranial calcification and CNS disease. *Am J Med Genet* 52: 58–65.

Remy P, Hosseini H, Degos JD, et al. (1995) Striatal dopaminergic denervation in pallidopyramidal disease demonstrated by positron emission tomography. *Ann Neurol* 38: 954–6.

Romanul FCA, Fowler HL, Radvany J (1977) Azorean disease of the nervous system. *N Engl J Med* 296: 1505–8.

Rosemberg S, Barbosa ER, Menezes-Neto JR, Santos CR (1995) Neuropathology of the eye of the tiger sign in Hallervorden–Spatz syndrome. *Dev Med Child Neurol* 37 (suppl 72): 108 (abstract).

Rosenberg RN, Nyhan WL, Coutinho P, et al. (1978) Joseph's disease: An autosomal dominant neurological disease in the Portuguese of United States and the Azores Islands. *Adv Neurol* 21: 33–57.

Ross ME, Jacobson IM, Dienstag JL, et al. (1985) Late-onset Wilson's disease with neurological involvement in the absence of Kayser–Fleischer rings. *Ann Neurol* 17: 411–3.

Rothfus WE, Hirsch WL, Malatck J, Bergman I (1977) Improvement of cerebral CT abnormalities following liver transplantation in a patient with Wilson's disease. *J Comput Assist Tomogr* 1: 415–8.

Rutledge JN, Hilal SK, Silver AJ, et al. (1987) Study of movement disorders and brain iron by magnetic resonance. *AJR* 149: 365–79.

Saito T (1981) An assessment of efficiency in potential screening for Wilson's disease. *J Epidemiol Community Health* 35: 274–80.

Savoiardo M, Halliday WC, Nardocci N, et al. (1993) Hallervorden–Spatz disease: MR and patho-logic findings. *AJNR* 14: 155–62.

Schaffert DA, Johnsen SD, Johnson PC, Drayer BP (1989) Magnetic resonance imaging in pathologically proven Hallervorden–Spatz disease. *Neurology* 39: 440–2.

Scheinberg IH, Sternlieb I (1999) *Wilson's disease. 2nd Edn.* Philadelphia: WB Saunders.

Schilsky ML, Scheinberg IH, Sternlieb Y (1994) Liver transplantation for Wilson's disease: Indications and outcome. *Hepatology* 19: 583–7.

Schulman S, Barbeau A (1963) Wilson's disease: A case with almost total loss of cerebral white matter. *J Neuropathol Exp Neurol* 22: 105–19.

Sener RN (1993a) Wilson's disease: MRI demonstration of cavitations in basal ganglia and thalami. *Pediatr Radiol* 23: 157.

— (1993b) The claustrum on MRI: Normal anatomy, and the bright claustrum as a new sign in Wilson's disease. *Pediatr Radiol* 23: 594–6.

Sethi KD, Adams RJ, Loring DW, El Gammal T (1988) Hallervorden–Spatz syndrome: Clinical and magnetic resonance imaging correlations. *Ann Neurol* 24: 692–4.

Simonati A, Dalla Bernardina B, Colombari R, Rizzutto R (1997) Ponto-cerebellar hypoplasia with dystonia: Clinico-pathological findings in a sporadic case. *Child's Nerv Syst* 13: 642–7.

Starosta-Rubinstein S (1995) Treatment of Wilson's disease. In: de Kurlan R (ed) *Treatment of Movement Disorders.* Philadelphia: JB Lippincott, pp. 115–51.

— Young AB, Kluin K, et al. (1987) Clinical assessment of 31 patients with Wilson's disease: Correlations with structural changes on magnetic resonance imaging. *Arch Neurol* 44: 365–70.

Stremmel W, Meyerrose KW, Niederau C, et al. (1991) Wilson disease: Clinical presentation, treat-ment, and survival. *Ann Med Interne* 115: 720–6.

Strisciuglio P, Sartorio R, Pecoraro C, et al. (1990) Variable clinical presentation of carbonic anhydrase II deficiency: evidence for heterogeneity? *Eur J Pediatr* 149: 337–40.

— Hu PY, Lim EJ, et al. (1998) Clinical and molecular heterogeneity in carbonic anhydrase II deficiency and prenatal diagnosis in an Italian family. *J Pediatr* 132: 717–20.

Swaiman KF (1990) Hallervorden–Spatz syndrome. *Int Pediatr* 5: 148–52.

— Smith SA, Trock GL, Siddiqui AK (1983) Sea-blue histiocytes, lymphocytic cytosomes, movement disorder and ^{59}Fe-uptake in basal ganglia: Hallervorden–Spatz disease or ceroid storage disease with abnormal isotope scan. *Neurology* 33: 301–5.

Takahashi H, Ohama E, Naito H, et al. (1988) Hereditary dentato-rubro-pallido-luysian atrophy: Clinical and pathologic variants in a family. *Neurology* 38: 1065–70.

Takashima S, Becker LE (1985) Basal ganglia calcification in Down's syndrome. *J Neurol Neuro-surg Psychiatry* 48: 61–4.

Tanzi RE, Petrukhin K, Chernov I, et al. (1993) The Wilson disease gene is a copper transporting ATPase with homology to the Menkes disease gene. *Nature Genet* 5: 344–50.

Taylor TD, Litt M, Kramer P, et al. (1996) Homozygosity mapping of Hallervorden–Spatz syndrome to chromosome 20p12.3–p13. *Nature Genet* 14: 479–81.

Thomas GR, Forbes JR, Roberts EA, et al. (1995) The Wilson disease gene: Spectrum of mutations and their consequences. *Nature Genet* 9: 210–7.

Tolmie JL, Shillito P, Hughes-Benzie R, Stephenson JPB (1995) The Aicardi–Goutières syndrome (familial, early onset encephalopathy with calcifications of the basal ganglia and chronic cerebro-spinal fluid lymphocytosis). *J Med Genet* 32: 881–4.

Tranchant C, Boulay C, Warter JM (1991) Le syndrome pallido-pyramidal: une entité méconnue. *Rev Neurol* 147: 308–10.

Tsukamoto H, Inui K, Taniike M, et al. (1992) A case of Hallervorden–Spatz disease: Progressive and intractable dystonia controlled by bilateral thalamotomy. *Brain Dev* 14: 269–72.

Uhl M, Pawlik H, Laubenberger J, et al. (1998) MRI findings in pontocerebellar hypoplasia. *Pediatr Radiol* 28: 547–51.

Urechia CI, Retezeano A, Maller O (1950) La maladie de Hallervorden–Spatz: deux cas de rigidité progressive familiale avec un examen anatomique. *Encephale* 39: 197–219.

Vakili S, Drew AL, Schuching S, et al. (1977) Hallervorden–Spatz syndrome. *Arch Neurol* 34: 729–38.

Van Caillie-Bertrand M, Degenhart HJ, Visser HK, et al. (1985a) Wilson's disease: assessment of D-penicillamine treatment. *Arch Dis Child* 60: 652–5.

— — — et al. (1985b) Oral zinc sulphate for Wilson's disease. *Arch Dis Child* 60: 656–9.

Venta PJ, Welty RJ, Johnson TM, et al. (1991) Carbonic anhydrase II deficiency syndrome in a Belgian family is caused by a point mutation at an invariant histidine residue (107 His→Tyr); Complete structure of a normal human *CAII* gene. *Am J Hum Genet* 49: 1082–90.

Verrips A, Hiel JAP, Gabreëls FJM, et al. (1997) The Aicardi–Goutières syndrome: Variable clinical expression in two siblings. *Pediatr Neurol* 16: 323–5.

Victor M, Adams RD, Cole M (1965) The acquired (non-Wilsonian) type of chronic hepato-cerebral degeneration. *Medicine* 44: 345–96.

Walshe JM (1956) Penicillamine. A new oral therapy for Wilson's disease. *Am J Med* 21: 487–95.

— (1986) Wilson's disease. In: Vinken PJ, Bruyn GW, Klawans HL (eds) *Handbook of Clinical Neurology. Vol. 5, no 49. Extrapyramidal Disorders.* Amsterdam: Elsevier, pp. 223–38.

— (1999) Penicillamine. The treatment of first choice for patients with Wilson's disease. *Mov Disord* 14: 545–50.

— Dixon AK (1986) Dangers of non-compliance in Wilson's disease. *Lancet* 1: 845–6.

Warner TT, Lennox GG, Janota I, Harding AE (1994a) Autosomal-dominant dentato-rubro-pal-lido-luysian atrophy in the United Kingdom. *Mov Disord* 9: 289–96.

— Williams L, Harding AE (1994b) DRPLA in Europe. *Nature Genet* 6: 225 (letter).

— — Walker RWH, et al. (1995) A clinical and molecular genetic study of dentatorubropalli-doluysian atrophy in four European families. *Ann Neurol* 37: 452–9.

Werlin SL, Grand RJ, Perman JA, Watkins JB (1978) Diagnostic dilemmas of Wilson's disease: Diagnosis and treatment. *Pediatrics* 62: 47–51.

Wiebers DO, Hollenhorst RW, Goldstein NP (1977) The ophthalmologic manifestations of Wilson's disease. *Mayo Clin Proc* 52: 409–16.

Williams FJ, Walshe JM (1981) Wilson's disease. An analysis of the cranial computerized tomo-graphic appearances found in 60 patients and the changes in response to treatment with chelating agents. *Brain* 104: 735–52.

Woods BE, Schaumburg HH (1972) Nigro-spino-dentatal degeneration with nuclear ophthalmo-plegia: A unique and partially treatable clinicopthological entity. *J Neurol Sci* 17: 149–66.

Yuh WTC, Flickinger FW (1988) Unusual MR findings in CNS Wilson disease. *AJR* 151: 834.

Zimmermann AW, Karimeddini MK, Ramsby GR, Zimme AE (1981) Hallervorden–Spatz syndrome: Increased cerebral uptake of ^{59}Fe and demonstration of striatal iron deposits on CT. *Neurology* 31 (suppl 2): 129 (abstract).

7
PAROXYSMAL MOVEMENT DISORDERS

INTRODUCTION AND CLASSIFICATION
Most movement disorders are permanent situations although short term variations of symptoms may occur. This chapter is concerned only with paroxysmal disturbances where movement is normal between the episodes. The paroxysmal character of the disorders studied here frequently results in a misdiagnosis of epilepsy, the more so as antiepileptic pharmaceuticals are often an effective treatment. Moreover, syndromes (Szepetowski et al. 1997, Guerrini et al. 1999) and cases with both epilepsy and paroxysmal movement disorder coexist. The normality of ictal EEG is a major differentiating characteristic, but the true nature of these paroxysmal dyskinesias is still debated (see Lombroso 2000).

Molecular genetic studies have permitted mapping of the genes for Mount and Reback paroxysmal dyskinesia (Fouad et al. 1996, Fink et al. 1997), paroxysmal choreoathetosis/spasticity (Auburger et al. 1996) and the interesting syndromes associating familial convulsions and paroxysmal dyskinesia (Szepetowski et al. 1997, Guerrini et al. 1999).

Two paroxysmal movement disorders (benign paroxysmal torticollis and paroxysmal tonic upgaze deviation) are transient disorders of infancy. In other paroxysmal conditions such as paroxysmal dyskinesia of Mount and Reback type, the disorder may last only a few years or be permanent. A classification of such disorders is shown in Table 7.1.

BENIGN PAROXYSMAL TORTICOLLIS OF INFANCY (BPT)
BPT was initially reported in 1969 by Snyder. Episodes of painless latero-, retro- or torticollis are the hallmark of this disorder.

Very often episodes appear in the morning (Hanukoglu et al. 1984), and they may be precipitated by changes in posture (Cataltepe and Barron 1993). Abnormal eye movements may herald an attack. At onset, most episodes are accompanied by irritability, pallor, vomiting and ataxia; then the infant remains quiet in the abnormal posture. The ataxia may be the dominant feature (Deonna and Martin 1981) and sometimes may become the only manifestation after several episodes of torticollis (Hanuklogu et al. 1984). Latero-, retro- or torticollis is the major feature but lateral incurvation of the trunk and extension of one lower limb are sometimes associated (Fig. 7.1) (Sanner and Bergstrom 1979, Deonna and Martin 1981). The duration of attacks may vary from minutes to several days and, rarely, up to two weeks. Cases of very short episodes of sudden deviation of the head and eye when the patient is moved from an upright to a supine

TABLE 7.1
Classification of paroxysmal movement disorders

Idiopathic
  Transient
    Benign paroxysmal torticollis of infantcy
    Paroxysmal tonic upgaze deviation of infancy
  Chronic
    Mount and Reback type (familial paroxysmal choreoathetosis)
    Kertesz type (paroxysmal kinesigenic choreoathetosis)
    Lance type (paroxysmal exercise-induced dystonia)
    Occurring during sleep
    Unclassified

Secondary

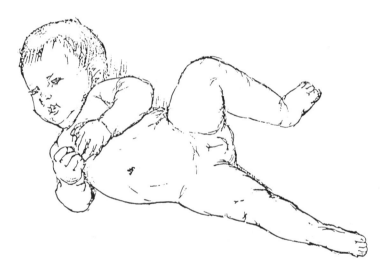

Fig. 7.1. Drawing of an episode of benign paroxysmal torticollis in a girl aged 9 months, showing torticollis and also curvature of the trunk and extension of the right leg. (Reproduced by permission from Sanner and Bergstrom 1979.)

position have been reported (Cataltepe and Barron 1993). Neurological examination between attacks is normal.

    In more than half the cases the episodes begin before 3 months of age (Fig. 7.2), sometimes as early as in the first week of life (Sanner and Bergstrom 1979, Hanukoglu et al. 1984) (Fig. 7.3) or as late as 30 months (Snyder 1969). Attacks tend to occur frequently at onset (every 2–4 weeks) and often with strikingly regular occurrence. They disappear spontaneously before the age of 5 years.

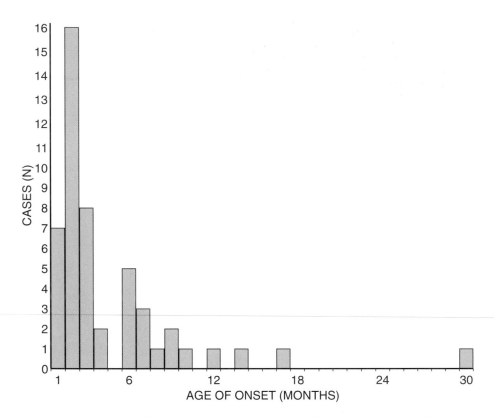

Fig. 7.2. Age of onset in 49 cases of benign paroxysmal torticollis [from cases reported by Snyder 1969, Sanner and Bergstrom 1979, Deonna and Martin 1981, Hanukoglu et al. 1984, Cataltepe and Barron 1993, and personal (EF-A) series].

Girls are more affected than boys (3:1). A few cases are familial (Lipson and Robertson 1978, Sanner and Bergstrom 1979, Deonna and Martin 1981, Roulet and Deonna 1988).

EEG and neuroimaging are normal. Auditory function and vestibular tests have been found to be abnormal by Snyder (1969), but normal by others (Deonna and Martin 1981).

Pathophysiology is unclear. Vestibular dysfunction is probable. Snyder's paper mooted "a possible form of labyrinthitis". Deonna and Martin (1981) followed patients with BPT in whom the episodes of torticollis were replaced by typical migraine or who developed migraine years after BPT, and some children later remembered having had headache during the episodes of torticollis. In at least one case, episodes of vomiting later followed by headache were observed (Roulet and Deonna 1988). Familial antecedents of migraine are frequent (Deonna and Martin 1981, Roulet and Deonna 1988). Some patients later develop benign paroxysmal vertigo (Dunn and Snyder 1976), suggesting a

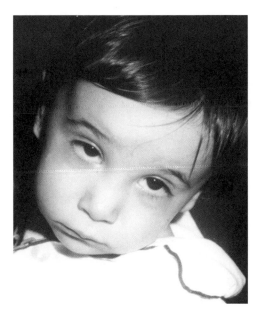

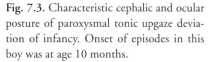

Fig. 7.3. Characteristic cephalic and ocular posture of paroxysmal tonic upgaze deviation of infancy. Onset of episodes in this boy was at age 10 months.

vestibular disturbance and a possible pathogenetic link with migraine (Eeg-Olofsson et al. 1982).

Differential diagnosis may be difficult in the first attack, especially if the disorder starts in the neonatal period, because BPT is not usually considered at this age. The differential diagnosis includes dystonic reactions to drugs (Casteels-van Daele 1979), posterior fossa tumours, cervical spine abnormalities, ocular coordination defects and Sandifer syndrome. When the episodic nature is confirmed and the child is neurologically normal between attacks, the diagnosis becomes easier.

Unless irritability and vomiting require symptomatic treatment, no drug therapy is necessary. Pharmacological treatment of dystonia is not useful. Clear explanation of the good prognosis of the disorder to the parents is essential.

PAROXYSMAL TONIC UPGAZE DEVIATION OF INFANCY
This entity was described in 1988 by Ouvrier and Billson. Thirty cases (Ahn et al. 1989, Deonna et al. 1990, Echenne and Rivier 1992, Campistol et al. 1993, Gieron and Korthals 1993, Sugie et al. 1995, Guerrini et al. 1998, Ruggieri et al. 1998) including one large series (Hayman et al. 1998) have been reported. The disorder is characterized by: (1) prolonged episodes lasting hours, rarely days (Deonna et al. 1990, Gieron and Korthals 1993) of sustained or intermittent upward gaze deviation; (2) occurrence of down-beating nystagmic jerks on attempts to look downward; (3) normal horizontal eye movements; (4) frequently, disappearance or alleviation with sleep; (5) aggravation during daytime with fatigue or infections; (6) onset in the first months of life (most cases between

4 and 10 months); and (7) spontaneous remission in a few years (30 months in the case of Deonna et al. 1990).

Some cases (Ouvrier and Billson 1988, Deonna et al. 1990) begin, in addition, with ataxia that may persist during the episodes (Echenne and Rivier 1992, Campistol et al. 1993, Apak and Topçu 1999). In one case, symptoms were more severe following sleep (Apak and Topçu 1999). Recurrences in a modified form have been reported (Hayman et al. 1998). Psychomotor retardation or language delay are present in up to 60–70% of cases (Hayman et al. 1998). The disorder disappears usually within one month to six years, but in one case lasted only two days (Hayman et al. 1998). Both autosomal dominant (Campistol et al. 1993, Guerrini et al. 1998) and recessive inheritance (Hayman et al. 1998) have been suggested. Cases with tonic upgaze without any other significant neurological disturbance present from birth and lasting some months have been reported (Mets 1990).

Laboratory, neurophysiological and neuroimaging examinations are normal. Only one case with MR images suggestive of periventricular leukomalacia despite a normal perinatal history has been reported (Sugie et al. 1995). Pathological study of one case was normal (Ouvrier and Billson 1988).

L-Dopa treatment (150 mg/d) (Ouvrier and Billson 1988, Campistol et al. 1993) resulted in disappearance of the episodes in a few patients (in 15 days and three months in the two cases of Campistol et al.) but has been ineffective in others (Hayman et al. 1998, Ruggieri et al. 1998).

PAROXYSMAL DYSKINESIAS

In 1940 Mount and Reback described a disorder characterized by sudden episodes of chorea or ballismus precipitated by ingestion of alcohol, coffee or tea and termed it 'familial paroxysmal choreoathetosis'. Similar cases were later reported under various names (Richards and Barnett 1968, Mayeux and Fahn 1982, Przuntek and Monninger 1983). Kertesz (1967) differentiated another form of episodic dyskinesia, distinct from that described by Mount and Reback, in which paroxysms were triggered by movement, for which he introduced the term 'kinesigenic'. Kertesz noted the beneficial effect of diphenylhydantoin. Because of the significant number of sporadic cases the term 'familial' was excluded from the name of this disease. This type is much more frequent than non-kinesigenic forms. Kinesigenic cases had previously been reported under a variety of names such as: 'periodic dystonia' (Smith and Heersema 1941). Because they were considered as a form of epilepsy (Lishman et al. 1962), terms such as 'reflex epilepsy' (Stevens 1966) or 'épilepsie bravais–jacksonienne réflexe' (Michaux and Granier 1945) have been used. A third form, described by Lance (1977), in which the episodes are induced by sustained exercise, is termed 'familial paroxysmal dystonia induced by exercise' (Plant et al. 1984) or 'intermediate type' (Buruma and Roos 1986). Characteristics of the three forms of paroxysmal dyskinesia are given in Table 7.2. In addition, secondary paroxysmal dyskinesias have also been reported (Table 7.3).

TABLE 7.2
Characteristics of the various types of paroxysmal dyskinesias*

	PDC (Mount and Reback)	PKC (Kertesz)	PDIE (Lance)
Localization	Extremities, face; uni/bilateral	Lower limbs	Unilateral
Duration	2 min–6 h	Generally <1 min; always<5 min	5–30 min
Frequency	2/y, occasionally 4/d	100/d–1/mo	1/d–2/mo
Age of onset	Generally from birth, in one case at 22 y	Infancy – 40 y	3–20 y
Inheritance	AD	AD, S, recessive?	AD
Male/female ratio	2:1	4:1	1:4
Precipiting movement	No	Abrupt movement	Continuous exercise
Other factors	Alcohol, coffee, chocolate, fatigue vibration	Stress, anticipated passive movements	Stress
Treatment	Clonazepam, oxazepam, haloperidol, valproic acid, acetazolamide	Phenytoin, phenobarbitone, carbamazepine, L-dopa	Clonazepam?

*Modified by permission from Buruma and Roos (1986).
PDC = paroxysmal dystonic choreoathetosis; PKC = paroxysmal kynesigenic choreoathetosis; PDIE = paroxysmal dystonia induced by exercise. AD = autosomal dominant; S = sporadic.

Several classifications have been proposed (e.g. Lance 1977, Goodenough et al. 1978), but the classification of Demirkiran and Jankovic (1995) based on precipitating circumstance is most useful, both to differentiate the forms and to predict the future course.

Common clinical features include episodic occurrence of choreic, dystonic, ballistic or mixed movements of sudden onset without disturbance of consciousness or postictal symptoms. The extent and localization are variable and may change with different attacks. During attacks the patients may be able to maintain some motor activities such as walking or swimming despite the dyskinesia. Attacks are often preceded by a feeling of fatigue or weakness on one side, and sometimes a sensation of being pinched (Lance 1977).

The paroxysms generally tend to increase in frequency during adolescence then to decrease gradually after age 20 years (Goodenough et al. 1978). Spontaneous cure has been reported (Hudgins and Corbin 1966). These diseases do not reduce life expectancy.

TABLE 7.3
Secondary paroxysmal dyskinesias

Antiepileptic drugs
  Hydantoins (Uriz and Fernández-Alvarez 1988)
  Gabapentin (Chudnow et al. 1997a)

Cranial trauma (Robin 1977, Drake et al. 1986)

Cystinuria (Cavanagh et al. 1974 – associated with mental retardation and epilepsy)

Hallervorden–Spatz disease (probable) (Hart et al. 1995)

Hartnup disease (Darras et al. 1989)

Hypoglycaemia (Newman and Kinkel 1984)

Idiopathic hypoparathyroidism (Tabae-Zadeh et al. 1972, Soffer et al. 1977)

Multiple sclerosis (Matthews 1958, Joynt and Green 1962, Osterman and Westerberg 1975, Berger et al. 1984, Nardocci et al. 1995)

Non-ketotic hyperglycinaemia (Brandt et al. 1976)

Perinatal hypoxia–ischaemia (Rosen 1964, Goodenough et al. 1978, Erickson and Chun 1987)

Pseudohypoparathyroidism (Micheli et al. 1989, Dure and Mussell 1998)

Pyruvate decarboxylase deficiency (Blass et al. 1971)

Thalamic infarct (Camac et al. 1990)

Thyrotoxicosis (Fishbeck and Layzer 1979)

Interictal neurological examination is normal, although in rare cases small involuntary movements such as mild dystonia and tremor have been recorded (Nardocci et al. 1989).

Familial forms are often transmitted as an autosomal dominant trait, but autosomal recessive inheritance predominates in familial cases of Lance-type paroxysmal dyskinesia. Apparently nonfamilial cases may arise due to incomplete penetrance of the gene or new mutation, or be diagnosed due to incomplete family data, or be truly secondary cases.

Neuroimaging and biochemical studies give normal results. Rare published cases, with cerebral neuroimaging abnormalities, should be considered as secondary (Watson and Scott 1979, Gilroy 1982).

Very few pathological data are available. Two nonkinesigenic cases of Lance (1977) were normal, and the cases of kinesigenic type reported by Stevens (1966) and Kertesz (1967) only 'suggested' a slight loss of neurons of the locus ceruleus or slight asymmetry of the substantia nigra.

PAROXYSMAL DYSKINESIA OF MOUNT AND REBACK
This disorder (alternatively known as paroxysmal dystonic choreoathetosis or paroxysmal nonkinesigenic dyskinesia) is characterized by episodes of dystonia or choreoathetosis frequently precipitated by ingestion of alcohol or other drinks or foods such as coffee, tea

or chocolate, and to a lesser extent by fatigue, hunger or emotional stress. They may begin very early in life, even in infancy. They are often bilateral but may be limited to one side of the body, affecting laryngeal or facial muscles producing dysarthria and dysphagia. Attacks may last 10–15 minutes or persist for several hours. The frequency of attacks varies from four per day to once monthly. The occurrence of abnormal eye movements (Przuntek and Monninger 1983) and of associated familial ataxia has been reported (Mayeux and Fahn 1982). In one case, the paroxysmal dystonia started at age 3 years and persistent dystonia followed at the age of 6 years (Bressman et al. 1988). Inheritance is autosomal dominant (Hudgins and Corbin 1966). Both the frequency and severity of paroxysms may vary even within the same family.

A gene for this type of paroxysmal dyskinesia has been mapped to chromosome 2q31–36 (Fouad et al. 1996, Fink et al. 1997).

Paroxysmal dyskinesia of Mount and Reback is more difficult to treat than the Kertesz type. The best therapeutic results have been obtained with benzodiazepines (clonazepam – Lance 1977, Mayeux and Fahn 1982; and oxazepam – Kurlan and Shoulson 1983), acetazolamide (Mayeux and Fahn 1982) and haloperidol (Coulter and Donofrio 1980). Usually the condition worsened or remained static with standard anticonvulsants (Lance 1977) but benefit with some antiepileptic drugs such as valproic acid (Przuntek and Monninger 1983), carbamazepine (Artigas and Lorente 1989) and gabapentin has been reported (Chudnow et al. 1997b).

PAROXYSMAL DYSKINESIA, KERTESZ TYPE

This form (also known as paroxysmal kinesigenic choreathetosis) has its onset usually between 6 and 15 years (Bressman et al. 1988). The abnormal movements are mainly dystonic with an athetoid component. Attacks last only seconds or minutes [usually less than five minutes, although Demirkiran and Jankovic (1995) reported cases with attacks lasting up to several hours] and are frequent (up to 100 times daily). They are mostly unilateral but may alternate in side or become bilateral. They are provoked by a rapid movement or an abrupt muscular effort, especially following a period of rest. In rare cases, orofacial movements such as yawning (Demirkiran and Jankovic 1995) or sudden passive movements may also induce attacks (Stevens 1966, Loong and Ong 1973). Some patients can abort an attack by various manoeuvres applied at the time of the preliminary feelings. There are no postictal signs. Between episodes, mild hemiparesis (Burger et al. 1972) or pyramidal tract signs (Nishi et al. 1981) are only exceptionally found.

The EEG is normal in over 90% of cases, and ictal recordings have consistently failed to show epileptic discharges (Goodenough et al. 1978, Demirkiran and Jankovic 1995).

Cases suggesting both autosomal dominant (Hudgins and Corbin 1966) and autosomal recessive inheritance (Smith and Heersema 1941, Kertesz 1967) have been reported. Variable penetrance was apparent in some families. Sporadic cases are not rare (Demirkiran and Jankovic 1995).

The pathophysiology is unknown. No DNA linkage has been established in this type

of paroxysmal dyskinesia. In some cases with unilateral attacks, proton magnetic resonance spectroscopy has shown significant decrease of peak ratios of choline/creatine and
myoinositol/creatine in the contralateral basal ganglia, suggesting a dysfunction of the
cholinergic system (Kim et al. 1998).

Kinesigenic dyskinesia usually responds favourably to some antiepileptic agents, viz.
phenytoin (at doses lower than for treatment of epilepsy) (Kertesz 1967), phenobarbitone,
primidone, sodium valproate (Suber and Riley 1980) and carbamazepine (at very low
doses) (Kato and Araki 1969, Lance 1977). L-Dopa may be effective (Loong and Ong
1973), and Lou (1989) obtained an excellent response with flunarizine (5 mg/d) in one
patient.

PAROXYSMAL DYSKINESIA, LANCE TYPE

This disorder was first described by Lance (1977) under the term 'intermediate paroxysmal non-kinesigenic dystonic choreoathetosis'. Attacks are precipitated by continuous
exercise (walking or running), hence the alternative name of paroxysmal exercise-induced
dyskinesia (Demirkiran and Jankovic 1995). Stress and cold can be exacerbating factors
(see Table 7.2) (Demirkiran and Jankovic 1995). Episodes usually last 5–30 minutes and
preferentially involve the lower limbs, sometimes spreading to the upper limbs and face.
About a quarter of cases are unilateral (Wali 1992, Bhatia et al. 1997) (Fig. 7.4). The onset
is between 2 and 30 years of age. Several families with an autosomal dominant pattern
of inheritance have been reported (Lance 1977, Plant et al. 1984, Nardocci et al. 1989,
Kluge et al. 1998) but the majority of cases are sporadic (Nardocci et al. 1989, Bhatia et
al. 1997). Association with rolandic epilepsy and writer's cramp has been reported (Guerrini et al. 1999) (see later). Levodopa (Demirkiran and Jankovic 1995), carbamazepine
and trihexyphenidyl (Bhatia et al. 1997) have been used with good results in only some
cases.

PAROXYSMAL DYSKINESIA OCCURRING DURING SLEEP

Some patients with paroxysmal dyskinesia have both diurnal and nocturnal episodes (De
Saint-Martin et al. 1997) or exclusively nocturnal episodes (Veggiotti et al. 1993,
Demirkiran and Jankovic 1995). Most patients show an autosomal dominant inheritance
(Fish and Marsden 1994, Demirkiran and Jankovic 1995) but sporadic occurrence has
been described. Lee et al. (1985) reported on three members of a family who exhibited
paroxysms of 'tonic–choreoathetoid' movements at the ages of 2, 10 and 24 years respectively. These occurred during non-REM sleep especially following days of intense activity.
The ictal EEG did not record paroxysmal elements. Carbamazepine was only partially
effective, while clonazepam was useless.

Lugaresi and Cirignotta (1981) and Lugaresi et al. (1986) described a syndrome of
nocturnal paroxysmal dystonia characterized by the occurrence, exclusively during sleep,
of episodes of intense "choreoathetoid, dystonic and ballistic" movements. The episodes
were repeated several times each night. Two variants were possible, short attacks lasting

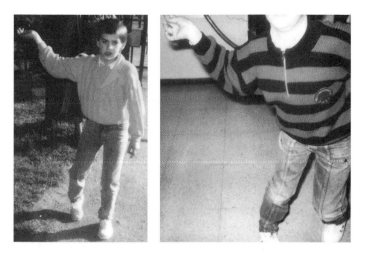

Fig. 7.4. Right hemidystonia precipitated by continuous exercise. This boy was born in 1978; there were no problems during pregnancy or delivery, nor any family history of neurological disorders. From day 25, he had episodes of head-turning to the right with rigidity of the right side of the body. At age 3 months a similar episode of long duration associated with ocular movements led to the use of phenobarbitone and phenytoin. EEG was normal. The attacks disappeared at age 2 years and treatment was discontinued at 4 years. At age 6, episodes of right-sided hemidystonia with abduction of right arm, supination and extension at the wrist began. There was abduction of the thigh and internal rotation of the foot. The episodes lasted minutes to hours and did not prevent walking. They were precipitated by walking or running for about 30 minutes and disappeared with carbamazepine treatment (400 mg/d).

15–40 seconds and long attacks lasting up to hours (Montagna et al. 1992). The onset in some of these patients was between 3 and 12 years of age. The disease tended to persist for years, although carbamazepine controlled the paroxysms. The nature of these episodes remains in doubt. They have many features reminiscent of those of frontal lobe seizures which are known to predominate during sleep and to occur frequently in the absence of definite EEG abnormalities. Most investigators now accept they are frontal lobe seizures (Tinuper et al. 1990, Oguni et al. 1992), especially the short-lasting attacks, but the subject remains controversial (Meierkord et al. 1992).

Scheffer et al. (1994) have described an autosomal dominant frontal lobe epilepsy with clusters of brief motor attacks occurring in sleep. Onset is usually in childhood. The gene has been localized in two families to chromosome 20q13.2 (Phillips et al. 1995) and cloned. This disease is frequently misdiagnosed as night terrors or paroxysmal nocturnal dystonia and closely resembles the cases described by Lugaresi et al. (1986).

OTHER PRIMARY PAROXYSMAL DYSKINESIAS
Two new clinical entities associating epilepsy and paroxysmal dyskinesia have been

recently described. *Infantile convulsions and paroxysmal choreoathetosis* is an autosomal dominant disorder associating infantile convulsions early in life with later (childhood or adolescence) paroxysmal choreoathetosis (Szepetowski et al. 1997). *Autosomal recessive rolandic epilepsy and paroxysmal exercise-induced dystonia and writer's cramp* (Guerrini et al. 1999) has been reported in three patients of a consanguineous family. The main symptoms are partial motor seizures of the rolandic type, dystonic writer's cramp of the right hand and, from age 2–3 years to 8–11 years, dystonic attacks involving the trunk or either hemibody appearing after exercise. Interestingly, in spite of the different type of inheritance both disorders have been linked to closely placed regions of chromosome 16, suggesting that they may be caused by a defect in the same gene.

Paroxysmal choreoathetosis with clinical characteristics reminiscent of those of non-kinesigenic paroxysmal dyskinesia of Mount and Reback but associated in some cases with spasticity has been described under the term of *autosomal dominant paroxysmal choreo-athetosis/spasticity syndrome*. Linkage to chromosome 1p has been demonstrated (Auburger et al. 1996).

Paroxysmal dystonia of infancy is discussed in Chapter 5.

SECONDARY PAROXYSMAL DYSKINESIAS

Secondary paroxysmal dyskinesias of any type (kinesigenic – Hwang et al. 1998, Mirsattari et al. 1999; non-kinesigenic – Kimura and Nezu 1999) can occur with many diseases (see Table 7.3) (Fig. 7.5) and cannot be correlated with a specific focal lesion in the CNS, as these can involve only the basal ganglia or the cerebral cortex, and sometimes also the brainstem or spinal cord (Riley 1996). In many cases the cause remains unde-termined, as in a patient of Micheli et al. (1986) who also had calcifications of the basal ganglia, a case of Kimura and Nezu (1999) with bilateral lesions in the globus pallidus and substantia nigra, and in two patients of Andermann et al. (1995) who presented with hypotonia of early onset. Because of the age of onset, generalized hypotonia, triggering of attacks by excitation and the secondary appearance of hemiplegic episodes in one child, the authors of this last report felt that these may have been atypical cases of alternating hemiplegia of childhood.

Paroxysmal tremor has been reported (see Chapter 3).

The response to therapy of secondary paroxysmal dyskinesias is variable. Micheli et al. (1987) mentioned the favourable effect of trihexyphenidyl (Artane) in a patient with mental retardation and a long history of neuroleptic drugs.

NOSOLOGY AND DIFFERENTIAL DIAGNOSIS OF PAROXYSMAL MOVEMENT DISORDERS

Because of the variety in expression and types of movement, the term dyskinesia seems preferable to those of choreathetosis or dystonia (Goodenough et al. 1978, Demirkiran and Jankovic 1995). The mechanism of production of paroxysmal movement disorders is unknown.

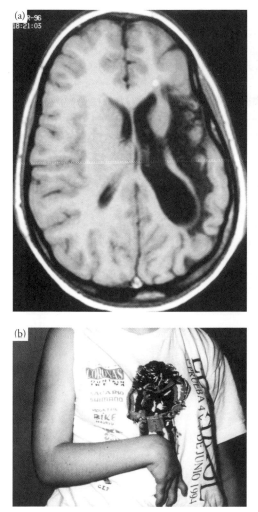

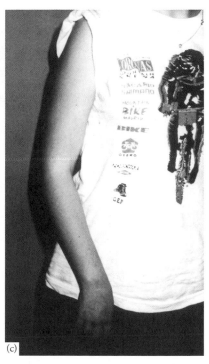

Fig. 7.5. Girl of 15 years with right-sided congenital hemiplegia. (a) MRI shows extensive lesion in the territory of the left sylvian artery. From 14 years onwards, she had repeated episodes of tonic flexion of the right upper limb (b) without impairment of consciousness lasting 4–6 hours. Interictal and ictal EEGs were normal. Diazepam i.v. suppressed the dystonia (c).

Their relationship with epileptic disorders is unclear. Their episodic paroxysmal stereotyped occurrence, often preceded by an aura, their response to antiepileptic drugs, and their frequent association with undoubtedly epileptic seizures supports an epileptic nature, but preservation of consciousness, even during bilateral episodes, and the absence of epileptiform activity in EEG recordings during attacks are strong arguments against the epileptic theory. Lombroso (1995, 2000) reported a case in which an epileptic discharge occurred at the same time as an episode of paroxysmal dyskinesia.

Several disorders must be considered in the differential diagnosis, as follows.

Alternating hemiplegia of childhood (see Chapter 5) must be considered in the differential diagnosis when paroxysmal dyskinesia occurs in infants.

Epilepsy. Frequent sensory prodromes and/or a family history of epileptic seizures (25% of the cases reported by Demirkiran and Jankovic 1995) can be misleading. Moreover, many types of epileptic seizures are not associated with unconsciousness, and dystonic epileptic movements or attitudes in partial complex seizures have been reported (Kotagal et al. 1989).

Startle provoked epileptic seizures (Chauvel et al. 1992) are common, especially in patients with congenital hemiplegia or other nonprogressive encephalopathies, and can closely resemble paroxysmal dyskinesia. The presence of interictal neurological signs and of spontaneous seizures is an important but inconstant differentiating feature (Manford et al. 1996). Movement-induced reflex epilepsy is very similar, and may be identical to kinesigenic paroxysmal dyskinesia.

Although the episodes of paroxysmal dyskinesia are clearly different from those of *episodic ataxias* (Gancher and Nutt 1986, Griggs and Nutt 1995), the distinction may be delicate in the absence of direct observation. The value of home videotaping should be emphasized in this regard. Both conditions share common features: autosomal dominant inheritance, lack of disturbance of consciousness, the facilitating effect of exercise and alcohol, and the beneficial effect of drugs such as acetazolamide (Griggs et al. 1978, Donat and Auger 1979). The presence of gait difficulties, ataxia and vertigo argues against paroxysmal dyskinesia.

Episodic ataxia type 1 may mimic paroxysmal kinesigenic dyskinesia because of the occurrence of brief attacks triggered by exercise and startle. However, there is interictal myokymia and spontaneous repetitive discharges (neuromyotonia) in the EMG. This disorder is due to point mutations on chromosome 12p (Browne et al. 1994).

In *type 2 episodic ataxia* or hereditary progressive ataxia, attacks are precipitated by emotional stress and exercise but not by startle. Interictal nystagmus is usually present on downgaze. Some of these patients develop progressive ataxia and dysarthria with vermian atrophy. The response to acetazolamide is generally dramatic. The gene is on chromosome 19p (Vahedi et al. 1995). This condition has been reported in association with paroxysmal dyskinesia in some patients (Mayeux and Fahn 1982, Gancher and Nutt 1986, Brunt and van Weerden 1990).

REFERENCES

Ahn JC, Hoyt WF, Hoyt CS (1989) Tonic upgaze in infancy. *Arch Ophthalmol* 107: 57–8.

Andermann F, Ohtahara S, Andermann E, et al. (1995) Infantile hypotonia and paroxysmal dystonia. A variant of alternating hemiplegia of childhood. In: Andermann E, Aicardi J, Vigevano F (eds) *Alternating Hemiplegia in Childhood.* New York: Raven Press, pp. 151–7.

Apak RA, Topçu M (1999) A case of paroxysmal tonic upgaze of childhood with ataxia. *Eur J Paediatr Neurol* 3: 129–31.

Artigas J, Lorente I (1989) Utilización de la carbamazepina en la coreoatetosis paroxística y en la corea de Sydenham. *An Esp Pediatr* 30: 41–4.

Auburger G, Ratlaff T, Lukes A, et al. (1996) A gene for autosomal dominant paroxysmal choreoathetosis/spasticity (CSE) maps to the vicinity of a potassium channel gene cluster on chromosome 1p, probably within 2 cM between D1S443 and D1S197. *Genomics* 31: 90–4.

Berger JR, Sheremata WA, Melamed E (1984) Paroxysmal dystonia as the initial manifestation of multiple sclerosis. *Arch Neurol* 15: 747–50.

Bhatia KP, Soland VL, Bhatt MH, et al. (1997) Paroxysmal exercise-induced dystonia: Eight new sporadic cases and a review of the literature. *Mov Disord* 12: 1007–12.

Blass JP, Kark RAP, Engel WK (1971) Clinical studies of a patient with pyruvate decarboxylase deficiency. *Arch Neurol* 25: 449–60.

Brandt NJ, Rasmussen K, Brante S, et al. (1976) D-Glyceric-acidaemia and non-ketotic hyperglycinaemia. Clinical and laboratory findings in a new syndrome. *Acta Pediatr Scand* 65: 17–22.

Bressman SB, Fahn S, Burke RF (1988) Paroxysmal nonkinesogenic dystonia. In: Fahn S, Marsden CD, Calne DF (eds) *Advances in Neurology. Vol. 50. Dystonia 2.* New York: Raven Press, pp. 403–13.

Browne DL, Gancher ST, Nutt JG, et al. (1994) Episodic ataxia/myokymia syndrome is associated with point mutations in the human potassium channel gene, *KCNA1. Nature Genet* 8: 136–40.

Brunt EP, Van Weerden TW (1990) Familial paroxysmal kinesigenic ataxia and continuous myokymia. *Brain* 113: 1361–82.

Burger LJ, Lopez RI, Elliot FA (1972) Tonic seizures induced by movement. *Neurology* 22: 656–9.

Buruma OJS, Roos RAC (1986) Paroxysmal choreoathetosis. In: Vinken PJ, Bruyn GW, Klawans HL (eds) *Handbook of Clinical Neurology. Vol. 5, no. 49. Extrapyramidal Disorders.* Amsterdam: Elsevier, pp. 349–58.

Camac A, Greene P, Khandji A (1990) Paroxysmal kinesigenic dystonic choreoathetosis associated with a thalamic infarct. *Mov Disord* 5: 235–8.

Campistol J, Prats JM, Garaizar C (1993) Benign paroxysmal tonic upgaze of childhood with ataxia. A neuroophthalmological syndrome of familial origin? *Dev Med Child Neurol* 35: 436–9.

Casteels-van Daele M (1979) Benign paroxysmal torticollis in infancy. *Acta Paediatr Scand* 68: 911–2.

Cataltepe SU, Barron TF (1993) Benign paroxysmal torticollis presenting as "seizures" in infancy. *Clin Pediatr* 32: 564–5.

Cavanagh NPC, Bicknell J, Howard F (1974) Cystinuria with mental retardation and paroxysmal dyskinesia in 2 brothers. *Arch Dis Child* 49: 662–4.

Chauvel P, Trottier S, Vignal JP, Bancaud J (1992) Somatomotor seizures of frontal lobe origin. *Adv Neurol* 57: 185–232.

Chudnow RS Dewey RB, Lawson CR (1997a) Choreoathetosis as a side effect of gabapentin therapy in severely neurologically impaired patients. *Arch Neurol* 54: 910–2.

— Mimbela RA, Owen DB, Roach ES (1997b) Gabapentin for familial paroxysmal dystonic choreoathetosis. *Neurology* 49: 1441–2.

Coulter DL, Donofrio P (1980) Haloperidol for nonkinesigenic paroxysmal dyskinesia. *Arch Neurol* 37: 325–6.

Darras BT, Ampola MG, Dietz WH, Gilmore HE (1989) Intermittent dystonia in Hartnup disease. *Ped Neurol* 5: 118–20.

Demirkiran M, Jankovic J (1995) Paroxysmal dyskinesias: Clinical features and classification. *Ann Neurol* 38: 571–9.

Deonna T, Martin D (1981) Benign paroxysmal torticollis in infancy. *Arch Dis Child* 56: 956–9.

— Roulet E, Meyer HU (1990) Benign paroxysmal tonic upgaze of childhood. A new syndrome. *Neuropediatrics* 21: 213–4.

De Saint-Martin A, Badinand N, Picard F, et al. (1997) Dyskinésie paroxystique diurne et nocturne de jeune enfant: une nouvelle entité? *Rev Neurol* 153: 262–7.

Donat JR, Auger R (1979) Familial periodic ataxia. *Arch Neurol* 36: 568–9.

Drake ME, Jackson RD, Miller CA (1986) Paroxysmal choreoathetosis after head injury. *J Neurol Neurosurg Psychiatry* 49: 837–8.

Dunn DW, Snyder H (1976) Benign paroxysmal vertigo of childhood. *Am J Dis Child* 130: 1099–100.

Dure LS, Mussell HG (1998) Paroxysmal dyskinesia in a patient with pseudohypoparathyroidism. *Mov Disord* 13: 746–8.

Echenne B, Rivier F (1992) Benign paroxysmal tonic upward gaze. *Pediatr Neurol* 8: 154–5.

Eeg-Olofsson O, Odkvist L, Lindskog U, Andersson B (1982) Benign paroxysmal vertigo in childhood. *Acta Otolaryngol* 93: 283–9.

Erikson GR, Chun RWM (1987) Acquired paroxysmal movement disorders. *Pediatr Neurol* 3: 226–9.

Fink JK, Heders P, Mathay JG, Albin RL (1997) Paroxysmal dystonic choreoathetosis linked to chromosome 2q: Clinical analysis and proposed pathophysiology. *Neurology* 49: 177–83.

Fish DR, Marsden CD (1994) Epilepsy masquerading as a movement disorder. *Mov Disord* 3: 346–58.

Fishbeck KH, Layzer RB (1979) Paroxysmal choreoathetosis associated with thyrotoxicosis. *Ann Neurol* 6: 453–4.

Fouad GT, Servidei S, Durcan S, et al. (1996) A gene for familial paroxysmal dyskinesia (*FPD1*) maps to chromosome 2q. *Am J Hum Genet* 59: 135–9.

Gancher ST, Nutt JG (1986) Autosomal dominant episodic ataxia: A heterogeneous syndrome. *Mov Disord* 1: 239–53.

Gieron MA, Korthals JK (1993) Benign paroxysmal tonic upward gaze. *Pediatr Neurol* 9: 159.

Gilroy J (1982) Abnormal computed tomograms in paroxysmal kinesigenic choreoathetosis. *Arch Neurol* 39: 779–80.

Goodenough DJ, Fariello RG, Annis BL, Chun RWM (1978) Familial and acquired paroxysmal dyskinesias. A proposed classification with delineation of clinical features. *Arch Neurol* 35: 827–31.

Griggs RC, Nutt JG (1995) Episodic ataxias as channelopathies. *Ann Neurol* 37: 285–7.

— Moxley RT, Lafrance RA, McQuillen J (1978) Hereditary paroxysmal ataxia: Response to acetazolamide. *Neurology* 12: 1259–64.

Guerrini R, Belmante A, Corrozzo R (1998) Paroxysmal tonic upgaze of childhood with ataxia: A benign transient dystonia with autosomal dominant inheritance. *Brain Dev* 20. 116–8.

— Bonanni P, Naldocci N, et al. (1999) Autosomal recessive rolandic epilepsy with paroxysmal exercise-induced dystonia and writer's cramp: Delineation of the syndrome and gene mapping to chromosome 16p12–11.2. *Ann Neurol* 45: 344–52.

Hanukoglu A, Somekh E, Fried D (1984) Benign paroxysmal torticollis in infancy. *Clin Pediatr* 23: 272–4.

Hart YM, Farrell K, Tampieri D, et al. (1995) Symptomatic alternating paroxysmal dystonia and hemiplegia. In: Andermann E, Aicardi J, Vigevano F (eds) *Alternating Hemiplegia in Childhood*. New York: Raven Press, pp. 159–64.

Hayman M, Harvey AS, Hopkins IJ, et al. (1998) Paroxysmal tonic upgaze: A reappraisal of outcome. *Ann Neurol* 43: 514–20.

Hudgins RL, Corbin KB (1966) An uncommon seizure disorder: Familial paroxysmal choreoathetosis. *Brain* 89: 199–204.

Hwang WJ, Lu CS, Tsai JJ (1998) Clinical manifestations of 20 Taiwanese patients with paroxysmal kinesigenic dyskinesia. *Acta Neurol Scand* 98: 340–5.

Joynt RG, Green D (1962) Tonic seizures as a manifestation of multiple sclerosis. *Arch Neurol* 6: 293–9.

Kato M, Araki S (1969) Paroxysmal kinesigenic choreoathetosis: Report of a case relieved by carbamazepine. *Arch Neurol* 20: 508–13.

Kertesz A (1967) Paroxysmal kinesigenic choreoathetosis: An entity within the paroxysmal choreo-athetosis syndrome: Description of ten cases including one autopsied. *Neurology* 17: 680–90.

Kim ME, Im J-H, Choi CG, Lee MC (1998) Proton MR spectroscopic findings in paroxysmal kinesigenic dyskinesia. *Mov Disord* 13: 570–5.

Kimura S, Nezu A (1999) A case of paroxysmal non-kinesigenic dyskinesia associated with lesions of the globus pallidus and substantia nigra. *Eur J Paediatr Neurol* 3: 29–32.

Kluge A, Kettner B, Zschenderlein R, et al. (1998) Changes in perfusion pattern using ECD-SPECT indicate frontal lobe and cerebellar involvement in exercise-induced paroxysmal dystonia. *Mov Disord* 13: 125–34.

Kotagal P, Luders H, Morris HH, et al. (1989) Dystonic posturing in complex partial seizures of temporal lobe onset: A new lateralizing sign. *Neurology* 39: 196–201.

Kurlan R, Shoulson I (1983) Familial paroxysmal dystonic choreoathetosis and response to alter-nate day oxazepam therapy. *Ann Neurol* 13: 456–7.

Lance JW (1977) Familial paroxysmal dystonic choreoathetosis and its differentiation from related syndromes. *Ann Neurol* 12: 285–93.

Lee BI, Lesser RP, Pippenger CE, et al. (1985) Familial paroxysmal hypnogenic dystonia. *Neurology* 35: 1357–60.

Lipson EH, Robertson WC (1978) Paroxysmal torticollis of infancy: Familial occurrence. *Am J Dis Child* 132: 422–3.

Lishman WA, Symonds CP, Whitty CWM, Willison RG (1962) Seizures induced by movement. *Brain* 85: 93–108.

Lombroso CT (1995) Paroxysmal kinesigenic choreoathetosis: An epileptic or non-epileptic dis-order. *Ital J Neurosci* 16: 271–7.

— (2000) Nocturnal paroxysmal dystonia due to a subfrontal cortical dysplasia. *Epileptic Disord* 2: 15–20.

Loong SC, Ong YY (1973) Paroxysmal kinesigenic choreoathetosis: Report of a case relieved by L-dopa. *J Neurol Neurosurg Psychiatry* 36: 921–4.

Lou HC (1989) Flunarizine in paroxysmal choreoathetosis. *Neuropediatrics* 20: 20–112.

Lugaresi E, Cirignotta F (1981) Hypnogenic paroxysmal dystonia: Epileptic seizures or a new syndrome? *Sleep* 4: 129–38.

— — Montagna P (1986) Nocturnal paroxysmal dystonia. *J Neurol Neurosurg Psychiatry* 49: 375–80.

Manford MR, Fish DR, Shorvon SD (1996) Startle provoked epileptic seizures: Features in 19 patients. *J Neurol Neurosurg Psychiatry* 61: 151–6.

Matthews WB (1958) Tonic seizures in disseminated sclerosis. *Brain* 81: 193–206.

Mayeux R, Fahn S (1982) Paroxysmal dystonic choreoathetosis in a patient with familial ataxia. *Neurology* 32: 1184–6.

Meierkord H, Fish DR, Smith SJM, et al. (1992) Is nocturnal paroxysmal dystonia a form of frontal lobe epilepsy? *Mov Disord* 7: 38–42.

Mets M (1990) Tonic upgaze in infancy. *Arch Ophthalmol* 108: 482–3.

Michaux L, Granier M (1945) Epilepsie bravais–jacksonienne réflexe. *Ann Med Psychol* 103: 172–7.

Micheli F, Fernández-Pardal MM, Casas Parera IF, Giannaula RJ (1986) Paroxysmal dystonic choreoathetosis associated with basal ganglia calcifications. *Ann Neurol* 20: 750.

— — de Arbelaiz R, et al. (1987) Paroxysmal dystonia responsive to anticholinergic drugs. *Clin Neuropharmacol* 10: 365–9.

— — Parera IC, Giannula R (1989) Idiopathic hypoparathyroidism and paroxysmal kinesigenic choreoathetosis. *Ann Neurol* 26: 415.

Mirsattari SM, Berry ME, Holden JK, et al. (1999) Paroxysmal dyskinesias in patients with HIV infection. *Neurology* 52: 109–14.

Montagna P, Cirignotta F, Giovanardi Rossi P, Lugaresi E (1992) Dystonic attacks related to sleep and exercise. *Eur Neurol* 32: 185–9.

Nardocci N, Lamperti E, Rumi V, Angelini L (1989) Typical and atypical forms of paroxysmal choreoathetosis. *Dev Med Child Neurol* 31: 670–81.

— Zorzi G, Savoldelli M, et al. (1995) Paroxysmal dystonia and paroxysmal tremor in a young patient with multiple sclerosis. *Ital J Neurol Sci* 16: 315–9.

Newman RP, Kinkel WR (1984) Paroxysmal choreoathetosis due to hypoglycemia. *Arch Neurol* 41: 341–2.

Nishi K, Tanaka S, Narabayashi H (1981) Familial paroxysmal kinesigenic choreoathetosis. *Brain Nerve* 33: 981–8.

Oguni M, Oguni H, Kozasa M, Fukuyama Y (1992) A case with nocturnal paroxysmal unilateral dystonia and interictal right frontal epileptic EEG focus: A lateralized variant of nocturnal paroxysmal dystonia. *Brain Dev* 14: 412–6.

Osterman PO, Westerberg CE (1975) Paroxysmal attacks in multiple sclerosis. *Brain* 98: 189–202.

Ouvrier RA, Billson F (1988) Benign paroxysmal tonic upgaze of childhood. *J Child Neurol* 3: 177–80.

Phillips HA, Scheffer IE, Berkovic SS, et al. (1995) Localization of a gene for autosomal dominant nocturnal frontal lobe epilepsy to chromosome 20q13.2. *Nature Genet* 10: 117–8 (letter).

Plant GT, Williams AC, Earl CG, Marsden CD (1984) Familial paroxysmal dystonia induced by exercise. *J Neurol Neurosurg Psychiatry* 46: 275–9.

Przuntek H, Monninger P (1983) Therapeutic aspects of kinesigenic paroxysmal choreoathetosis and familial paroxysmal choreoathetosis of the Mount and Reback type. *J Neurol* 230: 163–9.

Richards RN, Barnett HJM (1968) Paroxysmal dystonic choreoathetosis: A family study and review of the literature. *Neurology* 18: 461–9.

Riley DE (1996) Paroxysmal kinesigenic dystonia associated with a medullary lesion. *Mov Disord* 11: 738–40.

Robin T (1977) Paroxysmal choreoathetosis following head injury. *Ann Neurol* 2: 447–51.

Rosen JA (1964) Paroxysmal choreoathetosis associated with perinatal hypoxic encephalopathy. *Arch Neurol* 11: 385–7.

Roulet E, Deonna T (1988) Benign paroxysmal torticollis in infancy. *Dev Med Child Neurol* 30: 407–12.

Ruggieri VL, Yepez LL, Fejerman N (1998) Síndrome de desviación paroxística benigna de la mirada hacia arriba. *Rev Neurol* 27: 88–91.

Sanner G, Bergstrom B (1979) Benign paroxysmal torticollis in infancy. *Acta Paediatr Scand* 68: 219–23.

Scheffer IE, Bhatia KP, Lopes-Cendes I, et al. (1994) Autosomal dominant frontal epilepsy misdiagnosed as sleep disorder. *Lancet* 343: 515–7.

Smith LA, Heersema PH (1941) Periodic dystonia. *Proc Mayo Clin* 16: 842–6.

Snyder CH (1969) Paroxysmal torticollis in infancy: A possible form of labyrinthitis. *Am J Dis Child* 117: 458–60.

Soffer D, Licht A, Yaar I (1977) Paroxysmal choreoathetosis as a presenting symptom in an idiopathic hypoparathyroidism. *J Neurol Neurosurg Psychiatry* 40: 692–4.

Stevens H (1966) Paroxysmal kinesigenic choreoathetosis. A form of reflex epilepsy. *Arch Neurol* 14: 415–20.

Suber DA, Riley TL (1980) Valproic acid and normal computerized scan in kinesigenic paroxysmal choreoathetosis. *Arch Neurol* 37: 327.

Sugie H, Sugie Y, Ito M, et al. (1995) A case of paroxysmal tonic upward gaze associated with psychomotor retardation. *Dev Med Child Neurol* 37: 362–9.

Szepetowski P, Rochette J, Berquin P, et al. (1997) Familial infantile convulsions and paroxysmal choreoathetosis: A new neurological syndrome linked to the pericentromeric region of human chromosome 16. *Am J Hum Genet* 61: 889–98.

Tabae-Zadeh MJ, Frame B, Kapphahn K (1972) Kinesigenic choreoathetosis and idiopathic hypoparathyroidism. *N Engl J Med* 286: 762–3.

Tinuper P, Cerullo A, Cirignotta F, et al. (1990) Nocturnal paroxysmal dystonia with short-lasting attacks: Three cases with evidence for an epileptic frontal lobe origin of seizures. *Epilepsia* 31: 549–56.

Uriz MS, Fernández-Alvarez E (1988) Disquinesia paroxística. Un efecto secundario poco común de las hidantoinas. *Rev Esp Pediatr* 44: 413–5.

Vahedi K, Joutel A, van Bogaert P, et al. (1995) A gene for hereditary paroxysmal cerebellar ataxia maps to chromosome 19p. *Ann Neurol* 37: 289–93.

Veggiotti P, Zambrino CA, Balottin U, et al. (1993) Concurrent nocturnal and diurnal paroxysmal dystonia. *Child's Nerv Syst* 9: 458–61.

Wali GM (1992) Paroxysmal hemidystonia induced by prolonged exercise and cold. *J Neurol Neurosurg Psychiatry* 55: 236–7.

Watson RT, Scott WR (1979) Paroxysmal kinesigenic choreoathetosis and brain stem atrophy. *Arch Neurol* 36: 522.

8

MOVEMENT DISORDERS WITH MYOCLONUS AS THE MAIN CLINICAL MANIFESTATION*

INTRODUCTION AND CLASSIFICATION

The definition, semiological characteristics and types of myoclonus have been considered in Chapter 1. Two per cent of the cases in our (EF-A and colleagues) series of movement disorders in children showed this phenomenon as main manifestation (see Fig. 1.5, p. 19), and about 20% showed it associated to other movement disorders.

Myoclonus is a nonspecific sign of a large number of disorders of the nervous system, the detailed mechanisms of which are not yet clear and may be multiple. Many epileptic syndromes of infancy and childhood feature myoclonus as a prominent manifestation (Aicardi 1994).

There have been several attempts to classify myoclonus, mainly on physiological and aetiological bases.

Halliday (1967) divided myoclonus into three major categories depending on the electrophysiological characteristics: pyramidal, extrapyramidal and segmental. With few modifications this classification persists when exchanging the terms pyramidal for cortical, extrapyramidal for subcortical and segmental for spinal (Shibasaki 1996).

Cortical myoclonus generally affects distal muscles and may be focal. It can be spontaneous or reflex in response to various stimuli. It can be provoked by movement or other stimuli (cortical reflex myoclonus), or be the manifestation of an epileptic discharge, in which case it is accompanied by paroxysmal EEG abnormalities. It is often associated with giant somatosensory potentials, and back-averaging techniques indicate that it is consistently preceded by a cortical discharge.

Subcortical myoclonus is usually generalized. It can be spontaneous or reflex or can be precipitated by rapid voluntary movements. Electrophysiological studies (Hallett 1985) indicate a likely brainstem origin with activation of muscle in both ascending (to facial and eye muscles) and descending (limb muscles) directions.

Segmental myoclonus involves muscle groups innervated by contiguous segments of the brainstem or spinal cord (brainstem or spinal myoclonus).

*Written in collaboration with Natalio Fejerman, Hospital Garrahan, Buenos Aires, Argentina.

TABLE 8.1
Aetiological classification of childhood myoclonus

Physiological myoclonus	Hallervorden–Spatz disease
Sleep jerks	Huntington disease
Anxiety-induced	Multiple carboxylase deficiency
Exercise-induced	Biotin deficiency
Hiccups	Viral encephalopathies
Benign myoclonus of early infancy	Subacute sclerosing panencephalitis
Benign neonatal sleep myoclonus	Herpes simplex encephalitis
Essential myoclonus	Postinfectious encephalitis
Hereditary	Toxic encephalopathies
Sporadic	Bismuth
Idiopathic epileptic myoclonus	Heavy metal poisoning
Symptomatic myoclonus	Drugs
Genetic	Others
Lafora body disease	Opsoclonus–myoclonus syndrome
Lipidosis	Hepatic failure
Sialidosis type I	Renal failure
Ceroid-lipofuscinoses	Dialysis syndrome
Friedreich ataxia	Hyponatraemia
Unverricht–Lundborg disease	Hypoglycaemia
Gaucher disease	Nonketotic hyperglycinaemia
Wilson disease	Posthypoxic (Lance–Adams syndrome)
Torsion dystonia	Tumour
Hereditary myoclonic dystonia	Trauma

Aetiological criteria can also be used to classify myoclonus (Marsden et al. 1982, Fahn et al. 1986). A classification based on the systems of Fahn et al. (1986) and Fejerman (1991a,b) is shown in Table 8.1.

Another classification frequently used distinguishes epileptic from nonepileptic myoclonus. It is based essentially on the presence or absence of an EEG paroxysm (usually spike–wave complexes) temporally linked with the clinical jerk and its electro-myographic correlates. This separation is of dubious pathophysiological significance as: (1) an EEG paroxysm may not be detected by routine recording techniques, being demonstrated only by more sophisticated methods (e.g. back-averaging of the EEG triggered by the EMG discharge); and (2) proven epileptic seizures can occur without EEG paroxysm recorded from the scalp.

However, distinguishing myoclonus that occurs in association with definite clinical and/or EEG epileptic manifestations ('epileptic myoclonus') from that in which such features are absent ('nonepileptic myoclonus') is of great practical significance for diagnosis, prognosis and treatment. This distinction will therefore be used in this chapter despite its limited physiological validity.

'Epileptic myoclonus' is in most cases of cortical origin (spontaneous or reflex). However, in some types (e.g. reticular reflex myoclonus), subcortical structures may be implicated.

'Nonepileptic myoclonus', which includes physiological and non-physiological cases, can originate from multiple levels of the central nervous system (basal ganglia, brainstem, spinal cord).

This chapter is divided into three sections: physiological myoclonus, nonepileptic myoclonus, and epileptic myoclonus. Although epileptic phenomena are not the topic of this book, epileptic disorders that feature myoclonus are an important part of myoclonic disorders and are therefore mentioned.

PHYSIOLOGICAL MYOCLONUS

A significant number of persons present myoclonus as a sporadic or dominant symptom without evidence of epilepsy or neurological signs or impairments.

Sleep myoclonus is a common phenomenon both in children and adults. It includes two types: myoclonic jerks, usually single and massive, at onset of sleep, also called 'sleep starts' or 'hypnagogic jerks' (Symmonds 1953); and an erratic type characterized by subtle sporadic contractions that are asynchronous and asymmetrical, and involve principally individual muscles of the hands and face. The latter type is seen mainly during REM sleep (Gastaut 1968, Fahn et al. 1986). Fusco et al. (1999) have reported in neurologically impaired infants a phenomenon closely related to sleep myoclonus with a repetitive character during the transition between wakefulness and sleep. They consider that children with epilepsy could suffer an intensification of the otherwise normal hypnagogic jerks. These episodes can easily be mistaken for epileptic seizures.

Partial or localized myoclonias in the waking state are rare physiological phenomena that occur usually after muscular fatigue or in certain postures, implying a slight tonic contraction of the muscles. Affected muscles may vary, but in each episode the myoclonus is repetitive and remains localized to the same muscle or group of muscles during seconds or a few minutes. The concomitant EEG is normal and a possible spinal origin has been mooted (Gastaut 1968).

Startle responses while awake — called "curtrait diurne" in the French literature (Gastaut 1968) – are a kind of slight bilateral or massive nonepileptic myoclonus appearing as a surprise reaction to a sudden sensory stimulus.

Exaggerated physiological myoclonus is a term that tries to encompass the cases in which physiological myoclonus (e.g startle response) may become so intense or frequent that the boundaries between normal and pathological get blurred.

NONEPILEPTIC MYOCLONUS
BENIGN NEONATAL SLEEP MYOCLONUS
In 1982 Coulter and Allen reported three infants with sleep myoclonus that began in the first month of life. Myoclonic jerks were described as bilateral, repetitive, and located primarily in the distal parts of the upper extremities. Neurological examination and

critical EEG were normal and remained normal during follow-up. They coined the term 'benign neonatal sleep myoclonus' (BNSM).

During the following years some small series of cases with relatively short follow-ups were published, emphasizing the importance of differential diagnosis with neonatal seizures (Resnick et al. 1986, Tardieu et al. 1986). The condition is probably frequent, as three series included respectively 10, 19 and 12 patients (Daoust-Roy and Seshia 1992, Donat and Wright 1992, Di Capua et al. 1993).

Clinical features
BNSM appears in term newborn infants during the first weeks of life; the earliest onset was registered at five hours postnatally (Coulter and Allen 1982). Because intensity and frequency of jerks increase up to the third week of life, more subtle myoclonus appearing in the early days may go unnoticed.

Myoclonic jerks in BNSM are mainly present during quiet sleep, and the phenom-enon is less frequent or absent altogether during REM sleep (Di Capua et al. 1993). In most cases jerks are predominant in the upper limbs, especially distally, but myoclonus in the facial, axial and abdominal muscles has also been rarely reported (Resnick et al. 1986, Daoust-Roy and Seshia 1992, Di Capua et al. 1993). The jerks may be bilateral or localized, rhythmical or arrhythmical, and even migratory or multifocal. BNSM frequently occurs in clusters of several jerks repeating at a rhythm of 1–5 per second during several seconds. These bouts of myoclonic jerks usually recur irregularly in series lasting 20–30 minutes (Di Capua et al. 1993) or up to 90 minutes (Blennow 1986), so BNSM was mistaken in some cases for convulsive status (Alfonso et al. 1995). Sleep state does not change during the episodes, and waking up always stops the jerks. Occasionally BNSM was shown to be stimulus sensitive, elicited for instance by noises (Coulter and Allen 1982). Its appearance after rocking the crib has been described as a diagnostic manoeuvre (Alfonso et al. 1995). Curiously, benzodiazepines were found to increase the intensity of BNSM (Resnick et al. 1986).

BNSM fades spontaneously from the second month onward, and usually disappears before the sixth month of life. Interictal and ictal EEG is normal in BNSM.

Aetiology
Genetic factors may be involved in the genesis of BNSM as two affected siblings have been reported in two small series of patients (Tardieu et al. 1986) and a history of jerks during sleep in one of the parents was also suggested in several cases.

Differential diagnosis
Often BNSM is misdiagnosed as epileptic seizures. The relationship of the attacks with quiet sleep, normal clinical and developmental status of the infant, and the normality of the EEG are important clues to BNSM diagnosis. Other diagnoses include physiological myoclonus, jitteriness (see Chapter 3), motor automatisms and tonic posturing. Motor

automatisms – such as pedalling, stepping, rotary arm movements and complex purpose-less movements – and other movements including tonic posturing and even focal or fragmentary myoclonus in the neonate may not be associated with EEG seizure discharges (Mizrahi 1987). Benign myoclonus of early infancy never starts in newborn infants and generally occurs in the waking state (Fejerman 1976, 1984, 1991a).

BENIGN MYOCLONUS OF EARLY INFANCY

In 1976 Fejerman presented ten infants with a disorder he termed 'benign myoclonus of early infancy' (BMEI), comprising fits somehow resembling infantile spasms but with clinical, EEG and evolutive features allowing clear differential diagnosis from West syndrome (Fejerman 1976, Fejerman and Medina 1997). These cases were subsequently included in another report (Lombroso and Fejerman 1977), and several cases have been reported since (Dravet et al. 1986, Caviedes Altable et al. 1992). Fejerman has now followed for two to 27 years a total of 41 cases (26 male, 15 female). All patients were seen because of repeated jerks of neck or upper limb muscles leading to abrupt flexion or rotation of the head and extension with abduction of limbs.

In 20 patients the movements were described as shuddering of the head and shoulders, in a few extending to the upper limbs and in three seen only in the upper limbs. In some cases the only feature was symmetrical or asymmetrical extension with abduction of the upper limbs. Isolated cases presented with head rotation and extension of one upper limb or with head drops. In the cases of Pachatz et al. (1999) the attacks were usually triggered by excitement or frustration.

In 14 patients these 'myoclonic' jerks repeated in series, but whether in series or isolated, the fits occurred several times daily in 40% of the cases. Consciousness was not affected during fits. In Fejerman's series no case was detected during sleep, but two patients with BMEI having jerks while asleep have been reported by Dravet et al. (1986).

The age at onset ranged from 1 to 12 months, and was between 3 and 9 months in 90% of cases. Neurological examination was normal in all cases, and repeated EEG during waking and sleep showed no abnormalities. Ictal EEG has also been shown to be normal (Pachatz et al 1999). Video/polygraphic recordings indicate that the motor phenomenon is not a myoclonic but a tonic contraction (Pachatz et al. 1999).

Most children were developmentally normal. The frequency of fits tended to increase in the weeks following onset, but was considerably reduced after several months. Most of the children are free of attacks in the course of the second year of life. One patient developed benign myoclonic epilepsy at 19 months of age, and another presented crypto-genic partial epilepsy at 6 years.

The mechanism is unknown but seems to be related to tics (Pachatz et al. 1999). Rare cases in siblings are on record (Galletti et al. 1989).

ESSENTIAL MYOCLONUS

This disorder was first reported by N Friedreich in 1881 under the name of 'paramyoclonus multiplex'. Since then cases with autosomal dominant inheritance (Daube and Peters 1966, Mahloudji and Pikielny 1967, Korten et al. 1974) and sporadic cases have been described (Bressman and Fahn 1986). According to Mahloudji and Pikielny (1967), criteria for diagnosis of the hereditary cases include: (1) onset of symptoms in the first or second decade of life; (2) a benign course, often variable but compatible with a normal life; (3) absence of seizures, dementia, gross ataxia and other neurological defects; and (4) a normal EEG.

The myoclonus is arrhythmical and diffusely distributed. It is frequently exacerbated by action and disappears in sleep. The clinical expression is variable between individuals even in the same pedigree, and in the same individual at different times (Korten et al. 1974). The course is nonprogressive or only very slowly progressive.

The resulting disability depends on the intensity of the myoclonus and affects mostly fine movements and those that require precise manipulation, such as drinking from a glass.

In some cases, a mild dystonia may be present. A relationship between hereditary essential myoclonus and essential tremor has been suggested (Korten et al. 1974).

Sporadic cases are more frequent than hereditary ones. Onset in sporadic cases is more variable than in hereditary ones but was before 18 years in five of 15 patients reported by Bressman and Fahn (1986). Sporadic cases may present with myoclonic discharges of a variety of types: waxing and waning amplitude [termed by Fahn and Singh (1981) 'oscillatory myoclonus'], segmental myoclonus, rhythmical or arrhythmical or multifocal arrhythmical myoclonus as in hereditary cases. The areas most involved are the trunk and proximal part of limbs. There is often an initial worsening followed by stability or improvement.

In hereditary cases the diagnosis is quite easy but differentiation from benign hereditary chorea (see Chapter 3) can be difficult. Other familial conditions featuring myoclonus such as Unverricht–Lundborg or Lafora diseases can easily be distinguished by their malignant course, seizures, mental regression and recessive mode of inheritance, but diagnosis at onset can be difficult. Clinical characteristics of myoclonic dystonia are discussed in Chapter 5.

HYPEREKPLEXIA

Hyperekplexia or startle disease is a rare disorder that is often misdiagnosed as epilepsy. Most cases are familial with autosomal dominant transmission (Andermann et al. 1980) but at least one family with proven autosomal recessive inheritance has been reported (Rees et al. 1994). Other cases are sporadic (Gastaut and Villeneuve 1967). One autosomal recessive case (Rees et al. 1994) and many autosomal dominant ones are due to mutations in the $\alpha 1$ subunit of the glycine receptor (GLRA1) in the short arm of chromosome 5 (Ryan et al. 1992, Shiang et al. 1995, Tijssen et al. 1995), but mutations were not identified in other patients with associated atypical features such as developmental language delay or seizures (Shiang et al. 1995).

Hyperekplexia is characterized by a strikingly excessive response to tactile, auditory, visual and other sudden sensory stimuli. It can occur in two forms. In the 'minor' form, the startle response is excessive but without additional symptoms. It consists of flexion of the head with extension, elevation and abduction of the upper limbs after a sudden unexpected noise. In the 'major' form, infants present from birth with exaggerated startle response induced by unexpected auditory or tactile stimuli, and marked muscular hypertonia. This form is probably identical to the 'hereditary stiff-baby syndrome' (Ryan et al. 1992). Touching the tip or the dorsum of the nose elicits, more easily than with other parts of the body, a symmetrical jerk of all four limbs and a tonic fit with apnoea, so that occasionally death from apnoea may result (Kurczynski 1983). This type of attack can be arrested by forced flexion of the head and legs, as described by Vigevano et al.(1989), which can be a life-saving manoeuvre. When children grow up, the startle response may cause falling. Tonic generalized attacks with cyanosis may occur during sleep. In prolonged attacks a few clonic movements can occur.

Periodic movements during sleep occur in some cases (Andermann and Andermann 1988).

Hypertonia without pyramidal signs decreases with time but can provoke hip subluxation (Chevrel et al. 1995) or hernias. Affected children walk by 2–3 years of age and often present with mild mental retardation.

Diagnosis of hyperekplexia is essentially clinical. Molecular DNA studies can firmly confirm or exclude the diagnosis but are expensive and rarely available. In a large family with both typical and supposed 'minor' forms, molecular studies later showed that the 'minor' cases in this family were in fact misinterpretation of normal startle in unaffected persons (Tijssen et al. 1995). Clinical diagnosis requires a consistent response to effective stimuli that does not habituate with their repetition. The condition should be distinguished from the so-called *secondary hyperekplexia* that can occur with some CNS disorders such as perinatal encephalopathy (Brown et al. 1991). In such cases, the response to the stimuli is less consistent and often shows habituation.

The course of the illness may be variable. Usually it is a lifelong disease, but improvement may occur after the first years of life so that the disease becomes stationary in adult life.

Clonazepam is the drug of choice, clearly reducing both the paroxysmal episodes that occur during sleep and drop attacks due to stimulus-induced contractions (Ryan et al. 1992, Fejerman and Medina 1997).Valproate and piracetam (Fejerman 1991b) have been also used with success (Obeso et al. 1986).

Because of their stiffness, severe cases are often misdiagnosed as having spastic quadriparesis with stimulus-sensitive myoclonic epilepsy, and it is easy to consider movement artefacts in the EEG as abnormal discharges.

It is interesting that despite its designation as 'startle disease' hyperekplexia has no proven relation to the normal human startle response, and it has been suggested that it can be akin to reticular reflex myoclonus (Matsumoto et al. 1992).

OPSOCLONUS–MYOCLONUS SYNDROME (OMS)

Many other terms have been used to designate this syndrome, among them those of 'dancing eyes syndrome' (Ford 1966), 'infantile polymyoclonia' (Dyken and Kolar 1968), 'acute cerebellar encephalopathy' (Bray et al. 1969), 'oculocerebellomyoclonic syndrome' (Lemerle et al. 1969), RIMEL (rapid irregular movements of eyes and limbs) (Pampiglione and Maia 1972), 'ataxic–opsoclonic–myoclonic syndrome' (Pinsard et al. 1980) and 'Kinsbourne syndrome' (Brandt et al. 1974).

The syndrome was identified by Paul Sandifer and reported by Kinsbourne (1962) as 'myoclonic encephalopathy of infants'. Kinsbourne described six cases with onset between 9 and 20 months of age of uncoordinated, irregular movements of the trunk and limbs, myoclonus and chaotic ocular movements. Four of these patients received ACTH with improvement. A few similar cases, generally attributed to encephalitis or poliomyelitic infection, had been previously reported (Cogan 1954, Arthuis et al. 1960). Although isolated observations had been previously reported, attention was drawn to the frequent association of OMS with neural tumours by the independent reports of Solomon and Chutorian (1968) and of Dyken and Kolar (1968). Subsequent reports have amply confirmed the association.

Clinical features

OMS is a disorder of infants and young children. The average age at onset is 17–19 months (Fernández-Alvarez et al. 1978, Boltshauser et al. 1979, Hammer et al. 1995), ranging between 4 months and 6 years.

The four main symptoms are irritability, tremor, incoordination and ocular dyskinesia. Often initial symptoms appear within one or two weeks of a viral infection or immunization and the clinical picture is completed in a few more days.

A change in behaviour (irritability, agressivity), without decrease of the level of consciousness, and some instability are rapidly followed by severe incoordination and generalized tremor. The infants are unable to stand or sit without help. Walking with support is disorganized with excessive flinging of the legs. Simultaneously or a few days later, ocular dyskinesia is obvious. The most characteristic ocular abnormalities consist of chaotic, rapid, irregular bursts of movement occurring generally in a horizontal plane. These ocular abnormal movements were termed opsoclonus by K Orzechowski. Opsoclonus is often intermittent and may be associated with fast palpebral movements (flutter) reminiscent of the wing motion of insects. Other abnormal ocular movements may include vertical or horizontal lightning eye move-ments (Atkin and Bender 1964). These are sometimes the only ocular abnormality. Eye movements may be perceived under closed eyelids during sleep.

Myoclonic jerks of the face, trunk and limbs are the fourth component of the syndrome. They are brief, sudden muscle contractions that may be of small amplitude and may escape recognition due to associated tremor. They predominantly involve the eyebrows and lips. In the limbs they are mostly proximal. In the lower limbs they may become manifest when the child walks on all fours as sudden elevation of one limb disorganizes the pattern.

Manipulation of objects is disturbed both by tremor and myoclonic jerks similar to the action and/or intention myoclonus described by Lance and Adams (1963) following hypoxic episodes.

Evolution

Two different forms can be observed: relapsing and non-relapsing. Non-relapsing forms have been reported in association with immunization (Tuchman et al. 1989) or viral infections such as coxsackie B3 virus (isolated in CSF or faeces, or serologically demonstrated), mumps (Ichiba et al. 1988), togavirus (Estrin 1977, Kuban et al. 1983, Herve et al. 1988), Epstein–Barr virus (Sheth et al. 1995) and poliomyelitis (Arthuis et al. 1960). In such cases onset is usually after 3 years of age. The duration of an attack in such forms is between 6 and 15 days, only exceptionally lasting for months (Tuchman et al. 1989). Most reports on patients with the non-relapsing form indicate systemic illness on presentation. Some such cases may be only a first episode of the classic type as reported follow-ups have often been short.

Neuroblastoma and OMS

Approximately 50% of published cases of OMS are associated with neuroblastoma. However, such cases may be preferentially published (Lott and Kinsbourne 1986) and in several large series the proportion of neuroblastoma cases was lower (Kinsbourne 1962, Boltshauser et al. 1979, Pinsard et al. 1980, Fernández-Alvarez 1989). A more recent series (Hammer et al. 1995) found a higher proportion of cases associated with neuroblastoma, probably due to improvement in imaging techniques, and the true frequency may be very high.

Seventy-two per cent of the sympathetic tumours associated with OMS are neuroblastomas and 27% ganglioneuroblastomas (Farrelly et al. 1984). OMS is more frequent with mediastinal tumours (40%), whereas this localization is only found in 10% of the cases of neuroblastoma in general (Altman and Buehner 1976, Farrelly et al. 1984)

Without treatment the disorder persists and leads to severe motor and cognitive impairment (Chiba et al. 1970). Even with treatment, a very frequent feature of OMS is its propensity to relapse, often related to viral infections.

Ancillary investigations

Except for findings related to neuroblastoma – when it is detected – the ancillary investigations are usually normal. The normality of the EEG is particularly remarkable and serves to separate OMS from some other diseases with action or intention myoclonus. A CSF pleocytosis is frequent in viral cases. Increased immunoglobulins in CSF and minimal increase in size of the fourth ventricle (Bray et al. 1969, Pampiglione and Maia 1972, Dyken and Kolar 1968, Moe and Nellhaus 1970), or the presence of pontine or cerebellar

TABLE 8.2
Forms of opsoclonus–myoclonus syndrome

'Classical' form

Onset: Acute (sometimes progressive). Age of onset: 6 mo–5 y

Clinical signs: Generalized tremor and incoordination, ocular dyskinesia (mainly opsoclonus), myoclonus and irritability. Incomplete forms (without opsoclonus or ataxia) have been reported

Therapy: Responsive to ACTH or corticosteroids

Evolution: Chronic *with exacerbations* (often related to viral infections)

Associated with sympathetic tumours
Variable evolution and response to tumour exeresis
Without demonstrated sympathetic tumours

Infectious (or parainfectious) form
Variable age of onset
Clinical signs as 'classical form'
Self-limited. No relapsing episodes

---

lesions (in postinfectious cases) (Willis et al. 1983, Hattori et al. 1988, Tuchman et al. 1989) have been exceptionally reported.

Brainstem auditory evoked potentials have shown pontine dysfunction in the acute phase with later normalization (Kalmanchey and Veres 1988).

Neuroblastoma must be intensively searched for in patients with OMS as detection of the tumour may be difficult. Catecholamine determination in urine is of limited value as it is within normal limits in 40% of cases (Senelick et al. 1973). Standard radiological studies can be negative (Koh et al. 1994) but CT scanning or MRI can diagnose neuroblastoma in cases in which the tumour had been missed previously. Currently, the diagnosis of tumour is made in more than 90% of cases by CT scanning or MRI (Koh et al. 1994). Scintigraphic visualization of neuroblastoma with MIBG (metaiodobenzylguanidine), a radioisotope, structurally an analogue of noradrenaline, selectively taken up and stored by tumours derived from the neural crest, is very useful (Parisi et al. 1993). Octreotide (a long-acting analogue of somatostatin) seems to be even more sensitive in localizing the neuroblastoma, and yields images of better quality (Posada and Tardo 1998).

Variants
Several clinical variants of OMS can occur (Table 8.2). In some cases incomplete manifestations may be present for up to several months before the full-fledged syndrome (Moe and Nellhaus 1970, Pampiglione and Maia 1972, Roberts and Freeman 1975, Fernández-Alvarez 1989).

Patients without opsoclonus are rarely observed; some have been reported as having *isolated postinfectious myoclonus syndrome* (Bhatia et al. 1992). Rare cases in adults with carcinoma or viral infection have been described (Anderson et al. 1988, Dropcho and

Payne 1986). Their response to ACTH is often incomplete or absent.

Cases following intranasal use of cocaine (Scharf 1989), hyperosmolar nonketotic coma (Pranzatelli 1992) and biotin-responsive multiple carboxylase deficiency (Parker et al. 1983) are also on record.

Outcome
Three-quarters of patients with the classical form or without neuroblastoma have long-term sequelae such as mental retardation, learning difficulties, delayed language development, persistent ataxia or marked clumsiness (Koh et al. 1994, Pohl et al. 1996). Evidence for improvement over time of important aspects of cognition and developmental progression of social–adaptive skills is common (Papero et al. 1995). In our experience (e.g. Fernández-Alvarez 1989) and that of others (Chiba et al. 1970), untreated or partially treated cases had a worse outcome, with severe mental difficulties, marked hypotonia and disturbances of ambulation, than correctly treated ones. In contrast with the relapsing cases, only one non-relapsing case had long-term residua in the form of persistent ocular dysmetria and palpebral flutter (Kuban et al. 1983).

Patients with OMS associated with neuroblastoma have a survival rate four times greater than that those with neuroblastoma in general (Altman and Baehner 1976, Koh et al. 1994). This may be due to an earlier diagnosis because of the neurological signs, but a strong immunological response to the tumour also manifesting against nervous system components, and/or the intrinsically lesser malignity of these tumours may be factors. Indeed, single copies of the *N-myc* gene are more common than multiple copies in cases with OMS (Cohn et al. 1988).

In one case myasthenia gravis has been reported as a late manifestation (Wilfong and Fernandez 1992), again suggesting the possible importance of immunological factors.

Differential diagnosis
Opsoclonus is distinct from nystagmus in lacking rhythmicity which by definition is necessary in the latter. OMS is easy to diagnose when the syndrome is fully developed. At onset, when only irritability, instability and tremor are present, diagnostic possibilities include: ingestion of toxic substances; posterior fossa neoplasm, which can be ruled out by neuroimaging studies; and cerebellar or brainstem parainfectious encephalitis. As suggested by Kinsbourne in his initial report (1962), "In the past, such cases may have been unrecognized and included in series of 'acute cerebellar ataxia'." However, the evolution is different since classical OMS has a chronic course with relapses and exacerbations usually in association with intercurrent infections. Metabolic diseases, mainly urea cycle disorders and aminoacidopathies, are also a cause of intermittent ataxia, irritability and nystagmus, but obnubilation is common, they are usually triggered by a catabolic state, and the presence of opsoclonus is exceptional. Myoclonic status epilepticus, the 'bad periods' in the course of Lennox–Gastaut syndrome or myoclonic epilepsies with associated erratic myoclonus and ataxia do not produce opsoclonus.

Pathology

Only a few pathological studies, mainly of cases associated with neuroblastoma, are available. Some gave normal results (Lemerle et al. 1969). Others (Moe and Nellhaus 1970, Ziter et al. 1979, Tuchman et al. 1989) found a decreased number of Purkinje cells and demyelination mainly affecting the cerebellar dentate nucleus. The cerebellum was normal in one personal case (EF-A), and only mild diffuse demyelination of the white matter was found in a second case.

Pathogenesis

OMS is probably due to various causes with a final common pathway involving neuro-immunological responses. The relationship with neuroblastoma does not seem to be dependent on the excretion of catecholamines by the tumour, although other unidentified humoral mediators might be at play (Nickerson and Hutter 1979). However, removal of the tumour and improvement are only occasionally related. Disturbances in the metabolism of 5-hydroxyindolacetic acid, the principal oxidative metabolite of 5-hydroxytryptamine (5-HT), and of homovallinic acid, a major dopamine metabolite, that have been found to be decreased in some patients under 4 years of age, have also been reported (Pranzatelli et al. 1995). Anti-Hu antibody was present in serum and CSF in a few cases (Fisher et al. 1994).

IgG and IgM autoantibodies against high-molecular-weight neurofilaments and Purkinje cell cytoplasm and axons have been demonstrated in the serum of patients with OMS when this has been tested early in the disease, subsequently diminishing with treatment (Connolly et al. 1997).

Because of the high frequency of sympathetic tumours in OMS it has been suggested that the apparently isolated cases of the syndrome may be due to such tumours that have spontaneously involuted (Brandt et al. 1974), and the possibility of the tumour remaining latent for long periods up to several months is known (Bray et al. 1969).

Treatment

Treatment with ACTH (10–40 UI/d) usually causes a quick disappearance of the clinical manifestations. Prednisone is also used but may be less effective than ACTH (Hammer et al. 1995). The maintenance dose should be adjusted to the individual patient's response. Treatment usually needs to be prolonged for months or even years (Tal et al. 1983, Fernández-Alvarez 1989, Papini et al. 1992). The dose of ACTH or corticosteroids should be tapered very slowly. Decreases of ACTH dose as small as 0.1 mg/d can result in relapses, and the minimum effective dose has to be determined for each case. Increased doses may be necessary at time of intercurrent infections. The necessity of continuing treatment has to be determined by periodically trying to decrease and eventually discontinue the drugs. Relapses often necessitate resumption of treatment even after months or years. Autoantibodies to ACTH have been found in one patient who developed tolerance to ACTH treatment (Pranzatelli et al. 1993).

In a few cases some measure of success was obtained with various other agents. Diaze-pam (Brissaud and Beauvais 1969), propranolol (Fowler 1976), L-5-HTP (Gobbi et al. 1986), azathioprine (an immunomodulating agent) (Penzien et al. 1993) and intravenous immunoglobulin G (Petruzzi and de Alarcon 1995, Eiris et al. 1997). One of us (EF-A) has tried carbamazepine, propranolol, primidone and immunoglobulin G with no benefit except in one case with carbamazepine treatment.

In cases with neuroblastoma one may wait for the results of surgical removal. However, ACTH/steroid treatment is usually necessary. Resection of the tumour has a variable effect on neurological symptoms: usually no improvement of symptoms results but dramatic improvement (Martin and Griffith 1971), or improvement and later reap-pearance (Brissaud and Beauvais 1969, Moe and Nellhaus 1970, Senelick et al. 1972, Nickerson and Hutter 1979) have been reported. The syndrome may even appear after surgical resection of the tumour (Lemerle et al. 1969, Deladieux et al. 1975).

OTHER DISORDERS WITH NON-EPILEPTIC MYOCLONUS
Spinal myoclonus is a rare type of myoclonus in children (Silfverskiöld 1962, Renault et al. 1995); in a review of 37 cases, Jankovic and Pardo (1986) found only one who was younger than 18 years. In most cases it involves muscles innervated by contiguous segments of the brainstem or spinal cord. It is often rhythmic and permanent and usually persists during sleep. Multiple causes can be responsible (trauma, demyelinating disorders, penicillin, herpes zoster, myelomeningocele, spinal tumours). The latency between appearance of myoclonus and discovery of a cause may be several years. In the case of Renault et al. (1995), myoclonic rhythmical contractions of the left hip were observed by the parents at 2 months of age, and at 3 years 8 months an intraspinal tumour was found.

Acute transient myoclonus of the upper extremities, trunk or abdominal musculature has been reported in association with β-haemolytic streptococcus infection: it has been considered as a possible variant of PANDAS (paediatric autoimmune neuropsychiatric disorder associated with streptococcal infection) (di Fazio et al. 1998).

Myoclonus can occur, as mentioned previously, in association with *idiopathic torsion dystonia* (ITD), but study of some families suggests that this may be the result of a coincidence between ITD and benign myoclonus (see Chapter 5).

Intention and action myoclonias are an essential feature of sialidosis type I, also known as the *cherry-red spot–myoclonus syndrome* (Rapin et al. 1978), of *galactosialidosis* (Suzuki et al. 1991) and of *Gaucher disease* (Mystri 1995). They may be associated with epileptic manifestations in such cases.

Mitochondrial diseases such as *MERRF* (mitochondrial epilepsy with ragged-red fibers, usually associated with a point mutation at nt8344 in the gene of the transfer RNA for lysine) or *Leigh disease* (see also Chapters 5–7) may be associated with myoclonus. In MERFF, myoclonus may be increased by action, intention or closure of the eyes (Jackson et al. 1993). Calcification or hypodensity of the basal ganglia is frequent.

EPILEPTIC MYOCLONUS

Myoclonic jerks are a component of many forms of epileptic seizures, including tonic–clonic attacks. Myoclonus in the form of isolated or repetitive jerks is a common feature of several types of epilepsy. Only when myoclonic jerks are the predominant manifestation of an epilepsy is it customary to term it myoclonic epilepsy.

Several types of myoclonic jerks may occur in various epilepsy syndromes.

Most jerks are axial or massive. They involve the muscles of the neck, the shoulders, and sometimes the hip flexors and trunk muscles in a symmetrical way. They often affect also eyelid and eye muscles, and the territory may be very extensive. Less commonly, they may involve the lower limbs and result in falls. Each jerk includes a brief contraction phase of 50 ms or less, followed by a period of loss of muscle tone that may be of variable duration (50–400 ms). When long enough, the resulting atonia may also be the cause of an atonic fall (Oguni et al. 1993).

Such myoclonic jerks occur in many forms of epilepsy including juvenile myoclonic epilepsy in which the upper extremities are frequently most affected (Dravet et al. 1982, Aicardi 1994), some cases of absence seizures, in which they can be very intense (myoclonic or clonic absences), and the various types of myoclonic epilepsy, either as the only type of seizure or in association with other types (Aicardi 1994). When the atonic component of individual myoclonias is prominent, the clinical picture is that of the so-called myoclonic–astatic epilepsy (Doose 1992, Aicardi 1996). Such cases represent a generalized form of negative myoclonus (see below) and may be paradoxically facilitated by some antiepileptic agents (especially carbamazepine and vigabatrin) (Guerrini et al. 1999).

Such myoclonic jerks, regardless of whether the muscular phenomena are active or passive, are associated with brief EEG discharges of spike–waves or polyspike–waves that are usually brief and irregular but may be rhythmical and longer in myoclonic absences.

A frequent type of bilateral myoclonia is eyelid myoclonia, often associated with eyeball deviation or jerk. This type occurs especially in the syndrome of eyelid myoclonia with absences (Jeavons and Harding 1975, Panayiotopoulos et al. 1996). In some cases, generalized myoclonus may occur continuously for long duration of up to several hours (status myoclonicus). Such events are sometimes seen in patients with juvenile myoclonic epilepsy and are not associated with complete loss of consciousness. They also are observed in comatose patients following anoxic/hypoxic events and are then of very poor prognosis.

Myoclonic jerks can also occur in limited muscle groups or single muscles, sometimes in a fixed location, more commonly erratically fluctuating in many muscles. This erratic, fragmentary myoclonus is frequent in many degenerative epileptic disorders such as Lafora or Unverricht–Lundborg diseases (Roger 1992, Aicardi 1994) (Table 8.3), usually in association with massive myoclonus and generalized tonic–clonic attacks. It is associated with a cortical paroxysm (cortical myoclonus) which may be obvious or necessitate back-averaging of the EEG triggered by the EMG discharge for detection. Such paroxysms may be multifocal but usually are recorded preferentially over the motor strip

TABLE 8.3
Types and causes of myoclonic epilepsy

Idiopathic myoclonic epilepsies
Juvenile myoclonic epilepsy (adolescents and young adults)
Benign myoclonic epilepsy (infants and young children)
Myoclonic absence epilepsy
Severe myoclonic epilepsy[1]
Myoclonic–astatic epilepsy[2]

Symptomatic and probably symptomatic myoclonic epilepsies
Non-progressive
   Lennox–Gastaut syndrome[3]
   Associated with brain lesions, focal or diffuse
   Angelman syndrome
Progressive
   Lafora body disease
   Unverricht–Lundborg (Baltic and Mediterranean myoclonus)
   Sialidosis type 1 (cherry-red spot–myoclonus syndrome)
   Myoclonic epilepsy with ragged-red fibres (MERRF)
   Other mitochondrial diseases with myoclonus
   Alpers poliodystrophy
   Juvenile (type III) Gaucher disease
   Galactosialidosis (mucolipidosis type I)
   Juvenile neuroaxonal dystrophy
   Ceroid-lipofuscinosis (types 1, 2, 3, 5, 6, 7)
   Huntington chorea (myoclonic variant)
   Wilson disease
   Hexosaminidase deficiency
   Nonketotic hyperglycinaemia (glycine encephalopathy)
   D-Glyceric aciduria
   Biopterin deficiency

[1] Defined as cryptogenic or symptomatic by the International League Against Epilepsy.
[2] Some cases may belong to the 'probably symptomatic' group. Myoclonus is especially common during episodes of nonconvulsive status.
[3] Myoclonus is present in only 20% of cases but also occurs during episodes of nonconvulsive status.

on the opposite side (Guerrini et al. 1993). Erratic myoclonus in progressive myoclonic epilepsies is often stimulus-related. Precipitation by movement, sometimes only intended, or even the thought of movement, is common in Unverricht–Lundborg disease and in sialidosis type 1. The same phenomenon is observed in post-hypoxic myoclonus following cardiac arrest or other causes of hypoxic brain damage known as Lance–Adams syndrome.

In these cases it may not be associated with epileptic manifestations. Other reflex precipitants are also frequent such as touch, sound or light. Awakening is frequently a precipitant in many types of myoclonic epilepsy. Closure of the eyes would precipitate myoclonic activity in one patient with MERRF (Garcia Silva et al. 1987).

In some cases, the active part of the myoclonia is not obvious, and the clinical and EMG correlates of the EEG event are negative phenomena, i.e. atonia with suppression of tonic EMG activity that may be localized to a segment contralateral to the EEG discharge or generalized (Oguni et al. 1993, Guerrini et al. 1993). The atonia temporally corresponds to the slow-wave of the spike–wave discharge (Tassinari et al. 1971, Shewmon and Erwin 1988). This 'negative myoclonus' is observed in some cases of 'atypical partial benign epilepsy' (Aicardi and Chevrie 1982, Guerrini et al. 1993), in cases of continuous spike–waves of slow sleep (CSWS) previously known as 'electrical status epilepticus of slow sleep' (ESES), and in some chronic congenital encephalopathies, the most common being Angelman syndrome (Guerrini et al. 1996) in which it often occurs in episodes of status and is also responsible for the saccadic nature of movement that was the origin of the previously used term of 'happy puppet syndrome'. Negative myoclonus may have the same triggering factors as positive myoclonus.

Both positive and negative erratic myoclonus often occur in children with severe epilepsies, especially severe myoclonic (or polymorphic) epilepsy (Dravet 1992), myoclonic–astatic epilepsy or some cases of Lennox–Gastaut syndrome in association with confusion or obtundation lasting hours or days. Such episodes of status epilepticus with erratic twitching or atonic partial or generalized falls may be misinterpreted as part of a degenerative disease with epilepsy (Aicardi 1994).

SYMPTOMATIC TREATMENT OF MYOCLONUS

With the exception of the favourable results of ACTH in OMS (which are probably related to aetiology), the efficacy of pharmacological treatment of nonepileptic myoclonus is disappointing. Many drugs have been tried in the treatment of myoclonus: antiepileptic agents, baclofen (Menon 1980), benzodiazepines (Ryan et al. 1992). It seems that myoclonus is the only dyskinesia that may respond to serotoninergic drugs (Pranzatelli 1994).

Essential myoclonus has been reported to be sensitive to primidone (Pranzatelli 1996), valproate (Lefkowitz and Harpold 1985), propranolol (Ferro and Calhau 1977), L-5-hydroxytryptophan (van Woert 1983) and clonazepam (Gledhill and Willes 1977). Piracetam (2-oxo-pyrrolidineacetamide) is effective on both cortical and subcortical myoclonus (Obeso et al. 1986) although more on cortical myoclonus (Ikeda et al. 1996). The dose is between 8 and 18 g/day or more. It is usually well tolerated. Most of the side effects are gastro-intestinal (gastric discomfort, diarrhoea). Thrombocytopenia and leukopenia have been also reported (Ikeda et al. 1996).

Treatment of *epileptic myoclonus* is that of the epilepsy in general but certain drugs are known potentially to increase or even produce de novo epileptic myoclonus (e.g. vigabatrin, phenytoin or lamotrigine) and should be used only with care.

REFERENCES

Aicardi J (1994) *Epilepsy in Children, 2nd edn.* New York: Raven Press.

— (1996) Myoclonic epilepsies in childhood. *Int Pediatr* 1: 195–200.

— Chevrie JJ (1982) Atypical benign epilepsy of childhood. *Dev Med Child Neurol* 24: 281–92.

Alfonso I, Papazian O, Aicardi J, Jeffries HE (1995) A simple maneuver to provoke benign neonatal sleep myoclonus. *Pediatrics* 96: 1161–3.

Altman AJ, Baehner RL (1976) Favourable prognosis for survival in children with coincident opso-myoclonus and neuroblastoma. *Cancer* 37: 846–52.

Andermann F, Andermann E (1988) Startle disorders of man: Hyperekplexia, jumping and startle epilepsy. *Brain Dev* 10: 213–22.

— Keene DL, Andermann E, Quesney LF (1980) Startle disease or hyperekplexia. Further delineation of the syndrome. *Brain* 103: 985–97.

Anderson NE, Budden-Steffen C, Rosenblum MK, et al. (1988) Opsoclonus, myoclonus, ataxia, and encephalopathy in adults with cancer: A distinct paraneoplasic syndrome. *Medicine* 67: 100–9.

Arthuis M, Lyon G, Thieffry S (1960) La forme ataxique de la maladie de Heine–Medin. *Rev Neurol* 103: 329–40.

Atkin A, Bender MB (1964) Lighting eye movements (ocular myoclonus). *J Neurol Sci* 1: 2–12.

Bhatia K, Thompson PD, Marsden CD (1992) 'Isolated' postinfectious myoclonus. *J Neurol Neurosurg Psychiatry* 55: 1089–91.

Blennow G (1986) Benign infantile nocturnal myoclonus. *Acta Paediatr Scand* 74: 505–7.

Boltshauser E, Deonna T, Hirt HR (1979) Myoclonic encephalopathy of infants or "dancing eyes syndrome". Report of 7 cases with long-term follow-up and review of the literature. *Helv Paediatr Acta* 34: 119–33.

Brandt S, Carlsen N, Glenting P, Helweglarsen J (1974) Encephalopathia myoclonica infantilis (Kinsbourne) and neuroblastoma in children. A report of three cases. *Dev Med Child Neurol* 16: 286–94.

Bray PF, Ziter FA, Lahey ME, Myers GG (1969) The coincidence of neuroblastoma and acute cerebellar encephalopathy. *J Pediatr* 75: 983–90.

Bressman S, Fahn S (1986) Essential myoclonus. In Fahn S, Marsden CD, Van Woert MH (eds) *Advances in Neurology. Vol. 43. Myoclonus.* New York: Raven Press, pp. 287–94.

Brissaud HE, Beauvais P (1969) Opsoclonus and neuroblastoma. *N Engl J Med* 280: 1242.

Brown P, Rothwell JC, Thompson PD, et al. (1991) The hyperekplexias and their relationship to the normal startle reflex. *Brain* 114: 1903–28.

Cavledes Altable BE, Moreno Belzue C, Arteaga R, Herranz Fernández JL (1992) Mioclonías benignas de la infancia temprana. *An Esp Pediatr* 36: 496–7.

Chevrel J, Berthier M, Bonneau D, et al. (1995) L'hyperekplexie. *Arch Pediatr* 2: 469–72.

Chiba S, Motoya H, Shinoda M, Nakao T (1970) Myoclonic encephalopathy of infants: a report of two cases of "dancing eyes" syndrome. *Dev Med Child Neurol* 12: 767–71.

Cogan DG (1954) Ocular dysmetria, flutter-like oscillations of the eyes and opsoclonus. *Arch Ophthalmol* 51: 318–35.

Cohn SL, Salwen H, Herst CV, et al. (1988) Single copies of the N-myc oncogene in neuroblastomas from children presenting with the syndrome of opsoclonus–myoclonus. *Cancer* 62: 723–6.

Connolly AM, Pestronk A, Mehta S, et al. (1997) Serum antibodies in childhood opsoclonus–myoclonus syndrome: An analysis of antigenic targets in neural tissues. *J Pediatr* 130: 878–94.

Coulter DL, Allen RJ. (1982) Benign neonatal myoclonus. *Arch Neurol* 39: 191–2.

Daoust-Roy J, Seshia SS (1992) Benign neonatal sleep myoclonus. *Am J Dis Child* 146: 1236–41.

Daube JR, Peters HA (1966) Hereditary essential myoclonus. *Arch Neurol* 15: 587–94.

Deladieux E, Binger G, Maurus R, Szliwowski H (1975) Myoclonic encephalopathy and neuro-blastoma. *N Engl J Med* 292: 46–7.

Di Capua M, Fusco L, Ricci S, Vigevano F (1993) Benign neonatal sleep myoclonus: Clinical features and video-polygraphic recordings. *Mov Disord* 8: 191–4.

Di Fazio MP, Morales J, Davis R (1998) Acute myoclonus secondary to group A β-hemolytic streptococcus infection: A PANDAS variant. *J Child Neurol* 13: 516–8.

Donat JF, Wright FS (1992) Clinical imitators of infantile spasms. *J Child Neurol* 7: 395–9.

Doose H (1992) Myoclonic astatic epilepsy of early childhood. In: Roger J, Dravet C, Bureau M, et al. (eds.) *Epileptic Syndromes in Infancy, Childhood and Adolescence, 2nd edn.* London: John Libbey, pp. 103–14.

Dravet C (1992) Severe myoclonic epilepsy. In: Roger J, Dravet C, Bureau M, et al. (eds.) *Epileptic Syndromes in Infancy, Childhood and Adolescence.* London: John Libbey, pp. 67–74.

— Roger J, Bureau M, Dalla Bernardina B (1982) Myoclonic epilepsies in childhood. In: Akimoto H, Katzamatzuri H, Seina M, Ward AA (eds.) *Advances in Epileptology, XIIIth Epilepsy International Symposium.* New York: Raven Press, pp. 135–40.

— Giraud N, Bureau M, et al. (1986) Benign myoclonus of early infancy or benign nonepileptic infantile spasms. *Neuropediatrics* 17: 33–8.

Dropcho E, Payne R (1986) Paraneoplasic opsoclonus–myoclonus. Association with medullary thyroid carcinoma and review of the literature. *Arch Neurol* 43: 410–5.

Dyken P, Kolar O (1968) Dancing eyes, dancing feet: Infantile polymyoclonia. *Brain* 91: 305–20.

Eiris J, del Rio M, Castro-Gago M (1997) Immune globulin G for the treatment of opso-clonus–myoclonus syndrome. *J Pediatr* 129: 175 (letter).

Estrin WJ (1977) The serological diagnosis of St Louis encephalitis in a patient with the syndrome of opsoclonus, body tremolousness and benign encephalitis. *Ann Neurol* 1: 596–8.

Fahn S, Singh N (1981) An oscillating form of essential myoclonus. *Neurology* 31: 80.

— Marsden CD, van Woert MH (1986) Definition and classification of myoclonus. *Adv Neurol* 43: 1–5.

Farrelly C, Daneman A, Chan HSL, Martin DJ (1984) Occult neuroblastoma presenting with opsomyoclonus: Utility of computed tomography. *AJR* 142: 807–10.

Fejerman N (1976) Mioclonías benignas de la infancia temprana. Comunicación preliminar. Actas IV Jornadas Rioplatenses de Neurología Infantil. In: *Neuropediatría Latinoamericana.* Montevideo: Delta, pp. 131–4.

— (1984) Mioclonías benignas de la infancia temprana. *An Esp Ped* 21: 725–31.

— (1991a) Myoclonies et epilepsies chez l'enfant. *Rev Neurol* 147: 782–97.

— (1991b) Myoclonus and epilepsies. In: Ohtahara S, Roger J (eds.) *New Trends in Pediatric Epileptology.* Okayama: Department of Child Neurology, Okayama University Medical School, pp. 94–110.

— Medina CS (1997) Hiperekplexia. In: Fejerman N, Fernández-Alvarez E (eds.) *Neurología Pediátrica. 2nd edn.* Buenos Aires: Panamericana, p. 597.

Fernández-Alvarez E (1989) Encefalopatía mioclónica del lactante (síndrome de Kinsbourne). *Int Pediatr* 4 (suppl. 2): 44–6.

— Camino A, Pineda M, Bidegain I (1978) Enfermedad de Kinsbourne. Estudio de cuatro casos. *An Esp Pediatr* 11: 461.

Ferro JM, Calhau ES (1977) Treatment of familial essential myoclonus with propranolol. *Lancet* 2: 143 (letter).

Fisher PG, Wechsler DS, Singer HS (1994) Anti-Hu antibody in a neuroblastoma-associated para-neoplasic syndrome. *Pediatr Neurol* 10: 309–311.

Ford FR (1966) *Diseases of the Nervous System in Infancy, Childhood and Adolescence.* Springfield, IL: CC Thomas.

Fowler EW (1976) Propranolol treatment of infantile polymyoclonus. *Neuropediatrics* 7: 443–50.

Fusco L, Pachatz C, Cusmai R, Vigevano F (1999) Repetitive sleep starts in neurologically impaired children: An unusual non-epileptic manifestation of otherwise epileptic subjects. *Epileptic Dis* 1: 63–7.

Galletti F, Brinciotti M, Emanuelli O (1989) Familial occurrence of benign myoclonus of early infancy. *Epilepsia* 30: 579–81.

Garcia Silva MT, Aicardi J, Goutières F, Chevrie JJ (1987) The syndrome of myoclonic epilepsy with ragged-red fibers. Report of a case and review of the literature. *Neuropediatrics* 18: 200–4.

Gastaut H (1968) Sémiologie des myoclonies et nosologie analytique des syndromes myocloniques. In: Bonduelle M, Gastaut H (eds.) *Les Myoclonies.* Paris: Masson, pp. 1–30.

— Villeneuve A (1967) The startle disease or hyperekplexia. Pathological surprise reaction. *J Neurol Sci* 5: 523–42.

Gledhill RF, Willes CM (1977) Clonazepam and branchial myoclonus. *Ann Neurol* 1: 306–7.

Gobbi G, Melideo G, Giovanardi-Rossi P (1986) The effect of intravenous L-5HTP in the myo-clonic encephalopathy of children. *Neuropediatrics* 17: 63–5.

Guerrini R, Dravet C, Genton P, et al. (1993) Epileptic negative myoclonus. *Neurology* 43: 1078–93.

— de Lorey TM, Bonanni P, et al. (1996) Cortical myoclonus in Angelman syndrome. *Ann Neurol* 39: 699–708.

— Belmonte L, Parmeggiani L, Perruca E (1999) Myoclonic status epilepticus following high-dose lamotrigine therapy. *Brain Dev* 21: 420–4.

Hallett M (1985) Myoclonus: Relation to epilepsy. *Epilepsia* 26 (suppl. 1): S67–S77.

Halliday AM (1967) The electrophysiological study of myoclonus in man. *Brain* 90: 241–83.

Hammer MS, Larsen MB, Stack CV (1995) Outcome of children with opsoclonus–myoclonus regardless of etiology. *Pediat Neurol* 13: 21–4.

Hattori T, Hirayama K, Imai T, et al. (1988) Pontine lesion in opsoclonus–myoclonus syndrome shown by MRI. *J Neurol Neurosurg Psychiatry* 51: 1572–5.

Herve F, Soulier J, Berger JP (1988) Syndrome opsomyocloniquc ct Coxsackie B3. *Arch Fr Pédiatr* 45: 597–9.

Ichiba N, Miyake T, Sato K, et al. (1988) Mumps-induced opsoclonus myoclonus and ataxia. *Pediatr Neurol* 4: 224–7.

Ikeda A, Shibasaki H, Tashiro K, et al. (1996) Clinical trial of piracetam in patients with myo-clonus. Nationwide multiinstitution study in Japan. *Mov Disord* 11: 691–700.

Jackson MJ, Schaeffer JA, Johnson MA, et al. (1993) Presentation and clinical investigation of mitochondrial respiratory chain disease. A study of 51 patients. *Brain* 118: 339–57.

Jankovic J, Pardo R (1986) Segmental myoclonus. Clinical and pharmacological study. *Arch Neurol* 43: 1025–31.

Jeavons PM, Harding GFA (1975) *Photosensitive Epilepsy. Clinics in Developmental Medicine No. 56.* London: Spastics International Medical Publications.

Kalmanchey R, Veres E (1988) Dancing eyes syndrome. Brain acoustic evoked potential approach. *Neuropediatrics* 19: 193–6.

Kinsbourne M (1962) Myoclonic encephalopathy of infants. *J Neurol Neurosurg Psychiatry* 25: 271–6.

Koh PS, Raffensperger JG, Berry S, et al. (1994) Long-term outcome in children with opsoclonus–myoclonus and ataxia and coincident neuroblastoma. *J Pediatr* 125: 712–6.

Korten JJ, Notermans SLH, Frenken CWGM, et al. (1974) Familial essential myoclonus. *Brain* 97: 131–8.

Kuban KC, Ephros MA, Freeman RL, et al. (1983) Syndrome of opsoclonus–myoclonus caused by Coxsackie B3 infection. *Ann Neurol* 13: 69–71.

Kurczynski TW (1983) Hyperekplexia. *Arch Neurol* 40: 246–8.

Lance JW, Adams RD (1963) The syndrome of intention or action myoclonus as a sequel to hypoxic encephalopathy. *Brain* 86: 111–22.

Lefkowitz D, Harpold G (1985) Treatment of ocular myoclonus with valproic acid. *Ann Neurol* 17: 103–4.

Lemerle J, Lemerle M, Aicardi J, et al. (1969) Trois cas d'association à un neuroblastome d'un syndrome oculocerebellomyoclonique. *Arch Fr Pediatr* 26: 547–58.

Lombroso CT, Fejerman N (1977) Benign myoclonus of early infancy. *Ann Neurol* 1: 138–48.

Lott I, Kinsbourne M (1986) Myoclonic encephalopathy of infants. *Adv Neurol* 43: 127–36.

Mahloudji M, Pikielny RT (1967) Hereditary essential myoclonus. *Brain* 90: 669–74.

Marsden CD, Hallett M, Fahn S (1982) The nosology and pathophysiology of myoclonus. In: Marsden CD, Fahn S (eds.) *Movement Disorders.* London: Butterworth Scientific, pp. 196–248.

Martin ES, Griffith JF (1971) Myoclonic encephalopathy and neuroblastoma. *Am J Dis Child* 122: 257–8.

Matsumoto J, Fuhr P, Nigro M, Hallett M (1992) Physiological abnormalities in hereditary hyperekplexia. *Ann Neurol* 32: 41–50.

Menon MK (1980) Possible value of baclofen in myoclonus. *JAMA* 224: 239–40.

Mizrahi EM (1987) Neonatal seizures: Problems in diagnosis and classification. *Epilepsia* 28 (suppl. 1): 546–55.

Moe PG, Nellhaus G (1970) Infantile polymyoclonia–opsoclonus syndrome and neural crest tumors. *Neurology* 20: 756–64.

Mystri PK (1995) Genotype/phenotype correlation in Gaucher disease. *Lancet* 346: 982–3.

Nickerson BG, Hutter JJ (1979) Opsomyoclonus and neuroblastoma. Reponses to ACTH. *Clin Pediatr* 18: 446–8.

Obeso JA, Artieda J, Luquin MR, et al. (1986) Antimyoclonic action of piracetam. *Clin Neuropharmacol* 9: 58–64.

Oguni H, Imaizumi Y, Uehara T, et al. (1993) Electroencephalographic features of epileptic drop attacks and absence seizures: A case study. *Brain Dev* 15: 226–30.

Pachatz C, Fusco L, Vigevano F (1999) Benign myoclonus of early infancy. *Epileptic Dis* 1: 57–61.

Pampiglione G, Maia M (1972) Syndrome of rapid irregular movements of eyes and limbs in childhood. *BMJ* 1: 469–73.

Panayiotopoulos CP, Agathonikou A, Koutramandis M, et al. (1996) Eyelid myoclonia with absences: the symptoms. In: Duncan J, Panayiotopoulos CP (eds.) *Eyelid Myoclonia with Absences.* London: John Libbey, pp. 17–26.

Papero PH, Pranzatelli MR, Margolis LJ, et al. (1995) Neurobehavioral and psychosocial functioning of children with opsoclonus–myoclonus syndrome. *Dev Med Child Neurol* 37: 915–32.

Papini M, Pasquinelli A, Filippini A (1992) Steroid-dependent form of Kinsbourne syndrome: Successful treatment with trazodone. *Ital J Neurol Sci* 13: 369–72.

Parisi M, Hattner RS, Matthay KK, et al. (1993) Optimized diagnostic strategy for neuroblastoma in opsoclonus–myoclonus. *J Nucl Med* 34: 1922–6.

Parker WD, Goodman SI, Stumpf DA, Wolf B (1983) Biotin responsive opsoclonus–myoclonus syndrome. *Neurology* 33 (suppl.): 153 (letter).

Penzien JM, Speck S, Vasella F (1993) Opsoclonus polymyoclonia syndrome. *Acta Paediatr* 82: 319–20.

Petruzzi MJ, de Alarcon PA (1995) Neuroblastoma-associated opsoclonus–myoclonus treated with intravenously administered immune globulin G. *J Pediatr* 127: 328–9.

Pinsard N, Ponscerdan C, Mancini J, et al. (1980) Le syndrome ataxie–opsoclonies–myoclonies. *Ann Pediat* 27: 269–75.

Pohl E, Pritchard J, Wilson J (1996) Neurological sequelae of the dancing eye syndrome. *Neuropediatrics* 155: 237–44.

Posada JC, Tardo C (1998) Neuroblastoma detected by somatostatin receptor scintigraphy in a case of opsoclonus–myoclonus syndrome. *J Child Neurol* 13: 345–6.

Pranzatelli MR (1992) The neurobiology of the opsoclonus–myoclonus syndrome. *Clin Neuropharmacol* 15: 186–228.

— (1994) Serotonin and human myoclonus: Rationales for the use of serotonin receptor agonists and antagonists. *Arch Neurol* 51: 605–17.

— (1996) Antidyskinetic drugs therapy for pediatric movement disorders. *J Child Neurol* 11: 355–69.

— Kao PC, Tate ED, et al. (1993) Antibodies to ACTH in opsoclonus–myoclonus. *Neuropediatrics* 24: 131–3.

— Huang Y, Tate E, et al. (1995) Cerebrospinal fluid 5-hydroxyindolacetic acid and homovallinic acid in the pediatric opsoclonus–myoclonus syndrome. *Ann Neurol* 37: 189–97.

Rapin I, Goldfisher S, Katzman R, et al. (1978) The cherry-red spot myoclonus syndrome. *Ann Neurol* 3: 234–42.

Rees MI, Andrew W, Jawad S, et al. (1994) Evidence for recessive as well as dominant forms of startle disease (hyperekplexia) caused by mutations in the a1 subunit of the inhibitory glycine receptor. *Hum Mol Genet* 3: 2175–9.

Renault F, Flores-Guevara R, d'Allest A-M (1995) Segmental myoclonus in a child with spinal cord tumour. *Dev Med Child Neurol* 37: 354–61.

Resnick TJ, Moshe SL, Perotta L, Chambers HJ (1986) Benign neonatal sleep myoclonus. *Arch Neurol* 43: 266–8.

Roberts KB, Freeman JM (1975) Cerebellar ataxia and 'occult neuroblastoma' without opsoclonus. *Pediatrics* 56: 464–5.

Roger J (1992) Progressive myoclonus epilepsies of childhood and adolescence. In: Roger J, Genton P, Bureau M, Dravet C (eds.) *Epileptic Syndromes in Infancy, Childhood and Adolescence.* London: John Libbey, pp. 381–400.

Ryan SG, Sherman SL, Terry JL, et al. (1992) Startle disease or hyperekplexia: Response to clonazepam and assignment of the gene (*STHE*) to chromosome 5q by linkage analysis. *Ann Neurol* 31: 663–8.

Scharf D (1989) Opsoclonus–myoclonus following the intranasal usage of cocaine. *J Neurol Neurosurg Psychiatry* 52: 1447–8.

Senelick RC, Bray PF, Lahey ME, et al. (1973) Neuroblastoma and myoclonic encephalopathy: Two cases and a review of the literature. *J Pediatr Surg* 8: 623–31.

Sheth RD, Horwitz SJ, Aronoff S, et al. (1995) Opsoclonus myoclonus syndrome secondary to Epstein–Barr virus infection. *J Child Neurol* 10: 297–9.

Shewmon DA, Erwin RJ (1988) Focal spike-induced cortical dysfunction is related to the aftercoming slow wave. *Ann Neurol* 23: 131–7.

Shiang R, Ryan SG, Zhu Y-Z, et al. (1995) Mutational analysis of familial and sporadic hyperek-plexia. *Ann Neurol* 38: 85–91.

Shibasaki H (1996) Overview and classification of myoclonus. *Clin Neurosci* 3: 189–92.

Silfverskiöld BP (1962) Rhythmic myoclonus in three girls. *Acta Neurol Scand* 38: 45–9.

Solomon GE, Chutorian AM (1968) Opsoclonus and occult neuroblastoma. *New Engl J Med* 279: 475–7.

Suzuki Y, Sakuraba H, Ohsima A (1991) Clinical and molecular heterogeneity in hereditary beta-galactosidase deficiency. *Dev Neurosci* 13: 299–303.

Symmonds CP (1953) Nocturnal myoclonus. *J Neurol Neurosurg Psychiatry* 16: 166–71.

Tal Y, Jaffe M, Sharf B, Amir N (1983) Steroid-dependent state in a child with opsoclonus. *J Pediatr* 103: 420–1.

Tardieu M, Khoury W, Navelet Y, et al. (1986) Un syndrome spectaculaire et bénin de convulsions néonatales: les myoclonies du sommeil profond. *Arch Fr Pediatr* 43: 259–60.

Tassinari CA, Igagoubi S, Gambarelli F, et al. (1971) Relationships between EEG discharge and EEG phenomena. *Electroencephalogr Clin Neurophysiol* 31: 176–82.

Tijssen MA, Shiang R, van Deutekom J, et al. (1995) Molecular genetic reevaluation of the Dutch hyperekplexia family. *Arch Neurol* 52: 578–82.

Tuchman RF, Alvarez LA, Kantrowitz AB, et al. (1989) Opsoclonus–myoclonus syndrome: Correlation of radiographic and pathological observations. *Neuroradiology* 31: 250–2.

van Woert MH (1983) Myoclonus and L-5-hydroxytryptophan (L-5HTP). *Prog Clin Biol Res* 127: 43–52.

Vigevano F, di Capua M, Dalla Bernardina B (1989) Startle disease: an avoidable cause of sudden infant death. *Lancet* 1: 216.

Wilfong AA, Fernandez F (1992) Myasthenia gravis in a child with sequelae of opsoclonus–myoclonus syndrome. *Can J Neurol Sci* 19: 88–9.

Willis J, Collada M, Robertson HJ (1983) Cerebellar lesion in myoclonic encephalopathy of infants. *Arch Neurol* 40: 818–9.

Ziter FA, Bray PF, Cancilla PA (1979) Neuropathologic findings in a patient with neuroblastoma and myoclonic encephalopathy. *Arch Neurol* 36: 51–5.

9
TIC DISORDERS

INTRODUCTION AND CLASSIFICATION

The first medical notions about tics date from the beginning of the 19th century when J Bouteille differentiated some "facial grimaces" from choreic movements and termed them "false chorea". The term "tic" seems to be related to veterinary medicine in which it was used to describe the sudden movements of horses when they are restrained (Barabas 1988). Others think that the word tic is related to old French, German or Italian languages to describe an unsightly unusual caprice (Lees and Tolosa 1988).

Landmarks in our knowledge of tics have been the description by Georges Gilles de la Tourette in 1885 of the syndrome that bears his name, the discovery of the therapeutic efficacy of haloperidol (Shapiro and Shapiro 1968) and the recognition of the significance of associated disturbances.

Tics are the most frequent abnormal movements in children. This is one reason for their importance. Another reason is their relationship to fascinating disturbances of human behaviour such as compulsion and obsessions. Because of this relationship, Luria (quoted by Sacks 1987) stated that the importance of Tourette syndrome is exceptional because "any understanding of such a syndrome must vastly broaden our understanding of human nature in general". Tics may also be related to other movements such as mannerisms or repetitive gestures whose degree of volitional character may be questioned. In fact, tics are the most striking manifestations of a complex disturbance that includes anomalies of thought (e.g. obsessions), sensation (e.g. sensitive tics) and behaviours (e.g. attention deficit disorder). Limitation of the study of tics to their motor phenomenology is a reductionism that may have negative consequences on their management.

The term tic is used to designate both a symptom and a disease. As a symptom it has a wide variety of expression (see Chapter 1). Tic disease has even more varied manifestations (Table 9.1). It may be limited to simple transient tics manifested only for less than a year or, in Tourette syndrome (TS), include several types of chronic motor and phonatory tics, often together with obsessive–compulsive manifestations, attention deficit, behaviour disorders or sleep disturbances.

For comparative studies and therapeutic trials, an objective tool of quantification is necessary. Some of the proposed methods are shown in Table 9.2. The Tourette Syndrome Severity Scale (Shapiro et al. 1983) and the Yale Global Tic Severity Scale (Leckman et al. 1989) are both simple and rapid and can serve as semi-structured questionnaires in patient evaluations.

TABLE 9.1
Varieties of tic disease

Transient single motor tics
Transient multiple motor tics
Transient multiple phonic tics
Chronic single tics
Chronic multiple motor tics
Chronic multiple phonic tics
Gilles de la Tourette syndrome
Nonspecific tics

TABLE 9.2
Methods of assessment of tics and comorbid disorders

Tourette Syndrome Global Scale (Harcherik et al. 1984)
Goetz Tic Rating Scale (Goetz et al. 1987)
Johns Hopkins Tic Severity Scale (Walkup et al. 1992)
Yale Global Tic Severity Scale (Leckman et al. 1989)
Tourette Syndrome Severity Scale (Shapiro et al. 1983)
Leyton Obsessional Inventory (Cooper 1970)
Yale–Brown Obsessive–Compulsive Scale (Goodman et al. 1989a,b)

TABLE 9.3
DSM-IV criteria for tic disorders*

Common criteria
• The tics occur many times a day (usually in bouts) nearly every day
• The disturbance causes marked distress or significant impairment in social, occupational or other important areas of functioning
• Onset is before age 18 years
• The disturbance is not due to the direct physiological effects of a substance or a general medical condition

Tourette syndrome
• Both multiple motor and one or more vocal tics have been present at some time during the illness, although not necessarily concurrently, throughout a period of more than 1 year, and during this period there was never a tic-free period of more than three consecutive months

Chronic tic disorder
• Single or multiple motor or vocal tics, but not both, have been present at some time during the illness throughout a period of more than one year, and during this period there was never a tic-free period of more than three consecutive months

Transient tic disorder
• Single or multiple motor and/or vocal tics for at least four weeks but not longer than 12 consecutive months

Tic disorder not otherwise specified
• Cases that do not meet criteria for a specific tic disorder

*Adapted from APA (1994).

The DSM-IV criteria (Table 9.3) are almost universally accepted, but although DSM-IV separates Tourette disorder from other forms of tics for pragmatic and conceptual reasons, we think, like Golden (1978), Fahn (1982) and others, that tics form a continuum from the simple transient forms to full-fledged TS. For research purposes the DSM-IV classification was adopted by the TS Classification Study Group of the

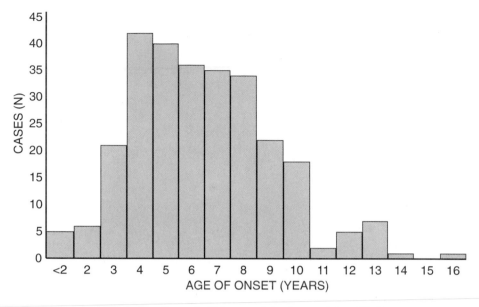

Fig. 9.1. Age of onset in 275 cases of tics (personal data, EF-A).

American Tourette Association, and each of the DSM-IV groups was divided into two categories, 'definite' and 'historical' (depending on whether or not the tics have been witnessed by a reliable observer); in addition, two further categories not covered by DSM-IV were added: *chronic single tic disorder*, and *probable Tourette syndrome* (Tourette Syndrome Classification Study Group 1993).

In this chapter, tics will be divided for management purposes into two main groups, viz. transient and chronic tics, the latter including Tourette.

AGE OF ONSET

It is sometimes difficult to know when tics start in a particular case because, for instance, blinking can easily go unrecognized. The average age of onset of tics is between 5 and 10 years (Fig. 9.1). Cases in children as young as 1 year have been reported (Rickards and Robertson 1997). Onset is before 15 years in over 99% of cases (Shapiro et al. 1988). Age of onset is not significantly different between the sexes.

EPIDEMIOLOGY

Transient and chronic single tics are very common in the childhood population, but epidemiological studies of tic disorder are difficult mainly because symptom intensity and expressivity vary greatly and subjects often do not recognize them. When family members of affected people were directly interviewed, the frequency of tics for which no medical advice was sought was high (Kurlan 1989). Other methodological difficulties are that often symptoms diminish with increasing age and that male subjects are more likely to exhibit tics (Tanner and Goldman 1997). Epidemiological studies in TS are less difficult. The annual *incidence* of TS in a population-based study was 0.46 per 100,000 persons (Lucas et al. 1982). A very complete study of *prevalence* (Apter et al. 1993) based on 16- to 17-year-old Israelis gave a sex-adjusted TS prevalence of 4.0 per 10,000. Considering that about one-third of TS cases are free of symptoms at age 17 years, the real incidence and prevalence of tics in the childhood population must be greater than these figures. This is in agreement with the finding in a mainstream school population (aged 13–14 years) of a prevalence estimate as high as 299 per 10,000 (Mason et al. 1998). In both these studies non-TS tics were not considered.

ASSOCIATED DISTURBANCES

Several 'behavioural disorders' are more frequent in patients with tics than in the general population. These are probably of more consequence than the tics (Comings 1995b, Lombroso et al. 1995). The genetic relationship between tics and associated disorders is not clear.

DSM-IV defines *obsessive–compulsive disorder* (OCD) as characterized by recurrent obsessions (persistent ideas, thoughts, impulses or images experienced as intrusive and inappropriate and causing marked anxiety or distress) and compulsions (repetitive behaviours such as hand washing, ordering, mental acts such as praying or counting, the goal of which is to prevent or reduce anxiety or distress). OCD is a heterogeneous disorder with some forms related to TS. OCD or obsessive–compulsive symptoms (OCS) are present in about half the patients (28 to 67% in various studies) (Nee et al. 1980, Pauls et al. 1986, Singer and Rosenberg 1989, Comings 1995b), and patients with OCD frequently have tics (Pitman et al. 1987). A need for symmetry, touching objects, tapping and rubbing are more common in patients with tics than in OCD without tics (Pitman et al. 1987, Leckman et al. 1995), whereas compulsions of cleanliness and verification of past gestures or words in spite of reasonable certainty that they have been performed or uttered are more common in OCD patients without tics (Holzer et al. 1994, Leckman et al. 1995). Sensory phenomena may precede obsessions in OCD patients with comorbid tics but not in OCD unassociated with tics (Miguel et al. 1997).

TS and primary OCD share many common clinical features (Como 1995), suggesting a common pathophysiological basis (Pauls et al. 1986). However, therapeutic effects differ between OCD and tics: obsessive–compulsive manifestations respond to antiserotoninergic drugs, tics to antidopaminergic agents. Obsessions in OCD patients with tics often benefit from combined therapy with serotonin reuptake inhibitors plus neuroleptics, while OCD without tics does not improve when neuroleptics are added (McDougle et al. 1994). Likewise, PET has shown in TS decreased metabolic activity in the frontal cingular and insular cortices (Chase et al. 1986), whereas in OCD there seems to be increased activity in the caudate and various cortical areas (Baxter et al. 1988, Swedo et al. 1990).

Attention deficit–hyperactivity disorder (ADHD) consists of "a persistent pattern of inattention and/or hyperactivity–impulsivity that is more frequent and severe than is typically observed in individuals at a comparable level of development" with "clear evidence of interference with developmentally appropriate social, academic, or occupational functioning" (DSM-IV, APA 1994). ADHD is present in 50–60% of children with TS, generally preceding the appearance of tics by 2–3 years (Comings and Comings 1984, Comings 1995a, Walkup et al. 1995).

Disturbances in cognitive processes such as learning or reading, writing and computing (Singer et al. 1995) are frequent (62% of patients according to Erenberg et al. 1987). Behaviour disturbances such as mythomania, shoplifting or vandalism may be more common than in the general population. A variety of soft neurologic signs, visual–perceptual disturbances, language disorders, and an increased frequency of sleep anomalies (12–62% of patients) such as sleep-walking, pavor nocturnus, nightmares and enuresis have been reported, especially when ADHD is associated with the tics (Nee et al. 1980, Comings and Comings 1987c, Allen et al. 1992).

An increased tendency to depression, anxiety, inappropriate sexual behaviour and oppositional defiant disorder (Comings 1995b) has been reported to be of higher frequency than in the general population. These may contribute to create problems with parents, siblings, teachers and peers (Stokes et al. 1991) and academic failure despite a normal level of intelligence. From 16% to 68% of children with TS have an educational level lower than their peers and the need for special educational services is five times greater than in the general population (Comings and Comings 1987a,b,c; Hagin and Kugler 1988).

From a practical point of view it is important to note that these associated disturbances often create difficulties in school. In one study (Abwender et al. 1996), 46 per cent of subjects with TS experienced a school-related problem. Since some major clinical features of associated disturbances such as ADHD and OCD are treatable, prompt recognition of the diagnosis and initiation of appropriate therapy could have a beneficial effect on school performance.

Ancillary investigations

The diagnosis of tics is clinical. Anomalies of neurotransmitters, if present, are not practically useful. The same applies to neuropsychological and neurophysiological tests, including EEG which may show nonspecific abnormalities in up to 34% of cases (Bergen et al. 1982). Morphologic neuroimaging studies give normal results (Demeter 1992), even though volumetric MRI in adults and children has shown a reduced volume of the left caudate nucleus in a few studies (Peterson et al. 1993, Singer et al. 1993, Hyde et al. 1995). SPECT studies have shown concordant results, with hypoperfusion in the left caudate nucleus (Moriarty et al. 1995).

Differential diagnosis
Isolated, simple motor tics can be difficult to differentiate from other abnormal move-

ments such as myoclonus, chorea and even non-propositive movements that are part of the behavioural repertoire of every individual. To arrive at a correct interpretation of tics, an overall assessment taking into account the psychological context and the evolution is required.

The diagnosis becomes easy after a child has presented for some time various tics with periods of variable intensity or if s/he can explain the compulsion. But because of the extreme variability of manifestations and the partial control that patients can exert on the movements, the clinical diagnosis may be difficult. Difficulties are mainly encountered in three situations: when the initial tics are uncommon, as for instance eyeball tic or retching (Rickards and Robertson 1997); when the dominant tics are complex movements; and in cases of acute onset with a 'storm of tics' and behavioural disturbances. In such cases, reinterpretation of previous phenomena that had appeared normal (e.g. throat clearing mistaken for cough), search for a family history of tics or obsessive disorder, and, in the patient, the presence of obsessive–compulsive features or ADHD or the 'premonitory urge' to perform the movement may help make the diagnosis. We have found that the capacity of the child to reproduce the tics is a useful clue as this is not found in any other movement disorder.

Tics rarely present as abnormal eyeball movements (Frankel and Cummings 1984, Binyon and Predergast 1991). Tics of the eyeballs are generally associated with other tics, but may occur alone and bear a resemblance to nystagmus or opsoclonus. When isolated, these should not be mistaken for oculogyric crises. The ability to reproduce the movement, awareness of its occurrence and a normal EEG differentiate tics from epileptic phenomena.

Differentiation of complex tics from other abnormal movements is usually straightforward. In contrast to chorea and myoclonus (the abnormal movements which share the most similarities with tics), tics do not alter volitional movements and therefore do not create disability, and they do not interfere with writing or other hand movements. Stereotypies, or ritual movements in OCD, may raise problems. Differentiating complex tics from compulsions is difficult, especially in young children. A compulsive component is present in some tics that are subjectively perceived as aiming to relieve an abnormal sensation (Pitman et al. 1987).

Differentiating tics from conversion reactions with 'pseudo-tics' may demand great diagnostic acumen (Dooley et al. 1994). A sample of the diagnostic problems raised by tics is given by the study of Feinberg et al. (1986) of patients with simultaneous abnormal movements of various types and disturbances of behaviour which proved resistant to pharmacological treatment.

Secondary tics are rare in children (see later). Neuroacanthocytosis (see Chapter 4) can present with tics but is almost exclusively a disorder of adults.

Inheritance
There is universal consensus that genetic factors play a role in tic disorders. Support for

a genetic component of TS comes from several lines of evidence, especially twin (Waserman et al. 1983, Hyde et al. 1992) and family studies (Kurlan et al. 1994, Walkup et al. 1996). A positive family history of chronic tics is present in one-third of patients (Golden 1978, Hanna et al. 1999). Data from epidemiological studies favour an auto-somal dominant inheritance of TS with variable expressivity (Pauls and Leckman 1986), bilineal transmission (Hanna et al. 1999), or a multifactorial inheritance (a major locus in combination with environmental factors) (Walkup et al. 1996). A search for the gene(s) associated with TS is under way at several centres.

The possibility that TS and OCD are alternative manifestations of the same genetic defect with predominant expression as tics in males and OCD in females has been entertained (Pauls and Leckman 1986, Pauls et al. 1986, Eapen et al. 1993).

In my series (EF-A), the frequency of a positive family history increases from 48% to 65% if relatives with OCD are included together with those with tics. No relationship with the HLA groups has been demonstrated.

Nongenetic factors seem also to be involved. In monozygotic twin pairs, the lighter at birth is more severely affected (Hyde et al. 1992). Central stimulant agents and neuro-leptics can produce tics in persons with genetic predisposition (Klawans et al. 1978, Bonthala and West 1983).

Pathology
The few pathological studies available have given normal results. Only minor abnor-malities of dubious significance have been found. Anomalies such as absence of dynor-phin reactivity in the pallidum (Haber et al. 1986) and reduction of cyclic AMP in the cortex (Singer et al. 1990) are difficult to interpret.

Pathogenesis
Tics are a good example of the interaction of genetic and environmental factors in the genesis of a disease (Cohen et al. 1982). They were initially considered as a neurotic mani-festation, but it is now generally recognized that organic factors are essential. Arguments for an organic origin include positive genetic findings, the persistence of tics during sleep, the therapeutic action of antidopaminergic drugs, the premovement potential studies (Obeso et al. 1981), and the decrease of metabolic activity in the frontal cingular and insular cortices and basal ganglia on PET studies (Chase et al. 1986, Stoetter et al. 1992). Evidence supporting a disturbance of neurotransmitters includes the absence of structural lesions, the variability of symptoms and the therapeutic effects of drugs, although the neurotransmitters involved, if any, have not been identified. Singer (1993) has postulated that tics result from increased dopaminergic transmission, whereas parkinsonism is due to severely decreased dopaminergic activity.

Other hypotheses implicate: (1) dopaminergic receptor hypersensitivity (Kurlan 1989); (2) imbalance between cholinergic and dopaminergic systems (Caine et al. 1984); (3) hyperactivity of alpha-adrenergic receptors (Leckman et al. 1992; and (4) participation of the endogenous opioid system (Kurlan et al. 1991). Although the anatomical location of such supposed biochemical abnormalities is not known, involvement of the basal ganglia appears probable.

The high incidence of tics (transient/chronic) and the comorbid disorders frequently associated raise the question as to whether they are an exaggeration of a normal human behaviour. Kurlan (1994) has suggested that they represent an excessive expression or abnormal persistence of a characteristic commonly occurring in normal childhood development.

TRANSIENT TICS

When transient, tics are usually simple. Most commonly, they involve orbicular muscle with uni- or bilateral blinking. They may, however, involve other territories, even occasionally the trunk and extremities. They can be multiple and include phonatory tics. They disappear by definition in less than one year (in 50% within 2–3 months), but there is no specific feature that allows prediction of their disappearance.

CHRONIC TICS

By definition (DSM-IV, APA 1994), chronic tics last over one year, even if they manifest intermittently. All combinations of single/multiple and motor/phonic tics can be observed, from chronic single motor tics or chronic single phonic tics, to the severe forms of TS.

Simple chronic tics are more common in adults. These are simple tics, virtually without fluctuation. They are often frequent and resistant to therapy.

GILLES DE LA TOURETTE SYNDROME (TS)

Gilles de la Tourette in 1885 described six personal cases and reviewed three from the literature (for an English translation of his report, see Goetz and Klawans 1982). A little later, Charcot gave the disorder the name of his student. Shapiro et al. (1988) set up criteria for diagnosis from a study of almost 400 cases. The association of multiple chronic tics and phonatory tics is required for the diagnosis. Often other manifestations, especially OCD and ADHD, are associated and can precede the onset of tics.

The first manifestations are variable (Table 9.4). Simple tics usually come first and vocalization appears within a few years. However, complex and/or phonatory tics may be the first manifestation. Commonly, parents tend to attribute the tics to psychological or local (e.g. conjuntivitis) causes. According to Bruun (1988), the onset is with facial tics in 66% and with phonatory tics in 13% of cases.

The course of the disorder is fluctuating with a tendency towards improvement with increasing age (Torup 1972). Symptoms may persist after puberty and even for a lifetime. According to Erenberg et al. (1987), 73% of patients have improved by 16 years of age and only 14% get worse. One-third of patients are symptom-free at the end of adolescence and a further third are ameliorated (Singer and Walkup 1991). No feature

TABLE 9.4
Form of onset of tic disorders in a personal series (N=238)*

Simple motor	
Palpebral	98 (42%)
Cephalic movements	47 (20%)
Ocular	15 (6%)
Shoulder/upper limb	15 (6%)
Facial/jaw	9 (4%)
Trunk	2 (1%)
Retching	2 (1%)
Other	6 (2%)
Multiple motor**	5 (2%)
Complex motor	13 (5%)
Phonatory	24 (10%)
'Storm'***	2 (1%)

*EF-A.
**More than two motor tics or motor and phonic tic.
***Sudden onset of multiple tics, obsessive–compulsive disorder and hyperactivity.

TABLE 9.5
Conditions that may cause or precipitate tics

Treatment with sympathicomimetic agents or psychostimulants (methylphenidate, pemoline, etc.) (Erenberg et al. 1985)

Tricyclic antidepressants, anticholinergic or antiepileptic drugs (Neglia et al. 1984, Burd et al. 1986, Kurlan et al. 1989, Sanchez-Ramos and Weiner 1993, Lombroso 1999)

Following discontinuation of neuroleptic treatment

Carbon monoxide intoxication (Pulst et al. 1983)

Following encephalitis (Northam and Singer 1991)

Following cardiopulmonary bypass and hypothermia (Singer et al. 1997)

Demyelinating, degenerative or metabolic diseases: Wilson disease, Huntington disease (Jankovic and Ashizawa 1995), porphyria, neurolipidosis, neuroacanthocytosis)

Head trauma (Eriksson and Persson 1969)

Chromosome abnormalities (Marskey 1974, Singh et al. 1982, Huret et al. 1988, Taylor et al. 1991)

---

appears to be predictive. Although the disorder is compatible with a normal life without physical disability (even though cervical myelopathy caused by tics involving the neck has been reported – Goetz and Klawans 1980), the chronic nature of the syndrome and the type of manifestations may have severe and incapacitating social and psychological consequences.

SECONDARY TICS

Some children develop transient or chronic tics, following or concurrent with various diseases or treatments. This situation is also called 'tourettism' or 'Tourette-like disorder'. This association does not imply causality, and the possibility exists of a coincidental association or of precipitating factors acting on predisposed persons (Kumar and Lang 1997) (Table 9.5).

Important, for practical reasons, is the controversy about the relationship between psychostimulants such as methylphenidate, a drug frequently used in the treatment of ADHD, and the development of tics. This is discussed later in this chapter.

Of special interest is the so-called PANDAS syndrome (paediatric autoimmune neuropsychiatric disorders associated with streptococcal infection). The basic hypothesis is that a group A β-haemolytic streptococcal infection may create antibodies that cross-react with basal ganglia neurons, as occurs in rheumatic chorea (Husby et al. 1976), producing or at least worsening TS or OCD (Kiessling et al. 1993, Swedo et al. 1994, Kurlan 1998). A significantly higher serum level of antibodies against putaminal neurons (but not caudate or globus pallidus) has been reported in children with TS (Singer et al. 1998), but no correlation was found between antibody level and clinical symptomatology of tics (age of onset, severity, etc.) or comorbid problems (ADHD or OCD). Some patients with tics or OCD and evidence of recent streptococcal infection who failed to respond to traditional pharmacotherapy improved following corticosteroids or immuno-modifying therapy (Tucker et al. 1996).

MANAGEMENT

Precise determination of the impact of tics and of associated disturbances on the individual patient's life is necessary to identify symptoms that require treatment. It is important to avoid considering only the disorder of movement out of the context of en-vironmental and psychological factors and to share management with other professionals such as psychologists. Treatment does not necessarily aim at suppressing the abnormal movements. Only a minority of children have tics of sufficient severity to justify such attempts. In spite of parental demands, it may be important to withhold pharmacological treatment when tics are reasonably tolerated by the child and, simultaneously, to inform the parents, school teachers and others involved of the nature of the disturbance, emph-asizing that tics are not a manifestation of mental disease. If pharmacological treatment is used, complete suppression of tics is not the goal because it is seldom attainable without the risk of intolerable side-effects.

The first effective drug used in the treatment of tics was haloperidol, a high-potency antidopaminergic and antinoradrenergic agent. It is effective in approximately 80% of cases (Erenberg et al. 1987, Shapiro et al. 1987). In children the usual starting dose is 0.25 mg/d. The dosage may be progressively increased by 0.25–0.5 mg increments every 4–7 days according to the response, to a maximum of 3 mg/d. Rarely does a patient require doses in the range of 5–10 mg/d (Chappell et al. 1995). The half-life of the drug allows once a day administration at bedtime. Side-effects are common and include drowsiness, difficulties of concentration, dysarthria, fatigue, dryness of the mouth, and dystonic and parkinsonian reactions (Erenberg et al. 1987, Shapiro et al. 1988). In the case of dystonic reaction, the dose should be lowered and antiparkinsonian agents may be added (e.g. biperidine). The long term risk of tardive dyskinesia (Golden 1985, Riddle et al. 1987) prevents its chronic use in children except in the most severe cases or as a last resort (Bharucha 1996).

New drugs with more selective antidopaminergic action and fewer side-effects have appeared in the past few years. One of the most effective is pimozide (Orap), which is an antidopaminergic agent but differs from haloperidol in that it has no antiadrenergic activity (Rose and Moldofsky 1977, Shapiro et al. 1987). The average initial dose is 0.5–1 mg/d. The dosage should be increased as tolerated to a maximum of 8 mg/d

(Regeur et al. 1986, Chappell et al. 1995). The potential side-effects of pimozide are the same as for haloperidol, and because pimozide may be cardiotoxic in a few patients (Cohen and Leckman 1984) an ECG should be done at baseline and at least at yearly intervals.

Tiapride (Eggers et al. 1988), fluphenazine (Goetz et al. 1984), chlorpromazine (Klawans et al. 1978) and tetrabenazine (Jankovic et al. 1984) have been also proposed. Alpha-2-adrenergic receptor agonists such as clonidine (Leckman et al. 1985) or guan-facine (Walkup et al. 1995) are effective drugs. The initial dose of clonidine is 0.05 mg/d, usually in the morning before school. This dosage should be increased by increments of 0.005 mg every 3–4 days to a maximum of 0.3 mg/d, divided into three or four doses. Its therapeutic effects may appear 2–4 weeks after onset of treatment (Chappell et al. 1995). Side-effects include sedation, insomnia and dryness of mouth. A withdrawal syndrome (agitation, rebound increase in tics, tachycardia and profuse sweating) can be associated with abrupt discontinuation of clonidine (Leckman et al. 1986). Clonidine may be also particularly effective on disturbances of behaviour (hyperactivity, inattention) when they are associated symptoms.

Many other drugs have been reported to be effective, including cholinergic agonists (Rosenberg and David 1982), clonazepam (Le Witt 1992) and flunarizine (Micheli et al. 1990). Naltrexone has been tried because of its interaction with endogenous opioids and dopamine, with contradictory results (Kurlan et al. 1991). More aggressive techniques such as botulinum toxin (Jankovic 1994, Salloway et al. 1996) or even leukotomy have exceptionally been used (Robertson et al. 1990). Pharmacotherapy is strictly palliative and most tics do not require it. It is wise to remember that a significant proportion of chronic tics and even TS will remit (Shapiro et al. 1988).

Behavioural treatment (Peterson et al. 1994), mainly *habit reversal*, is used in the treatment of chronic motor and vocal tics. Good results have been reported (Azrin et al. 1990), but in young children it is difficult to obtain enough motivation and collaboration with these therapies.

Treatment of associated disorders is as important as that of tics. OCD, if severe enough, may be in fact treated with clomipramine (Anafranil) (Flament et al. 1985) at a dose of 3 mg/kg/d. Side-effects include sedation, constipation, sweating and cardiovascular disturbances. Fluoxetine (Prozac) is useful (Riddle et al. 1990) at an initial dose of 5 mg/d (once a day) to a maximum of 40 mg/d (side-effects: sedation, dysphasia, anxiety or insomnia) (Riddle et al. 1991). Fluvoxamine is considered a good drug, and should be considered in the treatment of OCD; dose and duration of treatment must be longer than in depression.

Psychostimulant agents (methylphenidate, dextroamphetamine, pemoline) are the classical treatment of ADHD. It is commonly believed that stimulant drugs may precip-itate or exacerbate tics (Denckla et al. 1976, Lowe et al. 1982). Because ADHD usually precedes by some years the appearance of tics, it is possible that the development of tics in patients on psychostimulants may only be part of the natural history of tic disorders (Erenberg et al. 1985). Moreover, several controlled studies indicate that stimulants (such as methylphenidate, 0.3 mg/kg/d) are safe and effective for the treatment of ADHD in children with TS (Gadow et al. 1995).

Tricyclic antidepressants (imipramine, desipramine, nortriptyline) may have benefits if compared with stimulants (once-a-day dose, no detrimental effect on the ability to fall asleep, no association with decreases in appetite) and have been used to treat ADHD in TS with clear benefits (Spencer et al. 1993, Wilens et al. 1993). In children, desipramine doses are 25–100 mg/d, and nortriptyline doses 0.4–4.5 mg/kg/d.

REFERENCES

Abwender DA, Como PG, Kurlan R, et al. (1996) School problems in Tourette's syndrome. *Arch Neurol* 53: 509–11.

Allen RP, Singer HS, Brown JE, Salam MM (1992) Sleep disorders in Tourette syndrome: A primary or unrelated problem? *Pediatr Neurol* 8: 275–80.

APA (1994) *Diagnostic and Statistical Manual of Mental Disorders. 4th edn.* Washington DC: American Psychiatric Association.

Apter A, Pauls DL, Bleich A, et al. (1993) An epidemiological study on Gilles de la Tourette's syndrome in Israel. *Arch Gen Psychiatry* 50: 734–8.

Azrin NH, Peterson AL (1990) Treatment of Tourette syndrome by habit reversal: A waiting-list control group comparison. *Behav Ther* 21: 305–18.

Barabas G (1988) Tourette's syndrome: An overview. *Pediatr Ann* 17: 391–3.

Baxter LR, Schwartz JM, Mazziota JC, et al. (1988) Cerebral glucose metabolic rates in obsessive–compulsive disorder. *Arch Gen Psychiatry* 145: 1560–3.

Bergen D, Tanner C, Wilson R (1982) The electroencephalogram in Tourette syndrome. *Ann Neurol* 11: 382–5.

Bharucha KJ (1996) Pediatric movement disorders: Newer therapeutic strategies. *J Child Neurol* 11: 353–4.

Binyon S, Prendergast M (1991) Eye-movement tics in children. *Dev Med Child Neurol* 33: 352–5.

Bonthala CM, West A (1983) Pemoline induced chorea and Gilles de la Tourette's syndrome. *Br J Psychiatry* 143: 300–2.

Bruun RD (1988) The natural history of Tourette's syndrome. In: Cohen DJ, Bruun RD, Leckman JF (eds.) *Tourette's Syndrome and Tic Disorders: Clinical Understanding and Treatment.* New York: Wiley, pp. 21–40.

Burd L, Kerbeshian J, Fisher W, et al. (1986) Anticonvulsant medications: An iatrogenic cause of tic disorders. *Can J Psychiatry* 31: 419–23.

Caine ED, Ludlow CL, Polinsky RJ, Ebert MH (1984) Provocative drug testing in Tourette's syndrome: D-and L-amphetamine and haloperidol. *J Am Acad Child Psych* 23: 147–52.

Chappell PB, Leckman JF, Riddle MA (1995) The pharmacologic treatment of the tic disorders. *Child Adolesc Psychiatr Clin N Am* 4: 197–216.

Chase TN, Geoffrey V, Gillespie M, et al. (1986) Structural and functional studies of Gilles de la Tourette's syndrome. *Rev Neurol* 142: 851–5.

Cohen DJ, Leckman JF (1984) Tourette's syndrome: Advances in treatment and research. *J Am Acad Child Psychiatry* 23: 123–85.

— Detlor J, Shaywitz BA, Leckman JF (1982) Interaction of biological and psychological factors in the natural history of Tourette syndrome: A paradigm for childhood neuropsychiatric disorders. In: Friedhoff AJ, Chase TN (eds.) *Advances in Neurology. Vol. 35. Gilles de la Tourette Syndrome.* New York: Raven Press, pp. 31–4.

Comings DE (1995a) The role of genetic factors in conduct disorder based on studies of Tourette syndrome and attention-deficit hyperactivity disorder probands and their relatives. *Dev Behav Pediatr* 16: 142–57.

— (1995b) Tourette's syndrome: A behavioral spectrum disorder. In: Weiner WJ, Lang AE (eds.) *Advances in Neurology. Vol. 65. Behavioral Neurology of Movement Disorders.* New York: Raven Press, pp. 293–303.

— Comings BG (1984) Tourette's syndrome and attention deficit disorders with hyperactivity: Are they genetically related? *J Am Acad Child Psych* 23: 138–46.

— — (1987a) A controlled study of Tourette syndrome. I. Attention deficit disorder, learning disorders and school problems. *Am J Hum Genet* 41: 701–41.

— — (1987b) A controlled study of Tourette syndrome. II. Conduct. *Am J Hum Genet* 41: 742–60.

— — (1987c) A controlled study of Tourette syndrome. VI. Early development, sleep problems, allergies and handedness. *Am J Hum Genet* 41: 822–39.

— Himes JA, Comings BG (1990) An epidemiologic study of Tourette's syndrome in a single school district. *J Clin Psychiatry* 51: 463–9.

Como PG (1995) Obsessive–compulsive disorder in Tourette's syndrome. In: Weiner WJ, Lang AE (eds.) *Advances in Neurology. Vol. 65. Behavioral Neurology of Movement Disorders.* New York: Raven Press, pp. 281–91.

Cooper J (1970) The Leyton obsessional inventory. *Psychol Med* 1: 48–64.

Demeter S (1992) Structural imaging in Tourette syndrome. *Adv Neurol* 58: 201–6.

Denckla MB, Bemporad JR, Mac Kay MC (1976) Tics following methylphenidate administration: A report of 20 cases. *JAMA* 235: 1349–51.

Dooley JM, Stokes A, Gordon KE (1994) Pseudo-tics in Tourette syndrome. *J Child Neurol* 9: 50–1.

Eapen V, Pauls DL, Robertson MM (1993) Evidence for autosomal dominant transmission in Tourette's syndrome. United Kingdom Cohort Study. *Br J Psychiatry* 162: 593–6.

Eggers CH, Rothenberger A, Berhaus U (1988) Clinical and neurobiological findings in children suffering from tic disease following treatment with tiapride. *Eur Arch Psychiat Neurol Sci* 237: 223–9.

Erenberg G, Cruse RP, Rothner AD (1985) Gilles de la Tourette's syndrome: Effects of stimulant drugs. *Neurology* 35: 1346–8.

— — — (1987) The natural history of Tourette syndrome: A follow-up study. *Ann Neurol* 22: 383–5.

Fahn S (1982) The clinical spectrum of motor tics In Gilles de la Tourette syndrome. In: Friedhoff AJ, Chase TN (eds.) *Advances in Neurology. Vol. 35. Gilles de la Tourette Syndrome.* New York: Raven Press, pp. 341–4.

Feinberg TE, Shapiro AK, Shapiro E (1986) Paroxysmal myoclonic dystonia with vocalizations: New entity or variant of preexisting syndromes? *J Neurol Neurosurg Psychiatry* 49: 52–7.

Flament MF, Rapoport JL, Berg CJ, et al. (1985) Clomipramine treatment of childhood obsessive–compulsive disorder. A double-blind controlled study. *Arch Gen Psychiatry* 42: 977–83.

Frankel M, Cummings JL (1984) Neuro-ophthalmic abnormalities in Tourette's syndrome: Functional and anatomic implications. *Neurology* 34: 359–61.

Gadow KD, Nolan EE, Sprafkin J, Sverd J (1995) School observations of children with attention-deficit hyperactivity disorder and comorbid tic disorder: Effects of methylphenidate treatment. *Dev Behav Pediatr* 16: 167–76.

Goetz CG, Klawans HL (1980) Gilles de la Tourette syndrome and compressive neuropathies. *Ann Neurol* 8: 453 (letter).

— — (1982) Gilles de la Tourette on Tourette syndrome. In: Friedhoff AJ, Chase TN (eds.) *Advances in Neurology. Vol. 35. Gilles de la Tourette Syndrome.* New York: Raven Press, pp. 1–16.

— — Klawans HN (1984) Fluphenazine and multifocal tic disorders. *Arch Neurol* 41: 271–2.

— — Wilson RS, et al. (1987) Clonidine and Gilles de la Tourette's syndrome: Double blind study using objective rating methods. *Ann Neurol* 21: 210–4.

Golden GS (1978) Tics and Tourette's syndrome: A continuum of symptoms? *Ann Neurol* 4: 145–8.

— (1985) Tardive dyskinesia in Tourette syndrome. *Pediatr Neurol* 1: 192–4.

Goodman NK, Price LH, Rasmussen SA, et al. (1989a) The Yale–Brown obsessive–compulsive scale. I. Development, use, and reliability. *Arch Gen Psychiatry* 46: 1006–11.

— — — et al. (1989b) The Yale–Brown obsessive–compulsive scale. II. Validity. *Arch Gen Psychiatry* 46: 1012–6.

Haber SN, Kowall NW, Vonsattel JP, et al. (1986) Gilles de la Tourette's syndrome. A post-mortem neuropathological and inmunological study. *J Neurol Sci* 75: 225–41.

Hagin RA, Kugler J (1988) School problems associated with Tourette's syndrome. In: Cohen DJ, Bruyn RD, Leckman JF (eds.) *Tourette's Syndrome and Tic Disorders.* New York: John Wiley, pp. 223–36.

Hanna PA, Janjua FN, Contant CF, Jankovic J (1999) Bilineal transmission in Tourette syndrome. *Neurology* 53: 813–8.

Harcherik DF, Leckman JF, Detlor J, Cohen DJ (1984) A new instrument for clinical studies of Tourette's syndrome. *J Am Acad Child Psychiatry* 23: 153–60.

Holzer JC, Goodman WK, McDougle CJ, et al. (1994) Obsessive–compulsive disorder with and without a chronic tic disorder. A comparison of symptoms in 70 patients. *Br J Psychiatry* 164: 469–73.

Huret JL, Leonard C, Forestier B, et al. (1988) Eleven new cases of del(9p) and features of 80 cases. *J Med Genet* 25: 741–9.

Husby G, van de Rijn I, Zabriskie JB, et al. (1976) Antibodies reacting with cytoplasm of subthalamic and caudate nuclei neurons in chorea and acute rheumatic fever. *J Exp Med* 144: 1094–110.

Hyde TM, Aaronson BA, Randolph C, et al. (1992) Relationship of birth weight to the phenotypic expression of Gilles de la Tourette's syndrome in monozygotic twins. *Neurology* 42: 652–8.

— Stacey ME, Coppola R, et al. (1995) Cerebral morphometric abnormalities in Tourette's syndrome. *Neurology* 45: 1176–82.

Jankovic J (1994) Botulinum toxin in the treatment of tics. In: Jankovic J, Hallett M (eds.) *Therapy with Botulinum Toxin.* New York: Dekker, pp. 503–9.

— Ashizawa T (1995) Tourettism associated with Huntington's disease. *Mov Disord* 10: 103–5.

— Glaze DG, Frost JD (1984) Effect of tetrabenazine on tics and sleep of Gilles de la Tourette's syndrome. *Neurology* 34: 688–92.

Kiessling LS, Marcotte AC, Culpepper L (1993) Antineuronal antibodies in movement disorders *Pediatrics* 92: 39–43.

Klawans HL, Falk DK, Nausieda PA, Weiner WJ (1978) Gilles de la Tourette syndrome after long-term chlorpromazine therapy. *Neurology* 28: 1064–8.

Kumar R, Lang AE (1997) Secondary tic disorders. *Neurol Clin N Amer* 15: 309–31.

Kurlan R (1989) Tourette's syndrome: Current concepts. *Neurology* 39: 1625–30.

— (1994) Hypothesis II: Tourette's syndrome is part of a clinical spectrum that includes normal brain development. *Arch Neurol* 51: 1145–50.

— (1998) Tourette's syndrome and 'PANDAS'. Will the relation bear out? *Neurology* 50: 1530–4.

— Kersun J, Behr K, et al. (1989) Carbamazepine induced tics. *Clin Neuropharmacol* 12: 298–302.

— Majumdar L, Deeley C, et al. (1991) A controlled trial of propoxyphene and nantrolene in patients with Tourette's syndrome. *Ann Neurol* 30: 19–23.

— Eapen V, Stern J, et al. (1994) Bilineal transmission in Tourette's syndrome families. *Neurology* 44: 2336–42.

Leckman JF, Detlar J, Harcherik DF, et al. (1985) Short and long-term treatment of Tourette's syndrome with clonidine: A clinical perspective. *Neurology* 35: 343–51.

— Ort S, Carusa KA, et al. (1986) Rebound phenomena in Tourette's syndrome after abrupt withdrawal of clonidine. *Arch Gen Psychiatry* 43: 1168–76.

— Riddle MA, Hardin MT, et al. (1989) The Yale Global Tic Severity Scale: initial testing of a clinician-rated scale of tic severity. *Am J Child Adolesc Psychiatry* 28: 566–73.

— Pauls DL, Peterson BS, et al. (1992) Pathogenesis of Tourette syndrome: Clues from the clinical phenotype and natural history. In: Case TN, Friedhoff AJ, Cohen, DJ. (ed.) *Advances in Neurology. Vol. 58. Tourette Syndrome: Genetics, Neurobiology and Treatment.* New York: Raven Press, pp. 15–25.

— Grice DE, Barr LC, et al. (1995) Tic-related vs. nontic-related obsessive–compulsive disorder. *Anxiety* 1: 208–15.

Lees AJ, Tolosa E (1988) *Tics.* In: Jankovic J, Tolosa E (eds.) *Parkinson's Disease and Movement Disorders.* Baltimore: Urban & Schwarzenberg, pp 275–281.

Le Witt PA (1992) Therapeutics of Tourette syndrome. New medication approach. *Adv Neurol* 58: 263–70.

Lombroso CT (1999) Lamotrigine-induced tourettism. *Neurology* 52: 1191–4.

— Scahill LD, Chappell PB, et al. (1995) Tourette's syndrome: A multigenerational neuropsychiatric disorder. In: *Behavioral Neurology of Movement Disorders. Advances in Neurology. Vol. 65.* New York. Raven Press, pp. 305–318.

Lowe TL, Cohen DJ, Detlor J, et al. (1982) Stimulant medication precipitates Tourette's syndrome. *JAMA* 247: 1729–31.

Lucas AR, Behar CM, Rajput AH, Kurland LT (1982) Tourette syndrome in Rochester, Minnesota (1968–1979). In: Friedhoff AJ, Chase TN (eds.) *Advances in Neurology. Vol 35. Gilles de la Tourette Syndrome.* New York: Raven Press, pp. 267–9.

Marskey H (1974) A case of multiple tics with vocalization (partial syndrome of Gilles de la Tourette) and XYY karyotype. *Br J Psychiatry* 135: 593–4.

Mason A, Banerjee S, Eapen V, et al. (1998) The prevalence of Tourette syndrome in a mainstream school population. *Dev Med Child Neurol* 40: 292–6.

McDougle CJ, Goodman WK, Leckman JF, et al. (1994) Haloperidol addition in fluvoxamine-refractory obsessive–compulsive disorder. A double blind, placebo-controlled study in patients with and without tics. *Arch Gen Psychiatry* 51: 302–8.

Micheli F, Gatto M, Lekhuniec E, et al. (1990) Treatment of Tourette's syndrome with calcium antagonist. *Clin Neuropharmacol* 1: 77–83.

Miguel EC, Baer L, Coffey BJ, et al. (1997) Phenomenological differences appearing with repetitive behaviours in obsessive–compulsive disorder and Gilles de la Tourette's syndrome. *Br J Psychiatry* 170: 140–5.

Moriarty J, Campos Costa D, Schmitz B, et al. (1995) Brain perfusion abnormalities in Gilles de la Tourette's syndrome. *Br J Psychiatry* 167: 249–54.

Nee LE, Caine ED, Polinsky RJ, et al. (1980) Gilles de la Tourette syndrome: Clinical and family study of 50 cases. *Ann Neurol* 7: 41–9.

Neglia JP, Glaze DG, Zion TE (1984) Tics and vocalizations in children treated with carbamaze-pine. *Pediatrics* 73: 841–4.

Northam RS, Singer HS (1991) Postencephalitic acquired Tourette-like syndrome in a child. *Neurology* 41: 592–3.

Obeso JA, Rothwell JC, Marsden CD (1981) Simple tics in Gilles de la Tourette's syndrome are not prefaced by a normal premovement EEG potential. *J Neurol Neurosurg Psychiatry* 44: 735–8.

Pauls DL, Leckman JF (1986) The inheritance of Gilles de la Tourette's syndrome and associated behaviors: Evidence for autosomal dominant transmission. *N Engl J Med* 315: 993–7.

— Towbin KE, Leckman JF, et al. (1986) Gilles de Tourette's syndrome and obsessive–compulsive disorder: Evidence supporting a genetic relationship. *Arch Gen Psychiatry* 43: 1180–2.

Peterson AL, Campise RL, Azrin NH (1994) Behavioral and pharmacological treatments for tic and habit disorders: A review. *Dev Behav Pediatr* 15: 430–41.

Peterson BS, Riddle MA, Cohen DJ, et al. (1993) Reduced basal ganglia volume in Tourette's syndrome using three-dimensional reconstruction techniques from magnetic resonance images. *Neurology* 43: 941–9.

Pitman RK, Green RC, Jenike MA, et al. (1987) Clinical comparison of Tourette's disorder and obsessive–compulsive disorder. *Am J Psychiatry* 144: 116–7.

Pulst SM, Wakshe TM, Romero JA (1983) Carbon monoxide poisoning with features of Gilles de la Tourette's syndrome. *Arch Neurol* 40: 443–4.

Regeur L, Pakkenberg B, Fog R, Pakkenberg H (1986) Clinical features and long-term treatment with pimozide in 65 patients with Gilles de la Tourette syndrome. *J Neurol Neurosurg Psychiatry* 49: 791–5.

Rickards H, Robertson MM (1997) Vomiting and retching in Gilles de la Tourette syndrome: A report of ten cases and a review of the literature. *Mov Disord* 12: 531–5.

Riddle MA, Hardin MT, Towbin KE, et al. (1987) Tardive dyskinesia following haloperidol treat-ment for Tourette's syndrome. *Arch Gen Psychiatry* 44: 98–9 (letter).

— — King R, et al. (1990) Fluoxetine treatment of children and adolescents with Tourette's and compulsive disorders. *J Am Acad Child Adolesc Psychiatry* 29: 45–8.

— King R, Hardin MT, et al. (1991) Behavioral side effects of fluoxetine in children and adoles-cents. *J Child Adolesc Psychopharmacol* 1: 193–8.

Robertson M, Doran M, Trimble M, Lees AJ (1990) The treatment of Gilles de Tourette syndrome by limbic leucotomy. *J Neurol Neurosurg Psychiatry* 53: 691–4.

Rose MS, Moldofsky H (1977) Comparison of pimozide with haloperidol in Gilles de la Tourette syndrome. *Lancet* 1: 103 (letter).

Rosenberg GS, David KL (1982) Precursors of acetylcholine: Considerations underlying their use. In: Friedhoff AJ, Chase TN (eds.) *Advances in Neurology. Vol. 35. Gilles de la Tourette Syndrome.* New York: Raven Press, pp. 407–13.

Sacks O (1985) *The Man Who Mistook His Wife for a Hat.* New York: Gerald Duckworth.

Salloway S, Stewart CF, Israeli S, et al. (1996) Botulinum toxin for refractory vocal tics. *Mov Disord* 11: 746–8.

Sanchez-Ramos JR, Weiner WJ (1993) Drug-induced tics. In: Kurlan R (ed.) *Handbook of Tourette's Syndrome and Related Tics and Behavioural Disorders.* New York: Marcel Dekker, pp. 183–97.

Shapiro AK, Shapiro E (1968) Treatment of Gilles de la Tourette with haloperidol. *Br J Psychiatry* 114: 345–50.

— — Eisenkraft GJ (1983) Treatment of Gilles de la Tourette syndrome with pimozide. *Am J Psychiatry* 140: 1183–6.

— — Fulop G (1987) Pimozide treatment of tic and Tourette disorders. *Pediatrics* 79: 1032–9.

— — Young JG, Fenberg TE (1988) *Gilles de la Tourette Syndrome. 2nd edn.* New York: Raven Press.

Singer HS (1993) Tic disorders. *Pediatr Ann* 22: 22–9.

— Rosenberg LA (1989) The development of behavioral and emotional problems in Tourette syndrome. *Pediatr Neurol* 5: 41–4.

— Walkup JT (1991) Tourette syndrome and other tic disorders. *Medicine* 70: 15–32.

— Hahn IH, Krowiak E, et al. (1990) Tourette's syndrome: A neurochemical analysis of post-mortem cortical brain tissue. *Ann Neurol* 27, 443–6.

— Reiss AL, Brown JE, et al. (1993) Volumetric MRI changes in basal ganglia of children with Tourette's syndrome. *Neurology* 43: 950–956.

— Schuerholz LJ, Denckla MB (1995) Learning difficulties in children with Tourette syndrome. *J Child Neurol* 10 (suppl. 1): S58–S61.

— DeLa Cruz PS, Abrams MT, et al. (1997) A Tourette-like syndrome following cardiopulmonary bypass and hypothermia: MRI volumetric measurements. *Mov Disord* 12: 588–92.

— Giuliano JD, Hansen BH, et al. (1998) Antibodies against human putamen in children with Tourette syndrome. *Neurology* 50: 1618–24.

Singh DN, Howe GL, Jordan HW, Hara S (1982) Tourette's syndrome in a black woman with associated triple X and 9p mosaicism. *J Nat Med Assoc* 74: 675–82.

Spencer T, Biederman J, Kerman K, et al. (1993) Desipramine treatment of children with attention-deficit hyperactivity disorder and tic disorder or Tourette syndrome. *Am Acad Adolesc Psychiatry* 32: 354–60.

Stoetter B, Braun AR, Randolph C, et al. (1992) Functional neuroanatomy of Tourette syndrome: Limbic–motor interactions studied with FDG-PET. In: Chase TN, Friedhoff AJ, Cohen DJ (eds.) *Advances in Neurology. Vol. 58. Tourette Syndrome: Genetics, Neurobiology, and Treatment.* New York: Raven Press, 213–26.

Stokes A, Bawden HN, Camfield PR, et al. (1991) Peer problems in Tourette's disorder. *Pediatrics* 87: 936–42.

Swedo SE, Shapiro NE, Grady CL, et al. (1990) Cerebral glucose metabolism in childhood-onset obsessive compulsive disorder. *Arch Gen Psychiatry* 46: 518–23.

— Leonard HL, Kiessling LS (1994) Speculations on antineuronal antibody-mediated neuro-psychiatric disorders of childhood. *Pediatrics* 93: 323–6.

Tanner CM, Goldman SM (1997) Epidemiology of Tourette syndrome. *Neurol Clin N Amer* 15: 395–402.

Taylor LD, Krizman DB, Jankovic J, et al. (1991) 9p monosomy in a patient with Gilles de la Tourette's syndrome. *Neurology* 41: 1513–5.

Torup E A (1972) Follow-up study of children with tics. *Acta Paediatr Scand* 51: 261–8.

Tourette Syndrome Classification Study Group (1993) Definitions and classification of tic disorders. *Arch Neurol* 50: 1013–6.

Tucker DM, Leckman JF, Scahill L, et al. (1996) A putative post-streptococcal case of OCD with chronic tic disorder, not otherwise specified. *J Am Acad Child Adolesc Psychiatry* 35: 1684–91.

Walkup JT, Rosenberg IA, Brown J, Singer HS (1992) The validity of instruments measuring tic severity in Tourette's syndrome. *J Am Acad Child Adolesc Psychiatry* 30: 472–7.

— — Scahill LD, Riddle MA (1995) Disruptive behavior, hyperactivity, and learning disabilities in children with Tourette's syndrome. In: Weiner WJ, Lang AE (eds.) *Advances in Neurology. Vol. 65. Behavioral Neurology of Movement Disorders.* New York: Raven Press, pp. 259–72.

— Labuda MC, Singer HS, et al. (1996) Family study and segregation analysis of Tourette syndrome: Evidence for a mixed model of inheritance. *Am J Hum Genet 59*: 684–93.

Waserman J, Lal S, Gauthier S (1983) Gilles de la Tourette's syndrome in monozygotic twins. *J Neurol Neurosurg Psychiatry 46*: 75–7.

Wilens TE, Biederman J, Geist DE, et al. (1993) Nortriptyline in the treatment of ADHD: A chart review of 58 cases. *J Am Acad Child Adolesc Psychiatry 32*: 343–9.

10
DRUG-INDUCED MOVEMENT DISORDERS

Movement disorders caused by drugs are common. One hundred and forty of 410 child neurologists in the USA who answered a questionnaire had seen patients who had had such disorders during administration or following discontinuation of neuroleptic agents (Silverstein and Johnston 1987). In another study, 34 per cent of child and adolescent psychiatric patients treated with neuroleptics developed parkinsonism (Richardson et al. 1991). The characteristics of the abnormal movements are very variable. History is an important diagnostic cue, but a high index of suspicion is necessary as parents may often not be aware of or not remember any drug intake.

In this brief chapter we shall consider successively the disorders caused by neuroleptic agents, anti-epileptic drugs and other drugs.

MOVEMENT DISORDERS INDUCED BY NEUROLEPTIC AGENTS; OROLINGUAL DYSKINESIA
The term neuroleptic etymologically means 'that which grips the nerve' and is used to designate a broad group of antipsychotic and sedative drugs. Their main pharmacologic property is blockade of dopamine receptors, particularly the D2 subtype.

An *acute neuroleptic syndrome* induced by any of these drugs is common in children. It may present with dystonia (including torticollis or oculogyric crises), hypokinetic–rigid syndrome or akathisia. A single dose of haloperidol or prochlorpromazine is sometimes sufficient to cause it. It occurs within 96 hours of the initiation of neuroleptic therapy. Withdrawal of the drug and parenteral treatment with diazepam, diphenhydramide (Benadryl), orfenadrine or benztropine (Cogentin) results in disappearance of the symptoms in a few minutes. Acute akathisia can be treated with beta blockers or benzodiazepines (preferably clonazepam – Kutcher et al. 1987), but a single intravenous dose of diphenhydramine usually gives complete relief (Pranzatelli 1996).

Orolingual dyskinesia refers to repetitive movements of the tongue (twisting and protrusion), lip smacking or puckering, and chewing movements (Tolosa and Alom 1988). Children receiving chronic medication with neuroleptic agents may develop this type of dyskinesia. Random choreiform movements may be associated (Miyasaki and Lang 1995). Orolingual dyskinesia may occur some time after discontinuation of treatment (called then tardive dyskinesia), on sudden interruption of treatment (withdrawal syndrome) or less frequently on continued treatment.

The incidence of tardive dyskinesia in children is not known. It is observed mainly in children with previous brain damage. Three of 41 children and adolescents treated with various neuroleptic drugs developed tardive dyskinesia in one study (Gualtieri et al. 1984). Some children experience repetitive abnormal movements of the lips and tongue following drug ingestion. Such cases have been reported following ingestion of pemoline (a central stimulant with effects similar to D-amphetamine) (Nausieda et al. 1981) meto-clopramide (Putnam et al. 1992) or of methylphenydate (Weiner et al. 1978).

The pathophysiology of these disturbances is obscure. They may result from dys-function of the subcommissural part of the globus pallidus (Cools et al. 1989) or from a selective block of dopaminergic receptors. An idiosyncratic factor is probably involved.

The syndrome may not be disabling but the movements may be distressing for some patients and/or their family or teachers and require treatment. However, this is often ineffective although several medications (anticholinergics, reserpine, levodopa) have been tried. Emphasis should therefore be on prevention that consists of limitation to a minimum of the indications, duration and doses of the potentially responsible drugs.

Orolingual dyskinesia may be caused by anti-epileptic drugs such as carbamazepine (Joyce and Gunderson 1980) and phenytoin (Moss et al. 1994). I (EF-A) have observed six infants who developed orolingual dyskinesia during oral or i.v. administration of clonazepam (0.1–0.9 mg/kg/d). The symptoms appeared 2–30 days after onset of treat-ment. Lip movements were almost continuous, similar to those of a rabbit or a fish, associated with hypersalivation and frequent tongue protrusion. In some infants the movements prevented suction and swallowing, so that two required nasogastric feeding. Reduction of the dose of clonazepam or substitution of another benzodiazepine resulted in rapid resolution.

Abstinence syndrome (withdrawal dyskinesia) may occur within days of arrest of treatment (90% within 21 days). It is marked by chorea, dystonia, tremor or ataxia and sometimes vomiting. Symptoms disappear on reinitiation of treatment but this may require up to three months. Withdrawal dyskinesia is attributed to dopaminergic hyper-sensitivity (presynaptic denervation hypersensitivity).

The diagnosis of orolingual dyskinesia is usually easy. Rare cases of secondary dys-tonias, especially Hallervorden–Spatz disease, gangliosidosis and delayed-onset dyskinesia, may present with dystonia that affects mainly the face and tongue. Exceptional cases secondary to Wilson disease (Liao et al. 1991) or to a defect in biopterin synthesis (Factor et al. 1991) (see Chapter 3) are on record.

Treatment is with dopamine-depleting agents such as reserpine or tetrabenazine (Jankovic 1981)

Neuroleptic malignant syndrome is the most severe adverse reaction to neuroleptics. It bears no relationship to the dose or duration of treatment. Its incidence is estimated at around 0.5–2% of patients treated with neuroleptics (Kurlan et al. 1984, Guze and Baxter 1985). Piperazine, butyrophenones and haloperidol (Pranzatelli et al. 1994) are most often involved, although any neuroleptic can be the cause. Main symptoms are hyperthermia, muscular hypertonia, tremor, dystonic posturing, autonomic abnormalities (pallor, diaphoresis, unstable blood pressure, tachycardia) and a fluctuating level of consciousness (Guze and Baxter 1985). Laboratory findings include elevated levels of creatine kinase (may exceed 16,000 UI/L), liver enzymes, urea and creatinine; leukocytosis, hypocalcaemia and hypomagnesaemia may occur. The mortality rate is 20–30% and may be even higher with the use of depot forms of the responsible drug. The syndrome may occur at any age but it may be more common in children with previous brain damage (Corless and Buchanan 1965, Diamond and Hayes 1986).

The syndrome is probably due to a blockade of dopaminergic receptors (Henderson and Wooten 1981). Treatment must be aggressive. It includes discontinuation of neuroleptic(s), control of fever, correction of any metabolic disturbance, support of vital functions, and immediate administration of dantrolene sodium. Bromocriptine (2.5–10 mg, t.i.d.) (Guze and Baxter 1985, Dhib-Jalbut et al. 1987) and levodopa have also been used.

The main *differential diagnosis* is with malignant hyperthermia that follows exposure to inhaled halogenated anaesthetics and has similar features, but the circumstances of occurrence are different.

The use of *prophylactic medication* such as benzhexol (Artane) at onset of a neuroleptic therapy to prevent acute dystonia is controversial. It could be justified, if there is a high risk of acute dystonia, for instance if the patient has experienced a previous episode with other drugs. Some authors prefer to warn the family and give neuroleptic therapy without prophylactic drug.

MOVEMENT DISORDERS INDUCED BY ANTI-EPILEPTIC AGENTS

• *Phenytoin.* Various abnormal movements, viz. chorea (Nausieda et al. 1978), tremor, dystonia and asterixis, have been reported with this agent. They are often paroxysmal (Dravet et al. 1980) and tend to predominate in the face (orofacial dyskinesia) and upper limbs. When paroxysmal, the duration of attacks is variable. In one case (Uriz and Fernández-Alvarez 1988) they lasted from 30 minutes and two hours.

A majority of cases (54%) occur before 20 years of age. Approximately one-third of patients have plasma levels <20 mg/l (Harrison et al. 1993). In 18% of cases, dyskinesia was caused by a single i.v. dose of phenytoin. Most patients do not exhibit the usual toxic features (e.g. ataxia, nystagmus) of phenytoin toxicity (Shuttleworth et al. 1974).

Previous brain damage is commonly present (Dravet et al. 1980). Association of other anticonvulsant drugs and a family history of movement disorders such as rheumatic chorea seem to be predisposing factors (Nausieda et al. 1978).

The diagnosis may be difficult in children with severe epilepsy and encephalopathy. The abrupt onset, and the efficacy of diazepam, may erroneously suggest an epileptic origin. However, consciousness is preserved during the episodes.

The mechanism is unknown. It may be related to an interaction of phenytoin with dopaminergic receptors D2 (Shuttleworth et al. 1974). Previous dysfunction of the basal ganglia (Logan and Freeman 1969) may play a role.

• *Valproate.* Valproate produces a postural tremor similar to exaggerated physiological tremor (Hyman et al. 1979, Karas et al. 1982). It occurs mainly with blood levels in excess of 100 mg/L (or 700 mM) and usually disappears on decreasing the dose. Chorea (Lancman et al. 1994) and hemiparkinsonism (Alvarez-Gomez et al. 1993) have also been reported in patients with valproate treatment.

• *Carbamazepine.* Carbamazepine may, rarely, induce tremor (Wallace 1996) and dystonia in children with brain damage (Crosley and Swender 1979). Neglia et al. (1984) suggested that carbamazepine can trigger Tourette disease in susceptible patients but this remains unproved.

• *Ethosuximide.* Ethosuximide can produce acute chorea that follows its introduction and resolves after withdrawal or after administration of parenteral diphenhydramine (Miyasaki and Lang 1995).

• *Gabapentin.* Aggravation of a preexisting choreoathetosis by gabapentin has been reported (Khurana et al. 1996).

In general the management of hyperkinesias induced by anti-epileptic drugs depends on recognition of their toxic role. Determination of serum levels is often useful, but a correct therapeutic serum level does not rule out the diagnosis with some drugs such as phenytoin.

MOVEMENT DISORDERS CAUSED BY OTHER DRUGS
Bronchodilators (mainly beta-adrenergic agents) can produce tremor (Mazer et al. 1990, Scalabrin and Naspitz 1993).

D-*Amphetamine* can produce chorea (Mattson and Calvery 1968, Lundh and Tunving 1981).

Both *lithium* (Walevski and Radwan 1986) and *contraceptives* (Nausieda et al. 1979) can cause chorea, status dystonicus (Manji et al. 1998) or recurrence of previous rheumatic chorea.

Calcium channel blockers may mimic the toxic effects of the neuroleptics (Miyasaki and Lang 1995).

Chlorpromazine, thiorodazine, fluphenazine, trifluoroperazine and flunarizine (Marti-Maso et al. 1985, Chouza et al. 1986, Micheli et al. 1987) can cause hypokinetic–rigid syndrome.

REFERENCES
Alvarez-Gomez MJ, Vaamonde J, Narbona J, et al. (1993) Parkinsonism syndrome in childhood after sodium valproate administration. *Clin Neuropharmacol* 16: 451–5.
Chouza C, Camaño JL, Aljanati R, et al. (1986) Parkinsonism, tardive dystonia, akathisia and depression induced by flunarizine. *Lancet* 1: 1023–34.

Cools AR, Spooren W, Bezemer R, et al. (1989) Anatomically distinct output channels of the caudate nucleus and orofacial dyskinesia: Critical role of the subcommissural part of the globus pallidus in oral dyskinesia. *Neuroscience* 33: 535–42.

Corless JD, Buchanan DS (1965) Phenothiazine intoxicaction in children. *JAMA* 194: 565–7.

Crosley CJ, Swender PT (1979) Dystonia associated with carbamazepine administration: Experience in brain-damaged children. *Pediatrics* 63: 612–5.

Dhib-Jalbut S, Hesselbrock R, Mouradian MM, et al. (1987) Bromocriptine treatment of neuroleptic malignant syndrome. *J Clin Psychiatry* 48: 69–73.

Diamond JM, Hayes DD (1986) A case of neuroleptic malignant syndrome in a mentally retarded adolescent. *J Adolesc Health Care* 7: 419–22.

Dravet C, Dalla Bernardina B, Masdjian E, et al. (1980) Dyskinésies paroxystiques au cours des traitements par la diphénylhydantoine. *Rev Neurol* 136: 1–14.

Factor SA, Coni RJ, Cowger M, Rosenblum EL (1991) Paroxysmal tremor and orofacial dyskinesia secondary to a biopterin synthesis defect. *Neurology* 41: 930–2.

Gualtieri CT, Quade D, Hicks RE, et al. (1984) Tardive dyskinesia and other clinical consequences of neuroleptic treatment in children and adolescents. *Am J Psychiatry* 141: 20–3.

Guze BH, Baxter LR (1985) Neuroleptic malignant syndrome. *N Engl J Med* 313: 163–6.

Harrison MB, Lyons GR, Landow ER (1993) Phenytoin and dyskinesias: A report of two cases and review of the literature. *Mov Disord* 8: 19–27.

Henderson VW, Wooten GF (1981) Neuroleptic malignant syndrome. A pathogenetic role for dopamine receptor blockage? *Neurology* 31: 132–7.

Hyman NM, Dennis PD, Sinclair KG (1979) Tremor due to sodium valproate. *Neurology* 29: 1177–80.

Jankovic J (1981) Drug-induced and other orofacial–cervical dyskinesias. *Ann Intern Med* 94: 788–93.

Joyce RP, Gunderson CH (1980) Carbamazepine-induced orofacial dyskinesia. *Neurology* 30: 1333–4.

Karas BJ, Wilder BJ, Hammond EJ, et al. (1982) Valproate tremors. *Neurology* 32: 428–32.

Khurana DS, Riviello J, Helmers S, et al. (1996) Efficacy of gabapentin therapy in children with refractory partial seizures. *J Pediatr* 128: 829–33.

Kurlan R, Hamill R, Shoulson Y (1984) Neuroleptic malignant syndrome. *Clin Neuropharmacol* 7: 109–20.

Kutcher SP, Mackenzie S, Galarraga W, et al. (1987) Clonazepam treatment of adolescents with neuroleptic-induced akathisia. *Am J Psychiatry* 144: 823–4.

Lancman ME, Asconape JJ, Penry JK (1994) Choreiform movements associated with the use of valproate. *Arch Neurol* 51: 702–4.

Liao KK, Wang SJ, Kwan SY, et al. (1991) Tongue dyskinesia as an early manifestation of Wilson's disease. *Brain Dev* 13: 451–3.

Logan WJ, Freeman JM (1969) Pseudodegenerative disease due to diphenylhydantoin intoxication. *Arch Neurol* 21: 631–7.

Lundh H, Tunving K (1981) An extrapyramidal choreiform syndrome caused by amphetamine addiction. *J Neurol Neurosurg Psychiatry* 44: 728–30.

Manji H, Howard RS, Miller DH, et al. (1998) Status dystonicus: The syndrome and its management. *Brain* 141: 243–52.

Marti-Masso JF, Carrera N, de la Fuente E (1985) Posible parkinsonismo por cinaricina. *Med Clin* 85: 614–6.

Mattson R, Calvery JR (1968) Dextramphetamine-sulfate-induced dyskinesias. *JAMA* 204: 108–10.

Mazer B, Figueroa-Rosario W, Bender B (1990) The effect of albuterol aerosol on fine-motor performance in children with chronic asthma. *J Allergy Clin Immunol* 86: 243–8.

Micheli F, Pardal MF, Gatto M, et al. (1987) Flunarizine and cinarizine-induced extrapyramidal reactions. *Neurology* 37: 881–4.

Miyasaki JM, Lang AE (1995) Treatment of drug-induced movement disorders. In: Kurlan R (ed.) *Treatment of Movement Disorders.* Philadelphia: J.B. Lippincott, pp. 429–74.

Moss W, Ojukwu C, Chiriboga CA (1994) Phenytoin-induced movement disorder. *Clin Pediatr* 33: 634–8.

Nausieda PA, Koller WC, Klawans HL, Weiner WY (1978) Phenytoin and choreic movements. *N Engl J Med* 298: 1093–4.

— — Weiner WJ, Klawans HL (1979) Chorea induced by oral contraceptives. *Neurology* 29: 1605–9.

— — — — (1981) Pemoline-induced chorea. *Neurology* 31: 356–60.

Neglia JP, Glaze DG, Zion TE (1984) Tics and vocalizations in children treated with carbamazepine. *Pediatrics* 73: 841–4.

Pranzatelli MR (1996) Antidyskinetic drug therapy for pediatric movement disorders. *J Child Neurol* 11: 355–69.

— Mott SH, Pavlakis SG, et al. (1994) Clinical spectrum of secondary parkinsonism in childhood: A reversible disorder. *Pediatr Neurol* 10: 131–40.

Putnam PE, Orenstein SR, Wessel HB, Stowe RM (1992) Tardive dyskinesia associated with use of metoclopramide in a child. *J Pediatr* 121: 983–5.

Richardson MA, Hauland G, Craig TJ, (1991) Neuroleptic use, parkinsonian symptoms, tardive dyskinesia, and associated factors in child and adolescent psychiatric patients. *Am J Psychiatry* 148: 1322–8.

Scalabrin DM, Naspitz CK (1993) Efficacy and side effects of salbutamol in acute asthma in children: Comparison of oral route and two different nebulizer systems. *J Asthma* 30: 51–9.

Shuttleworth E, Wise G, Paulson G (1974) Choreoathetosis and diphenylhydantoin intoxication. *JAMA* 230: 1170–1.

Silverstein FS Johnston MV (1987) Risks of neuroleptic drugs in children. *J Child Neurol* 2: 41–3.

Tolosa E, Alom J (1988) Drug-induced dyskinesias. In: Jankovic J, Tolosa E (eds.) *Parkinson's Disease and Movement Disorders.* Baltimore: Urban & Schwarzenberg, pp. 327–47.

Uriz MS, Fernández-Alvarez E (1988) Disquinesia paroxística. Un efecto secundario poco común de las hidantoinas. *Rev Esp Pediatr* 44: 413–5.

Walevski A, Radwan M (1986) Choreoathetosis as toxic effect of lithium treatment. *Eur Neurol* 25: 412–5.

Wallace SJ (1996) A comparative review of the adverse effects of anticonvulsants in children with epilepsy. *Drug Saf* 15: 378–83.

Weiner WJ, Nausieda PA, Klawans HL (1978) Methylphenidate-induced chorea. Case report and pharmacologic implications. *Neurology* 28: 1041–4.

11

MOVEMENT DISORDERS IN CEREBRAL PALSY; MISCELLANEOUS MOVEMENT DISORDERS IN CHILDHOOD

Movement disorders caused by non-progressive lesions in a developing brain are a common problem in children. This chapter will consider two main types: the dyskinetic form of cerebral palsy (CP) and a rare but interesting disturbance, delayed onset dyskinesia. We will also discuss a heterogeneous group in which motor disturbances differ from the five types of abnormal movements described in the preceding chapters.

MOVEMENT DISORDERS IN CEREBRAL PALSY*

CP is a chronic disturbance of movement or posture due to non-progressive defects or lesions in an immature brain.

Dyskinetic CP is the second most frequent form of CP, after the spastic and ahead of the ataxic forms. Its incidence is 0.21/1000 newborn infants (Hagberg et al. 1989) and it constitutes 8–15% of all cases of CP (Aicardi and Bax 1998, Hagberg et al. 1996).

CLINICAL FEATURES
According to Perlstein (1952), dyskinetic CP is characterized by involuntary movements and postures, fluctuations of muscle tone and abnormal persistence of archaic motor reactions. The essential defect is a disturbed capacity to organize and execute voluntary movements. Hagberg et al. (1975) and Kyllerman et al. (1982) distinguish two types, choreoathetotic and dystonic. The choreoathetotic type is marked by the predominance of involuntary movements that include proximal choreic and distal athetotic components. The dystonic type is characterized predominantly by disturbances of muscle tone resulting in abnormal dystonic postures that increase with intended voluntary movements, emotional stimuli or maintenance of attitudes. Persistence of active archaic reflexes is also an important feature. Abnormal movements are often present but are not in the forefront of the clinical picture.

In the first months of life, diagnosis may be difficult as the clinical manifestations are nonspecific with a predominance of hypotonia, brisk primary reflexes (especially

*This section written in collaboration with Pilar Póo, Neuropediatric Department, Hospital San Juan de Dios, Barcelona, Spain.

tonic asymmetrical neck reflexes), exaggerated startle responses and a tendency to neck and back hyperextension on stimulation. Excessive mouth opening and tongue protrusion may suggest the development of dyskinetic CP.

The full-blown picture generally begins to be highly suggestive around the first birthday. Strong tonic spasms on changes of posture or extreme postures of flexion or extension of the limbs are the most striking features. They may sometimes amount to 'dystonic storms' (Manji et al. 1998). In some children, tremor and myoclonus may be associated with dystonic and choreoathetotic movements.

In 44% of the dystonic and in 9% of the choreoathetotic forms, pyramidal tract signs are present and may realize a full picture of spastic tetraparesis (Kyllerman et al. 1982). Fixed contractures, scoliosis, and hip or even shoulder dislocation may compound the picture.

Mental retardation and/or learning difficulties are found in 30% of affected children (Kyllerman et al. 1982). Many others are wrongly considered as having mental problems because of motor and speech difficulties despite a normal cognitive level. Epilepsy, often relatively benign, is present in 20–25% of cases (Kyllerman et al. 1982, Aicardi and Bax 1998). Hypoacusis and visual problems, especially strabismus and abnormalities of re-fraction (Schenk-Rootlieb et al. 1992), are common, though less so since kernicterus has become a rare pathology.

The resulting disability is a lifelong one and is especially severe in the dystonic sub-group.

NEUROIMAGING

CT scan usually shows only nonspecific abnormalities such as ventricular dilatation and increased width of sulci suggestive of cerebral atrophy (Kulakowski and Larroche 1980). MRI in series of patients with CP of probable perinatal origin showed increased T_2 signal in the thalamus, putamen and/or hemispheral white matter (Yokochi et al. 1991, Hoon et al. 1997). In some cases thalamic signal is decreased, which may reflect destructive lesions.

Although there is no strict relationship between the clinical features and the seat of lesions, choreoathetosis may be associated mostly with caudate and putaminal involve-ment whereas dystonia would be more frequently associated with pallidal damage. Cog-nitive deficits might result from the frequently associated cortical lesions. However, the cortex may be normal in one-third of cases. In these cases, thalamic lesions are often found. A role of the basal ganglia in cognitive defects is suspected but still controversial.

DIAGNOSIS

Dopa-responsive dystonia and metabolic encephalopathies of early infantile onset (see Chapter 5) can be misdiagnosed as CP. Treatment with L-dopa must be tried in spastic or dystonic CP cases in which there is any doubt about the cause. Glutaric aciduria, Lesch–Nyhan disease, Pelizaeus–Merzbacher disease (the last two when the patient is male) and mitochondrial diseases are the metabolic diseases most frequently erroneously diagnosed as CP. Special attention has to be given when there is parental consanguinity, when there is another similarly affected sibling, or when no clear abnormality was observed in the perinatal period.

AETIOLOGY

Perinatal hypoxic–ischaemic encephalopathy (HIE) in term newborn infants was the cause of 65% of the cases of dyskinetic CP in the series of Brun and Kyllerman (1979). In up to 10% of such cases, the clinical manifestations in the neonatal period may have been relatively mild and transient (Rosenbloom 1994), although in the majority, there are difficulties in establishing spontaneous respiration and often a full-blown picture of HIE.

Kernicterus, a classical cause of CP, is now very rare in industrialized countries. The role of hyperbilirubinaemia unassociated with haemolytic disease remains controversial (Kyllerman 1977). It might play an additional role to hypoxia and other factors (Hagberg and Hagberg 1993). A role of prenatal factors is suggested by the relative frequency of preterm birth or low birthweight for term (Kyllerman 1983).

Pathological lesions may be of various types. The terms status dysmyelinatus and status marmoratus were coined by Vogt in 1920 (see Brun and Kyllerman 1979).

Status marmoratus applies to a glial scar with loss of neurons and hypermyelination responsible for a marbled appearance of the basal ganglia, especially the caudate, putamen and, sometimes, the thalamus (Friede 1989, Volpe 1995). It is commonly found in cases following perinatal HIE. Contrary to previous beliefs, hypermyelination is localized not to axons but to astrocytic process (Bignami and Ralston 1968, Borit and Herndon 1970). The lesion is more common in term newborn infants than in preterm ones.

Status dysmyelinatus is characterized by neuronal loss in the globus pallidus with consequent reduction in myelinated fibres (Friede 1989). It was the classical lesion of kernicterus. Status dysmyelinatus and status marmoratus are probably different degrees of the same lesional process (Christenson and Melchior 1967).

Cortical lesions are commonly associated. Ulegyria is signs a shrunken convolutions with a narrow atrophic base and a less severely involved crown, giving a mushroom-like appearance. Ulegyric convolutions are preferentially located in the central cortical areas bilaterally and probably explain the frequency of pyramidal tract signs in the lower limbs in post-axphyctic dyskinetic CP. Abnormal deposition of myelin occurs along astrocytic processes as in lesions of the basal nuclei (Borit and Herndon 1970).

In exceptional cases *cortical dysplasias* can be a cause of CP, especially the dystonic type. The dystonia can appear at a late age (Sans et al. 1997).

Lesions of the basal ganglia and thalamus are typically observed following acute hypoxic injury in term infants and are often associated with damage to brainstem nuclei (Pasternak and Gorey 1998, Roland et al. 1998).

The relationship between clinical features and type and location of lesions remains controversial. The most common finding is bilateral sclerosis of the globus pallidus.

MRI studies in the acute stage of HIE usually show extensive involvement of the basal nuclei and, often, of the thalamus (Rolland et al. 1998).

TREATMENT

Physiotherapy, speech therapy, prevention of contractures, and orthopaedic help to avoid secondary deformations and to promote verticalization or improvement in sitting posture, even though their results are not spectacular, are essential in the long-term management of children with dystonic CP. Because of their multiple disabilities these children require multidisciplinary care, and special attention should be given to nutrition, growth and communication. This last often necessitates the use of sign language, but new developments in computer science open the hope of better substitutes for verbal language.

Drug therapy (Pranzatelli 1996) has only a minor place in most patients. Currently a trial of L-dopa is indicated in all cases in which there is no obvious aetiological factor or in atypical cases. Some studies report a favourable response to L-dopa in cases of dyskinetic CP. Other antidystonic drugs may be of help. In 15 patients on trihexyphenidyl (10–15mg/d), I (EF-A) observed a moderate positive response; none of these had responded to L-dopa.

Continuous intrathecal baclofen infusion has been reported to reduce generalized dystonia in children with cerebral palsy (Albright 1996).

Some patients with dyskinetic CP develop 'dystonic storms' or 'status dystonicus' (Manji et al. 1998) spontaneously or following infectious and febrile disease. Treatment of this situation is considered in Chapter 5.

DELAYED-ONSET DYSKINESIA

Although the pathological substrate of CP is thought to remain unchanged with the passing of time, the clinical features do not necessarily stay unchanged. Spastic diplegia preceded by a hypotonic stage and the full picture of dyskinetic CP usually requires about two years to develop (Hanson et al. 1970).

Some authors have observed the late appearance of dystonia in patients who had had symptoms and signs of a fixed motor disorder for several years. Burke et al. (1980) described five children with antecedents of neonatal distress and signs of spastic CP who developed new manifestations of dystonia between the ages of 6 and 14 years. They coined the term 'delayed-onset dystonia' for such cases. New cases have since been reported (Montagna et al. 1981, Obeso et al. 1985, Fernández-Alvarez 1990, Saint-Hilaire et al. 1991, Fletcher and Marsden 1996).

The onset of the syndrome is not usually related to any exogenous factor. In particular, it does not coincide with the administration of drugs, with intercurrent infections or with other acute neurological symptoms.

In most cases, the initial lesion is acquired in the pre- or perinatal period. However, delayed-onset dystonia may also appear following an acquired insult, most commonly a cerebral infarct (Factor et al. 1988; personal cases, JA).

TABLE 11.1
Differential diagnosis of delayed-onset dyskinesia

Tardive dyskinesia
 Antecedents of prolonged neuroleptic treatment
Idiopathic torsion dystonia
 Absence of pre- or perinatal antecedents
 Absence of pyramidal tract symptoms and of mental retardation
 Normal neuroimaging
Hallervorden–Spatz disease
 Pallidal lesion on MRI
 Consanguinity
 Retinitis pigmentosa
 Acanthocytosis
Metabolic diseases (e.g. hexosaminidase A deficiency)

In such cases, manifestations similar to those of idiopathic torsion dystonia appear on top of a previous spastic syndrome. In some cases, other abnormal movements such as orolingual dystonia with continuous, light contractions, resembling those of a rabbit's mouth, are present. The voice is also dystonic, and usually athetoid-type movements are present in the hands. The disturbances are bilateral but usually asymmetrical.

Ancillary investigations give normal results except those that indicate the presence of a previous lesion.

Treatment is purely symptomatic and follows the same principles as that of torsion dystonia.

The *differential diagnosis* is summarized in Table 11.1.

Delayed-onset dyskinesia is of great interest as a manifestation of CNS plasticity following an insult, especially in terms of the time it takes to develop. The phenomenon might also suggest that some apparently primary dystonias could develop as a result of unrecognized old brain lesions.

Hemiparkinsonism–hemiatrophy syndrome, which begins with to an unilateral contralateral body hemiatrophy and a slowly progressive course with secondary development of dystonia, rest tremor and, eventually, parkinsonian features on the contralateral side (Buchman et al. 1988), may represent another syndrome of delayed-onset dyskinesia with adult onset (Giladi et al. 1990).

RHYTHMIC HABIT PATTERNS (RHP)
Repetitive patterns of movement, lacking practical purpose, are a normal part of the motor repertoire of children, and even of adults (leg shaking, foot tapping, finger drumming, etc.). The following terms have been used to designate these movements: motor rhythmias (Backwin and Backwin 1972), rhythmic patterns (Lourie 1949),

TABLE 11.2
Some patterns of repetitive movements in children

Predominantly in otherwise normal children
Hand sucking
Thumb sucking
Sucking of tongue with lips
Nail-biting
Trichotillomania
Body rocking
Head banging
Head rolling

Prevalent in children with mental retardation and/or
severe behaviour disorders (e.g. autism)
Hand biting (to the point of producing calluses)
Continuous tongue protrusion
Bruxism when awake
Hand washing, knitting stereotypies
Unmotivated applause and striking objects

---

rhythmic habit patterns (Kravitz and Boehm 1971), rhythmical stereotypies (Thelen 1979), habit spasms, mannerisms and automatisms. They are often observed in children with behavioural problems but can also occur in normal children. The limits of such motor activity are ill-defined.

Stereotypies can be transient (physiological) or persistent. Thelen (1979, 1980) has identified 49 patterns of stereotypies in the otherwise normal infant.

Some such patterns are grouped according to their predominance in normal and abnormal children in Table 11.2.

Stereotypies are repetitive, often rhythmical, voluntary (they can be initiated or interrupted by the subject) but non-purposeful movements. They are common in infants. The time spent in such activities is variable but increases progressively until the age of 6 months; it then decreases and at the same time its pattern becomes more varied (Thelen 1979).

Head banging occurs generally with the child is in the prone position or on all fours. It is particularly common just before sleep. It is observed in 5.1% (Sallustro and Atwell 1978) to 15.2% (de Lissovoy 1961) of otherwise normal infants, usually beginning around 9 months of age and lasting up to 3–4 years. It is more common in boys.

Body rocking is the back-and-forth motion of the body on hands and knees or in the sitting position. *Head rolling* is a rhythmic oscillation of the head and is also common (6.3–19.1%) (Sallustro and Atwell 1978).

Persistent stereotypies are common in pathological subjects: blind or autistic children (Ritvo et al. 1968), children with mental retardation or emotional disturbances (Kaufman and Levitt 1965), and institutionalized infants (Spitz 1965). Stereotypies of hand or thumb biting or other frightening autoaggressive behaviours are frequent in children with mental retardation. In Lesch–Nyhan disease they are a characteristic symptom.

Rocking stereotypies are common with various types of autism. In Rett syndrome, a progressive disease limited to girls with mental regression, autism, ataxia and frequently epilepsy, the hand movements (hand-washing, kneading or knitting) involve both hands, usually in the midline, with complex intertwining of individual digits. They may be associated with rigidity and dystonic postures, and involvement of the central grey matter has been demonstrated in some cases (Hagberg et al. 1983).

In children without mental retardation or autism the peak performance of rocking stereotypies is at 12–17 months and they can persist for years (Werry et al. 1983). Hyperactive behaviour or attention-deficit problems are frequently associated (Tan et al. 1997). The stereotypies are usually performed when the child is in a state of excitement or stress but can also occur when the child is bored or in intense concentration.

The neurophysiological basis of stereotypies is unknown. A relationship with hyperactivity and akathisia is possible (Gillberg 1995). They seem to be linked to the dopaminergic system, as dopamine agonists (such as amphetamine or apomorphine) (Castall et al. 1977) can induce them and they are blocked by certain lesions in the basal ganglia (Gillberg 1995).

These movements may occasionally be confused with *complex partial seizures* but there is no disturbance of consciousness and the children can interrupt the stereotypy if they are aroused. In rare children, stereotypies appear to be an integral part of epileptic seizures as shown by their regular association with paroxysmal EEG activity. *Complex tics* resemble stereotypies but are often accompanied by simple tics and are associated with an uncomfortable feeling of tension when trying to suppress the movements. The *bobbing-head doll syndrome* (see Chapter 3) resembles a stereotypy but its circumstances of occurrence in children with hydrocephalus makes it clearly different.

When stereotypies are not severe the only useful treatment is parental reassurance. When head banging or other potentially injurious stereotypies occur very frequently, behavioural modification may be necessary.

SYNKINESIAS AND MIRROR MOVEMENTS

Synkinesias are superfluous, non-propositive movements that occur in association with a propositive movement in another part of the body. Many of them are normal developmental phenomena and tend to disappear with maturation.

Contralateral imitation synkinesias, a tendency to reproduce in one side of the body voluntary movements performed by the other side, are a normal phenomenon until at least 12 years of age (de Ajuriaguerra and Stambak 1955) and in the case of fine finger movements can persist even longer.

Synkinesias are abnormal when they (1) persist beyond the usual age of disappearance, (2) are exaggerated, or (3) show a clear asymmetry.

TABLE 11.3
Disorders that can be associated with mirror movements

Klippel–Feil syndrome (Gunderson and Solitare 1968)
Arnold–Chiari malformation (Spillane et al. 1957)
Agenesis of the corpus callosum (Schott and Wyke 1981)
Friedreich ataxia (Heck 1964)
Kallman syndrome (hypogonadotrophic hypogonadism with anosmia) (Conrad et al. 1978)
Usher syndrome (Schott and Wyke 1981)
Congenital hemiplegia

MIRROR MOVEMENTS

Mirror movements are exaggerated imitation synkinesias (Cincotta et al. 1996). They are especially marked when the voluntary movement requires concentration. They may be genetically determined and transmitted as an autosomal dominant character (Haerer and Currier 1966, Regli et al. 1967, Rasmussen and Waldenstrom 1978, Paulson and Gill 1995), or sporadic (Artigas et al. 1989, Ruggieri et al. 1999) in otherwise normal subjects. They may also be associated with other neurological disturbances (Table 11.3).

They predominate in the hands and upper limbs, and only exceptionally affect the lower extremities with resulting difficulties in walking. In the upper limb they may considerably disturb alternating movements of the extremities such as climbing a ladder.

They tend to improve spontaneously and to some extent by exercise but may persist into adulthood.

In patients with Klippel–Feil syndrome with mirror movements, abnormalities of the posterior column and complete or partial absence of pyramidal decussation have been reported (Gunderson and Solitare 1968) or suspected clinically (Haerer and Currier 1966).

Walshe (1947) believed that mirror movements represent a defect of inhibition of the uncrossed pyramidal tracts, but study of the cortical potentials induced by movement suggest that the defect may be due to cortical dysfunction (Shibasaki and Nagae 1984). Transcranial magnetic stimulation has shown abnormal ipsilateral responses suggesting an abnormal cortical representation (Rasmussen 1993).

RESTLESS LEGS SYNDROME (RLS)

RLS consists of dysaesthesias or paraesthesias of ill-defined but unpleasant character, which involve the lower extremities (and sometimes also the arms — Michaud et al. 2000) and are referred to the depth of the limb rather than the skin. These sensations are associated with an irresistible urge to move the limbs by walking, rubbing or otherwise. Symptoms are worse at evening or night time, often resulting in insomnia or frequent sleep disruptions (Lugaresi et al. 1986).

RLS is traditionally considered a disease of middle to older age. There are a few reports of this syndrome in childhood and adolescence, usually familial cases with autosomal dominant inheritance (Montplaisir et al. 1985, Godbout et al. 1987, Walters 1995, Trenkwalder et al. 1996), but in a survey of 107 adult patients about 20% reported an onset before age 10 years (Walters et al. 1994). Symptomatic cases may be due to diabetes mellitus, uraemia or amyloidosis. The existence of an oligosymptomatic axonal neuropathy has been postulated (Iannaccone et al. 1995).

Diurnal or nocturnal repetitive myoclonus (Hening et al. 1986) and periodic leg movements in sleep (Brodeux et al. 1988, Walters et al. 1988a) may occur in association.

The course is stable in paediatric patients but can become progressive over the age of 50 years (Trenkwalder et al. 1996).

Treatment with benzodiazepines, carbamazepine (Telstad et al. 1984), bromocriptine (Walters et al. 1988b), L-dopa (Brodeux et al. 1988), opioids (Hening et al. 1986) and baclofen (Gilleminault and Flagg 1984) is of uncertain efficacy.

REFERENCES

Aicardi J, Bax M (1998) Cerebral palsy. In Aicardi J *Diseases of the Nervous System in Childhood.* 2nd edn. London: Mac Keith Press, pp. 210–39.

Albright AL (1996) Intrathecal baclofen in cerebral palsy movement disorders. *J Child Neurol* 11 (suppl.): S29–S35.

Artigas J, Fernández-Alvarez E, Lorente I (1989) Movimientos en espejo. Revisión de 11 observaciones. *An Esp Pediatr* 31: 559–63.

Backwin H, Backwin RM (1972) *Behaviour Disorders in Children.* Philadelphia: WB Saunders.

Bignami A, Ralston HJ (1968) Myelination of fibrillary astroglial processes in long term wallerian degeneration. The possible relationship to "status marmoratus". *Brain Res* 11: 710–3.

Borit A, Herndon RM (1970) The fine structure of plaques fibromyeliniques in ulegyria and in status marmoratus. *Acta Neuropathol* 14: 304–11.

Brodeux C, Montplaisir J, Godbout R, Marinier R (1988) Treatment of restless legs syndrome and periodic movements during sleep with L-dopa: A double-blind, controlled study. *Neurology* 38: 1845–8.

Brun A, Kyllerman M (1979) Clinical, pathogenetic and neuropathological correlates in dystonic cerebral palsy. *Eur J Pediatr* 131: 93–104.

Buchman AS, Goetz CG, Klawans HL (1988) Hemiparkinsonism with hemiatrophy. *Neurology* 38: 527–30.

Burke RE, Fahn S, Gold AP (1980) Delayed onset dystonia in patients with "static" encephalopathy. *J Neurol Neurosurg Psychiatry* 43: 789–97.

Castall B, Marsden CD, Naylor RJ, Pycock CJ (1977) Stereotyped behavior patterns and hyperactivity induced by amphetamine and apomorphine after discrete 6-hydroxydopamine lesions of extrapyramidal and mesolimbic nuclei. *Brain Res* 123: 89–111.

Christenson E, Melchior JC (1967) *Cerebral Palsy—A Clinical and Neuropathological Study. Clinics in Developmental Medicine No. 25.* London: Spastics International Medical Publications.

Cincotta M, Lori S, Gangemi PF, et al. (1996) Hand motor cortex activation in a patient with congenital mirror movements: A study of the silent period following focal transcranial magnetic stimulation. *EEG Clin Neurophysiol* 101: 240–6.

Conrad B, Kliebel J, Jetzel WD (1978) Hereditary bimanual synkinesis combined with hypogonadotrophic hypogonadism and anosmia in two brothers. *J Neurol* 218: 263–74.

de Ajuriaguerra J, Stambak M (1955) L'evolution des syncinésies chez l'enfant. *Presse Med* 63: 817–9.

De Lissovoy V (1961) Head banging in early childhood: A study of incidence. *J Pediatr* 58: 803–5.

Factor SA, Sanchez-Ramos J, Weiner WJ (1988) Delayed-onset dystonia associated with cortico-spinal tract dysfunction. *Mov Disord* 3: 201–10.

Fernández-Alvarez E (1990) Delayed-onset dyskinesia. In: Papini M, Paquinelli A, Gidoni EA (eds) *Development, Handicap, Rehabilitation: Practice and Theory.* Amsterdam: Elsevier, pp. 97–103.

Fletcher NA, Marsden CD (1996) Dyskinetic cerebral palsy: a clinical and genetic study. *Dev Med Child Neurol* 38: 873–80.

Friede RL (1989) *Developmental Neuropathology, 2nd edn.* Berlin: Springer-Verlag.

Giladi N, Burke RE, Kostic V, et al. (1990) Hemiparkinsonism–hemiatrophy syndrome: Clinical and neuroradiologic features. *Neurology* 40: 1731–4.

Gillberg C (1995) *Clinical Child Neuropsychiatry.* Cambridge: Cambridge University Press.

Gilleminault C, Flagg W (1984) Effects of baclofen on sleep-related periodic leg movements. *Ann Neurol* 15: 234–9.

Godbout R, Montplaisir J, Poirer G (1987) Epidemiological data in familial restless syndrome. *Sleep Res* 16: 338 (abstract).

Gunderson CH, Solitare GB (1968) Mirror movements in patients with the Klippel–Feil syndrome. *Arch Neurol* 18: 675–9.

Haerer AF, Currier, RD (1966) Mirror movements. *Neurology* 16: 757–65.

Hagberg B, Hagberg G (1993) The origin of cerebral palsy. In: David TJ (ed) *Recent Advances in Paediatrics. Vol. 11.* London: Churchill Livingstone, pp. 67–83.

— Hagberg G, Olow I. (1975) The changing panorama of cerebral palsy in Sweden 1954–1970. II. Analysis of the various syndromes. *Acta Paediatr Scand* 64: 193–200.

— Alcardi J, Dias K, Ramos O (1983) A progressive syndrome of autism, dementia, ataxia and loss of purposeful hand use in girls. Rett's syndrome: Report of 35 cases. *Ann Neurol* 14, 471–9.

— Hagberg G, Zetterström R (1989) Decreasing perinatal mortality. Increase in cerebral palsy morbidity. *Acta Paediatr Scand* 78: 664–70.

— Hagberg G, Olow I, Wendt LV (1996) The changing panorama of cerebral palsy in Sweden. VII. Prevalence and origin in the birth period 1987–90. *Acta Paediatr* 85: 954–60.

Hanson RA, Berenberg W, Byers RK (1970) Changing motor patterns in cerebral palsy. *Dev Med Child Neurol* 12: 309–14.

Heck AF (1964) A study of neural and extraneural findings in a large family with Friedreich's ataxia. *J Neurol Sci* 1: 226–30.

Hening WA, Walters A, Kavey N, et al. (1986) Dyskinesias while awake and periodic movements in sleep in restless legs syndrome: Treatment with opioids. *Neurology* 36: 1363–6.

Hoon AH, Reinhardt EM, Kelley RI, et al. (1997) Brain magnetic resonance imaging in suspected extrapyramidal cerebral palsy: Observations in distinguishing genetic–metabolic from acquired causes. *J Pediatr* 131: 240–5.

Iannaccone S, Zucconi M, Marchettini P, et al. (1995) Evidence of peripheral axonal neuropathy in primary restless legs syndrome. *Mov Disord* 10: 2–9.

Kaufman ME, Levitt H (1965) A study of three stereotyped behaviors in institutionalized mental defectives. *Am J Ment Def* 69: 467–73.

Kravitz H, Boehm J (1971) Rhythmic habit patterns in infancy: Their sequence, age of onset and frequency. *Child Dev* 42: 399–413.

Kulakowski S, Larroche JC (1980) Cranial computerized tomography in cerebral palsy. An attempt at anatomo-clinical and radiological correlation. *Neuropediatrics* 11: 339–53.

Kyllerman M (1977) Dyskinetic cerebral palsy. An analysis of 115 Swedish cases. *Neuropädiatrie* 8 (suppl.): 528–32.

— (1983) Reduced optimality in pre- and perinatal conditions in dyskinetic cerebral palsy. Distribution and comparison to controls. *Neuropediatrics* 14: 29–36.

— Bager B, Bensch J, et al. (1982) Dyskinetic cerebral palsy. I. Clinical categories, associated neurological abnormalities and incidences. *Acta Paediatr Scand* 71: 543–50.

Lourie RS (1949) The role of rhythmic patterns in childhood. *Am J Psychiatry* 105: 653–60.

Lugaresi E, Cirignotta F, Coccagna G, Montagna P (1986) Nocturnal myoclonus and restless legs syndrome. *Adv Neurol* 43: 295–307.

Manji H, Howard RS, Miller DH, et al. (1998) Status dystonicus: The syndrome and its management. *Brain* 141: 243–52.

Michaud M, Chabli A, Lavigne G, Montplaisir J (2000) Arm restlessness in patients with restless legs syndrome. *Mov Disord* 15: 289–93.

Montagna P, Cirignotta P, Gallassi R, Sacquegna T (1981) Progressive choreoathetosis related to birth anoxia. *J Neurol Neurosurg Psychiatry* 44: 957 (letter).

Montplaisir J, Godbout R, Boghen D, et al. (1985) Familial restless legs with periodic movements in sleep: Electrophysiological, biochemical, and pharmacological study. *Neurology* 35: 130–40.

Obeso JA, Vaamonde J, Barraquer Bordas L (1985) Delayed onset dystonia. *J Neurol Neurosurg Psychiatry* 48: 1190–1.

Pasternak JF, Gorey HT (1998) The syndrome of acute near-total intrauterine asphyxia. *Pediatric Neurol* 18: 391–8.

Paulson GW, Gill WM (1995) Congenital mirror movements. *Mov Disord* 10: 117–8.

Perlstein MA (1952) Infantile cerebral palsy: Classification and clinical correlations. *JAMA* 149: 30–4.

Pranzatelli MR (1996) Oral pharmacotherapy for the movement disorders of cerebral palsy. *J Child Neurol* 11 (suppl. 1): S13–S22.

Rasmussen P (1993) Persistent mirror movements: a clinical study of 17 children, adolescents and young adults. *Dev Med Child Neurol* 35: 699–707.

— Waldenstrom E (1978) Hereditary mirror movements. A case report. *Neuropädiatrie* 9: 189–94.

Regli F, Filippa G, Weisendanger M (1967) Hereditary mirror movements. *Arch Neurol* 16: 620–3.

Ritvo ER, Ornitz EM, La Franchis S (1968) Frequency of repetitive behaviors in early infantile autism and its variants. *Arch Gen Psychiatry* 19: 341–7.

Roland EH, Poskitt K, Rodriguez E, et al. (1998) Perinatal hypoxic–ischemic thalamic injury: Clinical features and neuroimaging. *Ann Neurol* 44: 161–6.

Rosenbloom L (1994) Dyskinetic cerebral palsy and birth asphyxia. *Dev Med Child Neurol* 36: 285–9.

Ruggieri V, Amartino H, Fejerman N (1999) Movimientos en espejo congénitos. Tres nuevos casos de una rara entidad. *Rev Neurol* 29: 731–5.

Sallustro F, Atwell CW (1978) Body rocking, head banging and head rolling in normal children. *J Pediatr* 93: 704–8.

Sans A, Gassio R, Lopez-Casas J, Fernández-Alvarez E (1997) Inicio tardío de paralisis pseudobulbar y distonía en un caso de displasia cortical hemisférica. *Rev Neurol* 25: 875–6.

Saint-Hilaire MH, Burke RE, Bressman SB, et al. (1991) Delayed-onset dystonia due to perinatal or early childhood asphyxia. *Neurology* 41: 216–22.

Schenk-Rootlieb AJF, van Nieuwenhuizen O, van der Graaf Y, et al. (1992) The prevalence of cerebral visual disturbance in children with cerebral palsy. *Dev Med Child Neurol* 34: 473–80.

Schott GD, Wyke MA (1981) Congenital mirror movements. *J Neurol Neurosurg Psychiatry* 44: 586–99.

Shibasaki H, Nagae K. (1984) Mirror movements: Application of movement-related cortical potentials. *Ann Neurol* 15: 299–301.

Spillane JD, Pallis C, Jones AM (1957) Developmental abnormalities in the region of foramen magnum. *Brain* 80: 11–48.

Spitz R (1965) *The First Year of Life*. New York: International University Press.

Tan A, Salgado M, Fahn S (1997) The characterization and outcome of stereotypic movements in nonautistic children. *Mov Disord* 12: 47–52.

Telstad W, Sorensen O, Larsen S, et al. (1984) Treatment of restless legs syndrome with carbamazepine: a double blind study. *BMJ* 288: 444–6.

Thelen E (1979) Rhythmical sterotypies in normal human infants. *Anim Behav* 27: 699–715.

— (1980) Determinants of amounts of stereotyped behaviour in normal human infants. *Ethol Sociobiol* 1: 141–50.

Trenkwalder C, Seidel VC, Gasser T, Oertel WH (1996) Clinical symptoms and possible anticipation in a large kindred of familial restless syndrome. *Mov Disord* 11: 389–94.

Volpe JJ (1995) *Neurology of the Newborn. 3rd edn*. Philadelphia: WB Saunders.

Walshe FMR (1947) On the role of the pyramidal system in willed movements. *Brain* 70: 329–54.

Walters AS (1995) Toward a better definition of the restless legs syndrome. *Mov Disord* 10: 634–42.

— Henning WA, Chokroverty S (1988a) Frequent occurrence of myoclonus while awake and at rest, body rocking and marching in place in a subpopulation of patients with restless legs syndrome. *Acta Neurol Scand* 77: 418–21.

— — Kavey N, et al. (1988b) A double-blind randomized crossover trial of bromocriptine and placebo in restless legs syndrome. *Ann Neurol* 24: 455–8.

— Hickey K, Maltzman J, et al. (1994) A questionnaire study of the clinical course in 107 patients with restless legs syndrome. *Neurology* 44: A217–A218.

Werry JS, Carlielle J, Fitzpatrick J (1983) Rhythmic motor activities (stereotypies) in children under five: Etiology and prevalence. *J Am Acad Child Psychiatry* 22: 329–36.

Yokochi K, Aiba K, Kodama M, Fujimoto S (1991) Magnetic resonance imaging in athetotic cerebral palsied children. *Acta Paediatr Scand* 80: 818–23.

12

ANCILLARY INVESTIGATIONS

SECTION 1: RECORDING OF ABNORMAL MOVEMENTS*

Fine analysis of abnormal movements requires recording. Electrical methods had long been limited to the investigation of peripheral neurons. During the last two decades, however, they have been successfully applied to the study of abnormal movements and to the excitability of reflexes. They have proved to be an indispensable component of clinical examination.

Indeed, clinical observation alone does not suffice to account for all the principal characteristics of an abnormal movement. It does not allow a satisfactory analysis of rapid phenomena and recognizes only imperfectly the rhythmical nature of movements with irregular amplitude. In the case of large amplitude movements, a high frequency is often erreneously attributed. Such errors are easily corrected by the use of electrical examination.

In addition, some peculiarities of involuntary movements go unrecognized even by trained examiners, e.g. cocontraction of agonists and antagonists. Likewise, clinical observation cannot appreciate precisely abnormal synchronization of several muscle groups. Arrest of muscle activity is entirely missed when brief, as is the case with negative myoclonus (Fig. 12.1).

Electrical examination is also important by providing a lasting document that may allow comparison at various times and assessment of evolution of symptoms spontaneously or with therapy. Analysis of tracings may also show similarities with other abnormal movements of different causes but that may share pathophysiological mechanisms. For example, tardive dyskinesia induced by neuroleptic agents shares some features with the abnormal movements induced by L-dopa in Parkinson disease (Fig. 12.2), indicating that the mechanisms are the same despite the different causes (Rondot and Ribadeau-Dumas 1972).

Recordings allow the study of the effect of various extrinsic activating or inhibiting factors on abnormal movements and may thus contribute to clarifying the pathophysiological mechanisms.

Hence, recording of abnormal movements is an important adjunct to clinical examination. It permits visualization of movement itself, its amplitude, velocity and acceleration, and the electromyographic activity that generates it.

In this section we will review the various methods used for description and analysis of abnormal movements and illustrate them by a few examples.

*Authored by Pierre Rondot (*formerly* Professor of Neurology, Hôpital Saint-Anne, Paris) and N Bathien (*formerly* Departments of Neurology and Clinical Neurophysiology, Hôpital Saint-Anne, Paris, France).

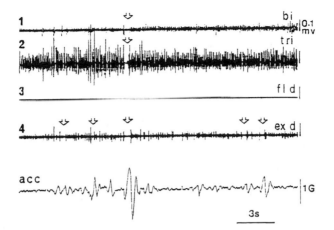

Fig. 12.1. Negative myoclonus.

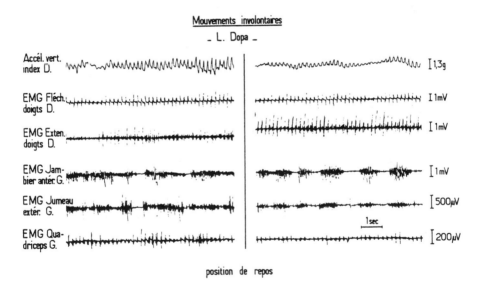

Fig. 12.2. L-Dopa dyskinesia.

ELECTROMYOGRAPHY (EMG)

EMG is a basic investigation that allows one to determine precisely the muscles where the abnormal activity is localized, its extension to other muscles and the nature of the activity (e.g. tremor, myoclonus).

Recording is usually with *surface electrodes* that show the overall pattern of muscle activity. Polygraphic examinations allow determination of the muscle first involved,

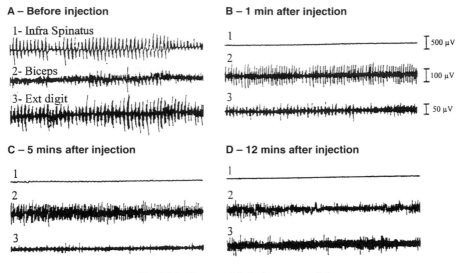

Fig. 12.3. Tremor with 'inductor muscle'.

which may be regarded as the 'inductor muscle' (Rondot et al. 1968; Fig. 12.3). Injection of alcohol or, more recently, of botulinum toxin into this muscle may suppress the movement for several weeks. In the upper limb, exploration of muscles of both the root and the extremity (flexors and extensors of the fingers, biceps and triceps, internal and external rotators of the shoulder, abductors and adductors of the arm) is imperative (Fig. 12.3). EMG investigation should be guided by the results of clinical examination.

Finer analysis of abnormal EMG activity requires the implantation of *coaxial electrodes* in the most active muscle. This is especially useful when the movements are of small amplitude. In this way it is possible to show that, in bursts of parkinsonian tremor, the same motor unit discharges only once when amplitude is small, but twice when the movement is of greater amplitude (Renou et al. 1970) (Fig. 12.4). Conversely, in spinal myoclonus, discharges of a single motor unit are much more numerous within each rhythmical burst (Garcin et al. 1966).

Recordings using coaxial electrodes are difficult when movements are large: the needle tends to move within the muscle explored, resulting in pain that may provoke a muscle contraction unrelated to the abnormal movement. Moreover, needle motion may injure muscle fibres and be responsible for more artefacts than with surface electrodes. Replacing the coaxial electrodes by *wire electrodes* inserted through a trocar electrode withdrawn after insertion may limit this problem. However, the wire may become displaced, thus preventing the follow-up recording of the same unit. *Multielectrodes*, in which several contacts are located on the same needle a few microns apart, may permit retrieval of a particular motor unit on a neighbouring lead when it has disappeared from the initial one, thanks to its unique morphology. This may be interesting for fine study of motor

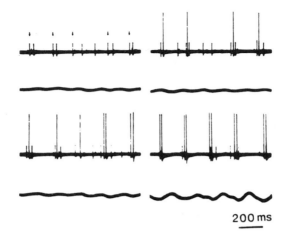

Fig. 12.4. 'Double' motor unit discharges in tremor.

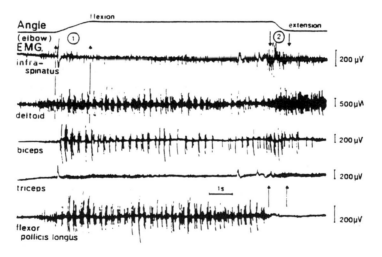

Fig. 12.5. Attitude tremor: note goniometer trace (top).

discharges. It allows visualization of the effects of stimulations or pharmacological agents on the abnormal activity.

RECORDING OF MOTION

Some abnormal movements become manifest clinically only at or above a certain amplitude of voluntary movement. This is especially the case for attitude tremor (Fig. 12.5). It is therefore of interest to record on the same document both the motion of a limb and the EMG of the corresponding muscles. It can also be useful to determine, during the movement, from which angle the EMG activity increases or decreases and from which angle it becomes manifest in the antagonists.

Such information may be of interest in both active and passive movements. The velocity of movement can be obtained by electronic differentiation of the analogical signal of displacement. A goniometer measures displacement. It includes a potentiometer attached to two levers placed as compass branches fixed to two segments of a limb on either side of an articulation. Variations in the compass opening generate variations in a resistance fed by a direct current. The latter are recorded polygraphically, together with the EMG tracings of the corresponding muscles.

RECORDING OF MOVEMENT ACCELERATION

Acceleration is a derivation of velocity. It is important to know in the case of fast, low-amplitude movements that often are below the sensitivity of the goniometer, in particular tremor.

Accelerometers register motion via a transducer tightly fixed to the moving segment of the body. They measure acceleration in the direction of movement, so the active axis of the transducer should be in the same direction as that of movement. In the case of complex movements, resulting from forces in various directions, several accelerometers are required, each assessing acceleration in the direction of its own active axis. Several types are used. Some of them, the piezoelectrical accelerometers, record the kinetic energy developed by the movement with a mass that generates a difference of potentials. Certain asymmetrical crystals (quartz, barium titanate, etc.) generate a difference of potential proportional to the applied constraint, when submitted to compression along their piezo-electrical axis. Other accelerometers are strain gauges. The electrical resistance of certain materials varies as a function of their lengthening. The force generated by movement is applied to a passive mass whose displacement in relation to an adjacent circuit induces modifications of resistance, capacity or reductance. The gauges are fixed to a metal strip selected so that its deformation is linear. Variable reductance accelerometers include a mobile mass in the air gap of a magnet. Movement of this mass generates a variation of potential in the circuit placed in the magnetic field, thus allowing measurement of movement acceleration.

When movement is oscillatory, accelerometer tracings allow immediate deduction of its frequency. This type of capter is especially indicated for recording of tremor (Fig. 12.6). When movement is not oscillatory, accelerometers allow demonstration of the finest variations of acceleration and also show clearly the discontinuity of movement (Fig. 12.7) and are particularly useful in the study of abnormal movements of cerebellar origin (Rondot et al. 1979). Volitional hyperkinesia is characterized by sudden jolts preventing the smooth continuity of coordinated movement. Accelerometer recordings can differentiate rhythmical hyperkinesias such as those of multiple sclerosis, from arrhythmical or myoclonic hyperkinesias (Fig. 12.7) such as those due to hypoxic encephalopathies or to toxins such as methyl bromide (Rondot et al. 1972).

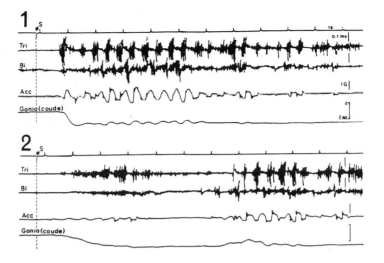

Fig. 12.6. Action tremor: note accelerometer (acc) trace.

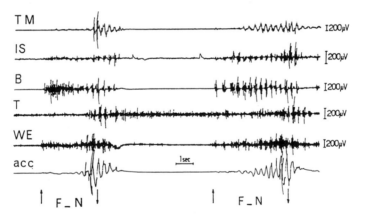

Fig. 12.7. Cerebellar movement, index-to-nose: EMG and accelerometer recording of the muscles teres major (TM), infraspinatus (IS), biceps (B), triceps (T) and extensor carpi radialis (WE).

MOVEMENT-RELATED CORTICAL POTENTIAL (MRP)

MRP is also called readiness potential (RP). Although its study is not directly concerned with involuntary movement, it may be interesting to verify whether the preparation of movement is normal or whether the abnormal movement proceeds from an abnormally excitable motor cortex, especially the supplementary motor area (SMA). The MRP is an event-related potential recorded in relation to a motor event, the initiation of movement. It consists of a cortical negativity preceding spontaneous voluntary movement by 1–1.5

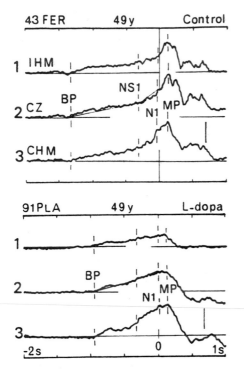

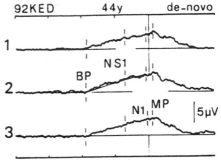

Fig. 12.8. Comparison of movement-related potentials recorded in a normal subject (Control), an untreated parkinsonian patient (de-novo) and a treated (L-dopa) patient of similar ages. Recordings at C2 level (2) and ipsilateral (1) and contralateral (3) motor cortex. (See text for explanation of gradients and abbreviations.)

seconds. Despite terminology differences, it is accepted that two components can be distinguished. An early negativity, often termed *Bereischaft Potential* (BP), begins about 1–1.5 s before the EMG activity accompanying the movement. It is of maximum amplitude at the vertex (CZ), followed by a slope NS^1 of greater gradient, maximum over the contralateral central area. It reaches a peak amplitude 10–50 ms before onset of the EEG activity. Recordings with subdural (Neshige et al. 1988, Ikeda et al. 1992) or intracerebral (Rektor et al. 1994) electrodes have shown that the MRP comes from multiple generators located in both the primary and the supplementary motor areas bilaterally. Studies of clinical models in which there is depressed function of the SMAs (Fève et al. 1994) or of the primary motor cortex as a result of cerebellar lesions (Shibasaki et al. 1986, Wessel et al. 1994) have evidenced a decreased amplitude of the MRP. No specific difference is observed in the components BP or NS^1 according to the anatomical location of the lesions. Figure 12.8 illustrates an example of the evolution of MRPs related to wrist movements in a patient with Parkinson disease before and after three months of L-dopa therapy.

OTHER METHODS
There are other methods of analysis of the circuits involved in abnormal involuntary movements, for example analysis of the reflex excitability of the motoneurons, but these are beyond the scope of this brief review.

SECTION 2: STUDIES WITH POSITRON EMISSION TOMOGRAPHY*

Various nonepileptiform movement disorders or dyskinesias comprise a significant portion of the caseload in paediatric neurology. Yet, there are relatively few tests available to make a specific diagnosis, which must therefore rely heavily on clinical impression. For most movement disorders in children, brain imaging with computed tomography (CT) and magnetic resonance imaging (MRI) are of limited value since macroscopic structural abnormalities are not present in the majority of these children. Functional brain imaging with positron emission tomography (PET) or single photon emission computed tomography (SPECT) is probably more likely to show abnormalities which can be related to the pathophysiology of the movement disorder or be applied for diagnostic purposes, but has not been adequately developed for these uses. In this section, we will review the potential applications of PET technology in the study of movement disorders occurring in children.

PET METHODOLOGY

PET is a quantitative imaging technique capable of measuring hundreds of local chemical functions in various body organs (Phelps et al. 1986). Like CT scanning, PET relies on reconstruction algorithms to produce tomographic images; however, unlike CT which uses an external X-ray beam, the source of radiation in PET is in the form of an administered chemical compound labelled with a positron emitting isotope. The most common applications of PET in neurology are the study of local cerebral glucose metabolism and blood flow, and neurotransmitter synthesis, uptake and binding. Less commonly used applications include the study of cerebral oxygen utilization, protein synthesis, amino acid transport, and various other biochemical and physiological processes (Phelps and Mazziotta 1985).

In a typical PET study of cerebral glucose metabolism, the child is fasted for four hours prior to administration of the tracer 2-deoxy-2[18F]fluoro-D-glucose (FDG). Venous access is obtained in either a hand or foot for administration of the FDG dose. It is important to minimize environmental effects on the distribution of glucose consumption in the brain, and therefore, during the FDG uptake period (first 30 minutes after injection), the child is kept awake, with minimal parent–child interaction. The lights in the room are dimmed, and visual, auditory and other sensory stimuli are kept to a minimum. After 30 minutes, sedation may be used if required, as sedation or natural sleep at this late period will no longer affect the cerebral distribution of the tracer since about 90% of the FDG, by this time, has been converted to FDG-6-phosphate which is trapped in brain tissue. Forty minutes after the FDG injection, scanning of the brain is performed and lasts about 30 minutes. The tomographic images usually are oriented parallel to the

*Authored by Harry T. Chugani and Diane C. Chugani (Departments of Pediatrics, Neurology and Radiology, Children's Hospital of Michigan, Wayne State University School of Medicine, Detroit, MI, USA).

canthomeatal plane, but any desired plane may be used. Furthermore, currently available software allows PET data to be resliced in any plane, and to be registered with the CT or MRI scans.

There has been an ongoing effort to minimize the invasiveness of PET in children, particularly with regard to quantification of function. Previously, it was necessary to collect arterial or arterialized (through hand warming in a small heated chamber) blood samples during the PET procedure and thus define the arterial input function to the brain in order to calculate the absolute rates of local cerebral glucose metabolism (Phelps et al. 1979). Due to recent advances in mathematical modelling, the arterial input function can now be defined based on dynamic imaging of the myocardium for 20 minutes following FDG administration and the collection of only three small venous blood samples (1 mL each) towards the end of the procedure from a different venous source than the one used for FDG injection. Although these less invasive modelling approaches have not yet been developed in the study of neurotransmitter function with PET, similar approaches are likely to be developed in the future.

MOVEMENT DISORDERS IN ADULTS

There have been many studies using PET in adults with various movement disorders, but an exhaustive review is beyond the scope of this chapter. Instead, selected examples in adults will be discussed only to illustrate potential applications in children. An attempt will be made also to discuss published studies in which some children were included as subjects.

The most widely studied movement disorder using PET in adults is parkinsonism. A number of studies performed during the early days of PET technology, when very few radiochemical probes had been synthesized for PET, indicated that FDG PET may not be sensitive enough to detect primary metabolic changes in patients with Parkinson disease (e.g. Rougemont et al. 1984). Still, FDG PET found several uses in the evaluation of patients with features of parkinsonism; for example, FDG PET can distinguish between Parkinson disease (normal striatal glucose metabolism) and striatonigral degeneration (decreased striatal glucose metabolism) (De Volder et al. 1989, Eidelberg et al. 1993). In addition, FDG PET can identify the parkinsonian patient with dementia (bilateral parietotemporal cortex hypometabolism) or depression (inferior frontal cortex hypometabolism) (Mayberg et al. 1990).

After the synthesis of several PET ligands designed to provide in vivo measurements of pre- and postsynaptic dopaminergic function, PET gained much more popularity in the study of pathophysiology and differential diagnosis of parkinsonism. PET with 18F-6-fluorodopa appears to provide a good index of the integrity of the nigrostriatal pathway (Pate et al. 1993) and has been used in several ways in patients with features of parkinsonism. For example, it can detect preclinical Parkinson disease (Brooks 1991), distinguish between parkinsonism and dopa-responsive dystonia (Turjanski et al. 1993), predict a favourable outcome in drug-induced parkinsonism (Burn and Brooks 1993), and evaluate the integrity and functional consequences of dopamine neuron transplantation in Parkinson disease (Sawle et al. 1992). Other PET ligands, e.g. licraclopride which labels the dopamine D2 receptors (Brooks et al. 1992) and 11C-L-deprenyl which labels monoamine oxidase B (Fowler et al. 1993), have not been as useful in the study of parkinsonism as in psychiatric diseases.

In contrast with the study of parkinsonism, FDG PET is quite sensitive in the evaluation of patients with Huntington disease. In asymptomatic subjects at risk for Huntington disease, FDG PET shows reduced glucose metabolism of the striatum (Mazziotta et al. 1987), and when used in conjunction with genetic testing, an accurate diagnosis can be made in most individuals at risk for the disease. Further studies comparing FDG PET with PET using the benzodiazepine receptor antagonist probe 11C-flumazenil found that striatal glucose hypometabolism preceded changes in receptor binding, and that benzodiazepine receptor binding decreases first in the caudate, followed by the putamen and thalamus (Holthoff et al. 1993).

The study of dystonia in adults with PET is highly relevant to paediatric neurology since the age of onset of dystonia is often during childhood. Glucose metabolism PET studies in dystonic subjects have shown hypometabolism in the caudate and lentiform nuclei, and in the frontal projection field of the mediodorsal thalamic nucleus (Karbe et al. 1992), thus supporting the notion that in dystonia there is an abnormal relationship between basal ganglia, thalamus and frontal association areas. PET studies with 18F-6-fluorodopa in patients with dopa-responsive dystonia have shown normal uptake; this finding suggests that dopa uptake, decarboxylation and storage mechanisms are intact in this condition (Snow et al. 1993).

In Friedreich ataxia, which typically presents in childhood, FDG PET studies have shown hypermetabolism across many brain structures early in the course of the disease; later, there is hypometabolism of all regions except the caudate and lenticular nuclei, particularly in nonambulatory patients (Gilman et al. 1990). It is unclear, however, whether the increased glucose metabolism seen early in the disease represents a persistence of the hypermetabolism normally seen in children and adolescents during development (Chugani et al. 1987). Nevertheless, these patterns of glucose metabolism are distinct from that in olivopontocerebellar atrophy, in which the cerebellar hemispheres, vermis and brainstem are hypometabolic on FDG PET (Gilman et al. 1988).

Several patients who developed palatal myoclonus (following stroke or infection, or idiopathic) were found to have increased glucose metabolism of the brainstem on FDG PET, but the resolution of PET did not allow visualization of specific brainstem nuclei responsible for this movement disorder (Dubinsky et al. 1991).

Finally, in patients with essential tremor, PET with radioactive water ($H_2{}^{15}0$) showed bilaterally increased cerebellar blood flow in the resting state; during arm extension, further abnormal increases of blood flow were seen in the cerebellum and in the red nucleus (Wills et al. 1994). These examples illustrate how PET has contributed towards our understanding of the pathophysiology of movement disorders in adults, and found its place in some clinical uses. There are currently many ongoing studies using PET with a variety of agents in adult patients with movement disorders and further progress is expected.

PET IN MOVEMENT DISORDERS IN CHILDREN

There have been far fewer studies using PET in children with movement disorders than in adult patients. These few studies will be reviewed next, with the hope that the potential important contributions of PET in elucidating the pathophysiology and developing new treatment strategies in children with movement disorders will be realized.

Juvenile Huntington disease

The pattern of cerebral glucose metabolism with PET scanning in the juvenile form of Huntington disease, characterized by intellectual decline, rigidity, seizures and behavioral difficulties, has been reported to be remarkably similar to that in the adult form; both forms show striatal hypometabolism (De Volder et al. 1988). This observation was partially confirmed in a subsequent study which reported hypometabolism also in the posterior thalamic nuclei (Matthews et al. 1989), consistent with neuropathological findings. These observations are likely to be of value in the differential diagnosis of juvenile Huntington disease, but require further study.

Systemic lupus erythematosus (SLE)

In children with chorea associated with SLE, we have found a dramatic increase in glucose metabolism of the striatum during the active phase, and a tendency to normalization upon resolution of the chorea. In a single patient with primary antiphospholipid syndrome and alternating hemichorea, contralateral striatal glucose hypermetabolism was seen (Furie et al. 1994). These patterns of glucose metabolism are clearly different from that of striatal hypometabolism seen in patients with neuroacanthocytosis (Dubinsky et al. 1989) and in patients with juvenile or adult Huntington disease (see above).

Tourette syndrome

We have not found any consistent abnormalities with FDG PET in children with Tourette syndrome. Furthermore, although it is widely assumed that disturbances in the dopamine system of the brain contribute to the pathophysiology of this common disorder, PET studies with 18F-6-fluorodopa and 11C-raclopride also have failed to show any consistent differences between patients and controls with either of these two markers for the dopamine system (Turjanski et al. 1994). Several ongoing studies are evaluating other aspects of dopaminergic transmission, as well as other neurotransmitters in Tourette syndrome.

Wilson disease

The typical pattern of glucose metabolism on FDG PET in patients with Wilson disease is hypometabolism of the lenticular nuclei (Hawkins et al. 1987). When studied with PET and 11C-raclopride, reduced uptake is seen in the striatum, which, following treatment with D-penicillamine, shows improvement suggesting that the defect in striatal neurons is reversible (Schwarz et al. 1994). This is an example of a disorder in which the effectiveness of therapy can be carefully monitored with PET, providing unique information not otherwise obtainable.

Subacute sclerosing panencephalitis (SSPE)
In a single child with the rapidly progressive form of SSPE, the absolute rates of glucose metabolism were markedly decreased in cortical grey matter structures, but normal in caudate and lenticular nuclei. In contrast, cerebral glucose metabolic rates were normal in another child who appeared to have slow progression of the disease (Yanai et al. 1987). There is one study suggesting that abnormal patterns of cerebral glucose metabolism may return to normal in SSPE following treatment with human interferon beta (Huber et al. 1989). These authors report a patient in whom, prior to such treatment, symmetric hypometabolism was seen in the thalamus, cerebellum and cortex (except the primary motor region) and hypermetabolism was present in the lentiform nuclei. Following treatment, which was associated with some clinical improvement, glucose metabolic rates returned to normal in the cerebral cortex. However, bilateral focal necrosis present in the putamen, as shown on CT and MRI scans, indicated disease progression. Persistent hypermetabolism was present in the caudate and the spared superoposterior portion of the putamen. The findings from this study are somewhat difficult to interpret, and must await confirmation and extension.

Spielmeyer–Vogt disease
Children with Spielmeyer–Vogt disease, the juvenile form of neuronal ceroid-lipo-fuscinosis, usually manifest cognitive and visual difficulties early in the disease, but may also show dystonia, seizures and dysarthria. By age 15–20 years, a parkinsonian syndrome emerges with akinesia, rigidity and cogwheeling. Our studies with PET in this disorder have shown decreased glucose metabolism in the calcarine cortex as an early finding, and the gradual rostral spread of glucose hypometabolism to other cortical areas as the disease progresses (Philippart et al. 1994). This pattern of metabolic abnormality appears to be different from those of other neurodegenerative diseases which have been studied with PET in both adults and children, and may therefore be of diagnostic value (Fig. 12.9).

Choreoathetoid/dystonic form of cerebral palsy
The term infant suffering from perinatal asphyxia may develop a movement disorder in the first year of life characterized by chorea, athetosis or dystonia. The neuropathological correlate of this disorder is usually gliosis and dysmyelination of the thalamus and basal ganglia, particularly the striatum. FDG PET studies in a number of such children have

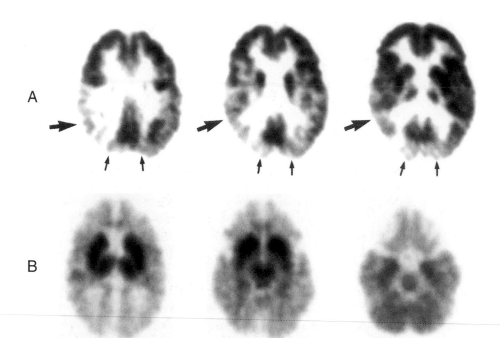

Fig. 12.9. PET images of cerebral glucose metabolism in two children with Spielmeyer–Vogt disease. (A) Early in the course, there is hypometabolism in the occipital cortex; as the disease progresses, hypometabolism is seen in other posterior cortical regions and may be asymmetric as shown in this child with occipital, right parietal and posterior temporal cortex hypometabolism (arrows). (B) Diffuse and severe cortical hypometabolism is seen in the late stages of the disease. Note the relative preservation of glucose metabolism in the basal ganglia, thalamus, brainstem and mesial temporal structures.

shown either absent or markedly depressed glucose metabolism in the thalamus and lentiform nuclei, with sparing of the caudate and lens (Kerrigan et al, 1991). The cerebral cortex is also relatively spared (Fig. 12.10), a finding that is consistent with the clinical observation that most of these children have relative preservation of cognitive function compared to their severe motor impairment. We currently use FDG PET on this group of children to evaluate their cognitive potential as a guide to early intervention.

Glutaric aciduria type I

We have studied a 3-year-old boy with glutaric aciduria type I who manifested right hemidystonia, horizontal nystagmus, and marked cognitive and motor delay. An FDG PET scan (Fig. 12.11) showed near absence of glucose metabolism in the striatum bilaterally, open opercula, and decreased cortical metabolic rates most pronounced in the frontotemporal regions, particularly in the left hemisphere (Awaad et al. 1996). The very

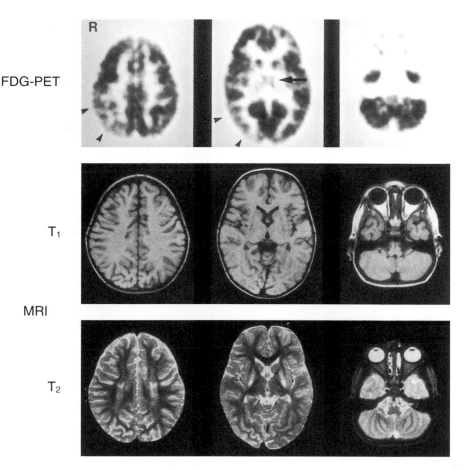

Fig. 12.10. MRI and PET images of a child with spastic diplegic cerebral palsy. The MRI shows irregular contour of the walls of the lateral ventricles and high-signal intensity in the periventricular white matter. The PET images reveal moderate hypometabolism in the right parieto-occipito-temporal cortex (arrows), which appears normal on MRI. In addition, there may be mild thalamic hypometabolism bilaterally.

selective involvement of the striatum may indicate that this region is particularly vulnerable to the endogenous toxins produced in this rare inborn error of metabolism

Alternating hemiplegia of childhood

Only a few children with alternating hemiplegia have been studied with PET [reviewed by Mikati and Fischman (1995)]. In between attacks, FDG PET studies have shown normal findings, except in one subject whose cerebellar glucose metabolic rate appeared to be lower than those of the other patients; however, it is unclear whether this was a true

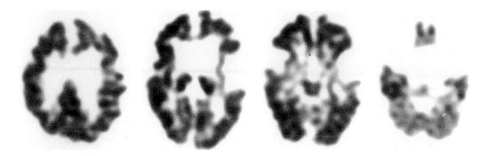

Fig. 12.11. PET images of a 3-year-old boy with glutaric acidaemia type 1. Note the virtual absence of glucose metabolism in the basal ganglia, and the open opercula with severe fronto-temporal atrophy.

abnormality or within the range of normal variation. An 11-year-old boy with alternating hemiplegia studied with PET during an acute episode of right hemiplegia was found to have slightly increased perfusion in the insula, putamen and claustrum in the left hemisphere (Tada et al. 1989). Although this has been interpreted as suggesting a vascular aetiology, we believe this is not necessarily the case because cerebral blood flow is tightly coupled to cerebral metabolism, and, therefore, intrinsic neuronal perturbations could also result in blood flow alterations.

OTHER POTENTIAL LIGANDS
There are many other PET ligands that have been developed for various research and clinical uses, some of which may be relevant in the study of childhood movement disorders. A few examples are listed below.
- 11C-cocaine (Volkow et al. 1994) and the cocaine analogue 11C-WIN 35,428 (Frost et al. 1993), both of which bind predominantly to dopamine transporter sites.
- 11C-SCH 23390, which binds to the D1 dopamine receptor (Tarde 1992).
- 11C homiferoine, which allows for the measurement of brain monaminergic uptake sites (Leenders et al. 1990).
- 11C-carfentanil, which is an agonist for the 'mu' subtype of the opiate receptor (Frost et al. 1989).
- 11C-α-methyltryptophan, which allows for the measurement of regional serotonin synthesis rate in brain (Diksic et al. 1991).

As these and other PET agents are applied to children with movement disorders, we can look forward to exciting new data that will enhance our understanding of these conditions. With this will come better methods to establish the diagnosis in affected individuals and carriers, as has already occurred in some movement disorders in adults. Finally, PET will be able to allow an objective monitoring of disease progression and response to various established and new treatment strategies.

SECTION 3: EXAMINATION OF BIOPSIED TISSUE*

Study of biopsed tissue in childhood movement disorders is limited to metabolic/degener-
ative diseases. Cerebral biopsies for the diagnosis of neurodegenerative diseases in infancy
and childhood are not performed, at present, in most neurological units. Appendicular and
rectal biopsies are indicated in some cases, whereas liver biospy is, usually, restricted to a
very small number of diseases (e.g. Wilson disease). The study of skin and conjunctival
biopsies is a useful tool in the diagnosis of certain metabolic and degenerative disease.

Appendicular and rectal biopsies allow the observation of lipid deposition in neurons
of the Meissner and Auerbach plexuses, and smooth muscle cells in different storage
diseases. Since complex lipids are also stored in fibroblasts, endothelial cells and other
dermal structures, skin and conjunctival biopsies are preferable to appendicular and
rectal biopsies in the diagnosis of the majority of neuronal storage diseases. Appendicular
and rectal biopsies have also been employed in the diagnosis of neuronal intranuclear
inclusion disease (see Chapter 2) (Goutières et al. 1990; and personal observations,
unpublished). No abnormalities in the skin and conjunctiva has been reported in this
disease.

Liver biopsies show intracytoplasmatic inclusions in metabolic storage diseases with
visceral involvement, including clear and polymorphic inclusions in hepatocytes in
different types of Niemann–Pick disease, and multiple cytosomes filled with tubules
measuring about $0.5–0.7\,\mu m$ in diameter in Gaucher cells in patients with glucocerebro-
sidosis. Liver biopsy may be useful in the diagnosis of Wilson disease (Chapter 6) as
microchemical methods can be used in the measurement of the levels of copper.

Electron microscopic examination of skin samples permits the visualization of abnormal cytosomes in fibroblasts, endothelial cells, pericytes, Schwann cells, axons, smooth
muscle cells, sweat glands and sebaceous glands. Moreover, fibroblasts can be separated
for culture, and enzymatic analysis can be carried out in cultured cells thus allowing the
identification of the metabolic disorder. The variety of cells is more limited in conjunctival biopsies than in skin biopsies since smooth muscle cells and glands are absent in the
conjunctiva.

Skin and conjunctival biopsies are useful in the diagnosis of neuronal storage disease,
including Niemann–Pick disease and ceroid-lipofuscinosis (Martin and Ceuterick 1978,
Libert and Danis 1979, Yamano et al. 1979, Arsenio-Nunes et al. 1981, Ceuterick and
Martin 1984). Skin biopsies are useful in the diagnosis of juvenile neuroaxonal dystrophy
(Schwendemann et al. 1987), but diagnosis of Hallervorden–Spatz disease through the
electronmicroscopic examination of the skin is not clear.

Neurologists must be concerned with the indications and limitations of the morphological study of the different types of biopsies. Electronmicroscopic examination by
expert neuropathologists is mandatory, and the interpretation of morphological data

---

*Authored by Isidro Ferrer, Ciutat Sanitaria Princeps d'Espanya, Department of Neuropathology,
Hospitalet, Barcelona, Spain.

must be done in combination with clinical data and results of other complementary examinations. Nonspecific intracellular inclusions may be secondary to therapy. In the present context of movement disorders in childhood, the examination of biopsied tissue is regrettably limited to a very small number of diseases.

Exemplary findings are shown in Figures 12.12–12.16.

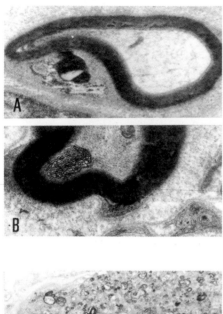

Fig. 12.12. Myelinated fibres in biopsies of the skin with adrenoleukodystrophy (A) and infantile neuroaxonal dystrophy (B). Clear spicular inclusions are found in Schwann cells in adrenoleukodystrophy. Tubular aggregates are seen in dystrophic axons in the patient with infantile neuroaxonal dystrophy.

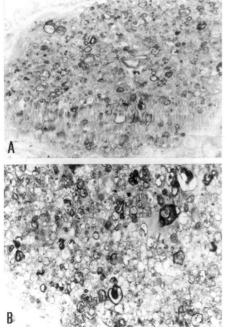

Fig. 12.13. Appendicular biopsy in a patient with juvenile GM2 gangliosidosis (A,B). The cytoplasm of a neuron is filled with membrane-bound membranous cytoplasmic bodies.

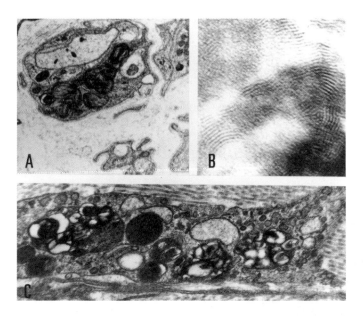

Fig. 12.14. Conjunctival biopsies in patients with GM1 gangliosidosis (A), Fabry disease (B) and Niemann–Pick disease type C (C). Membranous cytoplasmic bodies are seen in Schwann cells in the patient with juvenile GM1. Fingerprint profiles are observed in an endothelial cell in the patient with Fabry disease. Polymorphous inclusions, dense bodies and clear vacuoles are observed in fibroblasts in Niemann–Pick disease type C.

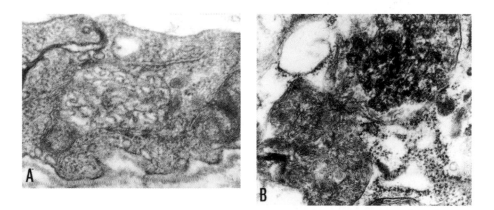

Fig. 12.15. Conjunctival biopsy in ceroid-lipofuscinosis. Cytosomes filled with curvilinear bodies are observed in an endothelial cell of a patient suffering from late infantile ceroid-lipofuscinosis (A). Cytosomes with dense granular inclusions and fingerprint inclusions are seen in a fibroblast of a patient with juvenile ceroid-lipofuscinosis (B).

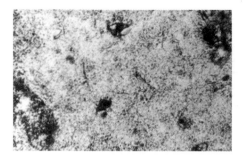

Fig. 12.16. Filamentous and granular non-membrane-bound inclusion is observed in a glandular cell of an apocrine gland in a patient with Lafora disease.

REFERENCES

Arsenio-Nunes ML, Goutières F, Aicardi J (1981) An electronmicroscopic study of skin and conjunctival biopsies in chronic neurological diseases of childhood. *Ann Neurol* 9: 163–73.

Awaad Y, Shamato H, Chugani H (1996) Hemidystonia improved by baclofen and PET scan findings in a patient with glutaric aciduria type I. *J Child Neurol* 11: 167–9.

Brooks DJ (1991) Detection of preclinical Parkinson's disease with PET. *Neurology* 41 (suppl. 2): 24–7.

— Ibanez V, Sawle GV, et al. (1992) Striatal D2 receptor status in patients with Parkinson's disease, striatonigral degeneration, and progressive supranuclear palsy, measured with 11C-raclopride and positron emission tomography. *Ann Neurol* 31: 184–92.

Burn, DJ, Brooks DJ (1993) Nigral dysfunction in drug-induced parkinsonism: An 18-F-dopa PET study. *Neurology* 43: 552–6.

Ceuterick C, Martin JJ (1984) Diagnostic role of skin and conjunctival biopsies in neurological disorders: An update. *J Neurol Sci* 65: 179–91.

Chugani, HT, Phelps ME, Mazziotta JC (1987) Positron emission tomography study of human brain functional development. *Ann Neurol* 22: 487–97.

De Volder AG, Bol A, Michel C, et al. (1988) Brain glucose utilization in childhood Huntington's disease studied with positron emission tomography (PET). *Brain Dev* 10: 47–50.

— Francart J, Laterre C, et al. (1989) Decreased glucose utilization in the striatum and frontal lobe in probable striatonigral degeneration. *Ann Neurol* 26: 239–47.

Diksic, M, Nagahiro S, Chaly T, et al. (1991) Serotonin synthesis rate measured in living dog brain by positron emission tomography. *J Neurochem* 56. 153 61.

Dubinsky RM, Hallett M, Levey R, Di Chiro G (1989) Regional brain glucose metabolism in neuroacanthocytosis. *Neurology* 39: 1253–5.

— Hallett M, Di Chiro G, et al. (1991) Increased glucose metabolism in the medulla of patients with palatal myoclonus. *Neurology* 41: 557–62.

Eidelberg D, Takikawa S, Moeller JR, et al. (1993) Striatal hypometabolism distinguishes striato-nigral degeneration from Parkinson's disease. *Ann Neurol* 33: 518–27.

Farde L (1992) Selective D1 and D2 dopamine receptor blockade both induces [sic] akathisia in humans—a PET study with [11C]SCH 23390 and [11C]raclopride. *Psychopharmacology* 107: 23–9.

Fève A, Bathien N, Rondot P (1994) Abnormal movement related potentials in patients with lesions of basal ganglia and anterior thalamus. *J Neurol Neurosurg Psychiatry* 57: 100–4.

Fowler JS, Volkow ND, Logan J, et al. (1993) Monoamine oxidase B (MAO B) inhibitor therapy in Parkinson's disease: The degree and reversibility of human brain MAO B inhibition by Ro 19 6327. *Neurology* 43: 1984–92.

Frost, JJ, Douglass KH, Mayberg HS, et al. (1989) Multicompartmental analysis of [11C]-carfentanil binding to opiate receptors in humans measured by positron emission tomography. *J Cereb Blood Flow Metab* 9: 398–409.

— Rosier AJ, Reich SG, et al. (1993) Positron emission tomographic imaging of the dopamine transporter with 11C-WIN 35,428 reveals marked declines in mild Parkinson's disease. *Ann Neurol* 34: 423–31.

Furie R, Ishikawa T, Dhawan V, Eidelberg D (1994) Alternating hemichorea in primary anti-phospholipid syndrome: Evidence for contralateral striatal hypermetabolism. *Neurology* 44: 2197–9.

Garcin R, Guiot G, Rondot P, et al. (1966) Myoclonies rythmées du membre supérieur droit: symptôme inaugural d'une tumeur intramédullaire cervicale. *Rev Neurol* 119: 985–6.

Gilman S, Markel DS, Koeppe RA, et al. (1988) Cerebellar and brainstem hypometabolism in olivopontocerebellar atrophy detected with positron emission tomography. *Ann Neurol* 23: 223–30.

— Junck L, Markel DS, et al. (1990) Cerebral glucose hypermetabolism in Friedreich's ataxia detected with positron emission tomography. *Ann Neurol* 28: 750–7.

Goutières F, Mikol J, Aicardi J (1990) Neuronal intranuclear inclusion disease in a child: Diagnosis by rectal biopsy. *Ann Neurol* 27: 103–6.

Hawkins RA, Mazziotta JC, Phelps ME (1987) Wilson's disease studied with FDG and positron emission tomography. *Neurology* 37: 1707–11.

Holthoff VA, Koeppe RA, Frey KA, et al. (1993) Positron emission tomography measures of benzodiazepine receptors in Huntington's disease. *Ann Neurol* 34: 76–81.

Huber M, Herholz K, Pawlik G, et al. (1989) Cerebral glucose metabolism in the course of sub-acute sclerosing panencephalitis. *Arch Neurol* 46: 97–100.

Ikeda A, Luders HO, Burgess RC, Shibasaki H (1992) Movement-related potentials recorded from supplementary motor area and primary motor area. Role of supplementary motor area in voluntary movements. *Brain* 115: 1017–43.

Karbe H, Holthoff VA, Rudolf J, et al. (1992) Positron emission tomography demonstrates frontal cortex and basal ganglia hypometabolism in dystonia. *Neurology* 42: 1540–4.

Kerrigan J, Chugani H, Phelps M (1991) Regional cerebral glucose metabolism in clinical subtypes of cerebral palsy. *Ped Neurol* 7: 415–25.

Leenders KL, Salmon EP, Tyrrell P, et al. (1990) The nigrostriatal dopaminergic system assessed in vivo by positron emission tomography in healthy volunteer subjects and patients with Parkinson's disease. *Arch Neurol* 47: 1290–8.

Libert J, Danis P (1979) Differential diagnosis of type A, B, and C Niemann–Pick disease by conjunctival biopsy. *J Submicrosc Cytol* 11: 143–57.

Martin JJ, Ceuterick C (1978) Morphological study of skin biopsy specimens: A contribution to the diagnosis of metabolic disorders with involvement of the nervous system. *J Neurol Neurosurg Psychiatry* 41: 232–48.

Matthews PM, Evans AC, Andermann F, Hakim AM (1989) Regional cerebral glucose metabolism differs in adult and rigid juvenile forms of Huntington disease. *Ped Neurol* 5: 353–6.

Mayberg HS, Starkstein SE, Sadzot B, et al. (1990) Selective hypometabolism in the inferior frontal lobe in depressed patients with Parkinson's disease. *Ann Neurol* 28: 57–64.

Mazziotta JC, Phelps ME, Pahl JJ, et al. (1987) Reduced cerebral glucose metabolism in asymptomatic subjects at risk for Huntington's disease. *N Engl J Med* 316: 357–62.

Mikati MA, Fischman AJ (1995) Positron emission tomography in children with alternating hemi-
    plegia of childhood. In: Andermann F, Aicardi J, Vigevano F (eds.) *Alternating Hemiplegia of
    Childhood.* New York: Raven Press, pp. 109–14.
Neshige R, Lüders H, Shibasaki H (1988) Recording of movement-related potentials from scalp
    and cortex in man. *Brain* 111: 719–36.
Pate BD, Kawamata T, Yamada T, et al. (1993) Correlation of striatal fluorodopa uptake in the
    MPTP monkey with dopaminergic indices. *Ann Neurol* 34: 331–8.
Phelps ME, Mazziotta JC (1985) Positron emission tomography: Human brain function and
    biochemistry. *Science* 228: 799–809.
— Huang SC, Hoffman EJ, et al. (1979) Tomographic measurement of local cerebral glucose
    metabolic rate in humans with (F-18)2-fluoro-2-deoxy-D-glucose: Validation of method. *Ann
    Neurol* 6: 371–88.
— Mazziotta JC, Schelbert HR (1986) *Positron Emission Tomography and Autoradiography.* New
    York: Raven Press.
Philippart M, Messa C, Chugani H (1994) Spielmeyer–Vogt (Batten, Spielmeyer–Sjogren) disease:
    Distinctive patterns of cerebral glucose utilization. *Brain* 117: 1085–92.
Rektor I, Fève A, Buser P, et al. (1994) Intracerebral recording of movement related readiness
    potentials: An exploration in epileptic patients. *Electroencephalogr Clin Neurophysiol* 90:
    273–83.
Renou G, Rondot P, Metral S (1970) Analyse des décharges itératives d'unités motrices au cours
    des bouffées de tremblement. *Rev Neurol* 122: 420–3.
Rondot P, Ribadeau-Dumas JL (1972) Dopamine et mouvements anormaux. *Rev Neurol* 127:
    99–113.
— Korn H, Scherrer J (1968) Suppression of an entire limb tremor by anesthetizing a selective
    muscular group. *Arch Neurol* 19: 421–9.
— Saïd G, Ferrey G (1972) Les hyperkinésies volitionelles. *Rev Neurol* 126: 415–26.
— Bathien N, Toma S (1979) Physiopathology of cerebellar movements. In: Massion J, Sasaki S
    (eds.) *Cerebro-cerebellar Interactions.* Amsterdam: Elsevier–North Holland, pp. 203–30.
Rougemont D, Baron JC, Collard P, et al. (1984) Local cerebral glucose utilization in treated and
    untreated patients with Parkinson's disease. *J Neurol Neurosurg Psychiatry* 47: 824–30.
Sawle GV, Bloomfield PM, Bjorklund A, et al. (1992) Transplantation of fetal dopamine neurons
    in Parkinson's disease: PET [18F]6-L-fluorodopa studies in two patients with putaminal
    implants. *Ann Neurol* 31: 166–73.
Schwarz J, Antonini A, Kraft E, et al. (1994) Treatment with D-penicillamine improves dopamine
    D-2-receptor binding and T2 signal intensity in de novo Wilson's disease. *Neurology* 44:
    1079–82.
Schwendemann G, Arendt G, Noth J (1987) Diagnosis of juvenile–adult form of neuroaxonal
    dystrophy by electron microscopy of rectum and skin. *J Neurol Neurosurg Psychiatry* 50: 818–21.
Shibasaki H, Barrett G, Neshige R, et al. (1986) Volitional movement is not preceded by cortical
    slow negativity in cerebellar dentate lesions in man. *Brain Res* 368: 361–5.
Snow BJ, Torbjoern G, Nygaard G, et al. (1993) Positron emission tomographic studies of dopa-
    responsive dystonia and early-onset idiopathic parkinsonism. *Ann Neurol* 34: 733–8.
Tada H, Miyake S, Yamada M, et al. (1989) A patient with alternating hemiplegia in childhood.
    No To Hattatsu 21: 283–8.
Turjanski N, Bhatia K, Burn DJ, et al. (1993) Comparison of striatal 18F-dopa uptake in adult-
    onset dystonia–parkinsonism, Parkinson's disease, and dopa-responsive dystonia. *Neurology*
    43: 1563–8.

— Sawle GV, Playford ED,et al. (1994) PET studies of the presynaptic and postsynaptic dopaminergic system in Tourette's syndrome. *J Neurol Neurosurg Psychiatry* 57: 688–92.

Volkow ND, Fowler JS, Wang GJ, et al. (1994) Decreased dopamine transporters with age in healthy human subjects. *Ann Neurol* 36: 237–9.

Wessel K, Verleger R, Nazarenus D, et al. (1994) Movement-related cortical potentials preceding sequential and goal-directed finger and arm movements in patients with cerebellar atrophy. *Electroencephalogr Clin Neurophysiol* 92: 331–41.

Wills AJ, Jenkins IH, Thompson PD, et al. (1994) Red nuclear and cerebellar but no olivary activation associated with essential tremor: A positron emission tomographic study. *Ann Neurol* 36: 636–42.

Yamano T, Shimada M, Okada S, et al. (1979) Electron microscopic examination of skin and conjunctival biopsy specimens in neuronal storage diseases. *Brain Dev* 1: 16–25.

Yanai K, Ilinuma K, Tada K, et al. (1987) Regional cerebral metabolic rate for glucose in subacute sclerosing panencephalitis. *Eur J Pediatr* 146: 288–9.

INDEX